"A marvelous contribution to the *book of Natural Healing* thoroughly systems of healing and the interre cellent resource for both the layper it fascinating, comprehensive and recommend it to all my students."

G000124364

...g. I'll certainly

Rosemary Gladstar
Founder of The California School of Herbal Studies
Co-founder of Traditional Medicinal Teas

Now, all the information that has been uncovered during the holistic health movement is compiled in this one volume in a concise and usable format. With this book you will acquaint yourself with the variety of natural therapies available as well as heal yourself and your family of most ailments.

Designed to function as a home reference guide (yet enjoyable and interesting enough to be read straight through), *The Complete Handbook of Natural Healing* addresses all natural healing modalities in use today:

- Dietary regimens
- Nutritional supplements
- Cleansing and detoxification
- Vitamins and minerals
- Herbology
- Homeopathic medicine
- Cell salts
- Traditional Chinese medicine
- Ayurvedic medicine
- Body work and exercise
- Mental and spiritual therapies
- Subtle and vibrational healing
- Color and music therapies
- Crystal healing
- Diagnostic techniques

In addition, a section of 41 specific ailments, including their physiological and psychological descriptions, outlines all natural treatments for everything from insect bites to varicose veins to AIDS.

About the Author

Marcia Starck is a medicine teacher, astrologer, consultant and lecturer. She is the founder of Earth Medicine Ways, a foundation that utilizes ancient rituals and modern spiritual elements.

Marcia has been a healer for over 20 years and has studied nutrition, herbs, homeopathy, Chinese medicine, Ayurvedic medicine, color therapy, crystals and radiesthesia. She wrote this book so that all this information would be in one comprehensive volume.

A medical astrologer as well as a healer, her research correlating the horoscope with disease factors is included in *Astrology: Key to Holistic Health* and *Earth Mother Astrology*.

Presently, Marcia works with Women's Rituals and rites of passage, which are the subject of her forthcoming book, *Women's Medicine Ways*.

Her educational background includes a B.A. in English Literature, Phi Beta Kappa, from Douglass College, Rutgers University, as well as graduate work at San Francisco State College and the University of California, Berkeley. She was born December 24, 1939 at 2:38 A.M. in Paterson, NJ.

To Write to the Author

We cannot guarantee that every letter written to the author can be answered, but all will be forwarded. Both the author and the publisher appreciate hearing from readers, learning of your enjoyment and benefit from this book. Llewellyn also publishes a bimonthly news magazine with news and reviews of practical esoteric studies and articles helpful to the student, and some readers' questions and comments to the author may be answered through this magazine's columns if permission to do so is included in the original letter. The author sometimes participates in seminars and workshops, and dates and places are announced in *The Llewellyn New Times*. To write to the author, or to ask a question, write to:

Marcia Starck
c/o THE LLEWELLYN NEW TIMES
P.O. Box 64383-742, St. Paul, MN 55164-0383, U.S.A.
Please enclose a self-addressed, stamped envelope for reply, or $1.00 to cover costs.

The Complete Handbook of Natural Healing

Marcia Starck

1991
Llewellyn Publications, Inc.
St. Paul, Minnesota, 55164-0383, U.S.A.

FIRST EDITION

Cover and interior illustrations by Rohmana D'Arezzo Harris

"Cycles of Nourishment & Control" (p. 177) and "Five Phase Correspondences" (p. 178) reprinted by permission, © John W. Garvy, Jr., Well Being Books, P.O. Box 396, Newtonville, MA 02160.
Iridology charts, pp. 241-42, reprinted with permission by Bernard Jensen, D.C.

Library of Congress Cataloging-in-Publication Data

Starck, Marcia.
     The complete handbook of natural healing / by Marcia Starck. —
  1st ed.
       p.   cm.
     Includes bibliographical references and index.
     ISBN 0-87542-742-1
     1. Alternative medicine. 2. Self-care, Health. I. Title.
     [DNLM: 1. Alternative Medicine. 2. Self Care. WB 890 S7946c]
R733.S834 1991
615.5—dc20
DNLM/DLC
for Library of Congress   91-14163
                                             CIP

Llewellyn Publications
A Division of Llewellyn Worldwide, Ltd.
P.O. Box 64383, St. Paul, MN 55164-0383

This book is dedicated to the memory of my father, Paul Rittenberg, whose death at an early age inspired me to explore the path of Natural Healing.

Other Books by Marcia Starck

Astrology: Key to Holistic Health
Earth Mother Astrology

Forthcoming Books

Women's Medicine Ways

ACKNOWLEDGMENTS

I wish to thank four people whose assistance made this book possible. First, my friend Gynne Stern, who encouraged me in publishing this book and typed the entire manuscript. Second, Matthew Wood, author of *Seven Herbs: Plants as Teachers*, whose critiques and careful analysis of the manuscript enabled me to transform it into an accurate and comprehensive book. Third, my editor at Llewellyn, Kathy Halgren, who thought of all the things I forgot and who paid such careful attention to the details. And finally, my friend Rohmana Harris who painted the beautiful cover and made the various drawings throughout the book.

I also would like to thank Terry Buske for designing the book and Nancy Mostad and the rest of the Llewellyn staff for their help. My deep appreciation goes to Stephen Bannister, M.D., of Nevada City, Calif. for his Foreword, and to Russell Klobas, L.Ac., of Hallowell, Maine and Jeffrey Friedman, D.C., of San Rafael, Calif. for their help and support.

CONTENTS

FOREWORD

As a physician interested in both traditional and alternative approaches to health and disease, I found Marcia Starck's book broadly informative and very thought-provoking. It is unusual to find one author who can skillfully explain the vast array of approaches currently available, but Marcia has done so. For laypersons or health professionals who want a concise, lucid explanation of homeopathy or radiesthesia, they will find it here. Many other healing systems, such as herbology, color therapy, and Chinese medicine, are also presented in a clear and understandable fashion.

Food and nutrition are discussed with a world view, as in the description of six other milks besides cow's milk which are used throughout the world. Such health-food-store items as "steel cut oats" and "pearled barley" are described, as well as supplements like evening primrose oil.

Marcia does more than list and clearly explain health techniques and therapies; she also ties the information together with her knowledge of the basics of holistic health as the mind-body-spirit link. (See the Huna system in chapter 1.)

For the layperson, then, this book is a valuable guide to the often bewildering array of health products and services currently obtainable. For the conventional practitioner of medicine or psychology, this book gives a broad introduction to non-traditional ways of viewing health and disease. The alternative practitioner will find it a handy reference for enhancing her/his present approach to many common conditions, such as asthma, candida, high blood pressure and headaches.

Whether one's interest is in learning more about an alternative health approach or in having access to details about individual vitamins and minerals, Marcia's book will provide a broad and useful reference.

—Stephen Bannister, M.D.
Nevada City, Calif.

INTRODUCTION

This book was written over a seven-year period—between 1982-1989. The 1980s have witnessed a flowering of many natural approaches to healing which were seeded in the '60s. In that decade, two of the three outermost planets in the solar system, Uranus and Pluto, were in Virgo, a sign which symbolizes health and healing. Natural childbirth, health food stores, vitamin supplements, herbs, and Chinese medicine began to surface. A "back to nature" approach, without chemicals and pesticides, became popular in farming, giving rise to organic farms, wild-crafted herbs, and ecological movements to preserve the land, plants and wildlife that are becoming extinct.

In the '60s we also experienced the blossoming of many Eastern spiritual practices such as yoga, tai chi, and meditation. Along with these practices there was much talk of the mind-body connection and the influence the emotions and stress have on our physical vehicles. In the early '70s certain meditative practices, such as visualization, gained recognition, while the late '70s saw the introduction of more subtle types of healing—crystals and gems, color therapy, flower essences, as well as body therapies like reiki, jin shinn do, and polarity therapy which work with electrical energy. The concept of healing was expanding to include our emotional and subtle bodies. Disease was not just a phenomenon confined to the physical body.

The 1970s also brought the Gaia hypothesis, the concept that our Earth, the planet on which we reside, is a living, breathing organism, and, in fact, is in need of much healing. Its rain forests are being destroyed, affecting the ozone layer and the quality of air we breathe; its oceans and streams are being polluted, affecting our wildlife, our fish, our plants and the entire food chain. Individual healing has become a part now of a greater whole—the healing of our planet.

With all these strands of healing, how, then, to weave a book that would incorporate the diverse strands, and how to crystallize this information so that it can be useful when there are constant changes? Each day there is new information about the effects of certain nutrients, the benefits of particular herbs, the subtleties of new crystals, not to mention the field of psycho-neuro-immunology, which is uncovering more information daily about the relation of stress to our immune system.

When I began writing this book, I chose to start with the basics—Cleansing, Elimination, Nutrition—and to move on from there to Herbology, Homeopathy, Traditional Chinese Medicine and the more subtle and esoteric forms of healing.

I have included a chapter on Diagnostic Techniques because it is important that we have some basis from which to determine how much of the disease being manifested stems from physical causes, how much from mental causes and how much from spiritual and psychic causes. We also need to know which organs and body systems are involved.

Paracelsus, the father of modern healing, believed that disease originated from one of five basic causes. First, sidereal and astral influences act upon the etheric or vital body, which sets in motion certain vibratory rates causing imbalance or chemical conflict. The second cause is the introduction into the body of impurities, poisonous or harmful substances (including medicines and drugs). This involves personal responsibility for taking care of one's self, which includes nutrition, body cleansing and hygiene. Paracelsus lists as the third cause incorrect physical habits, including excessive eating and drinking and the overuse of certain condiments or spices. For the fourth cause, Paracelsus cites the psychological realm when he speaks of "intemperance of the mind and emotions which corrupt man's psychic nature," thus being one of the first to insinuate the mind-body link. As the fifth, he notes spiritual causes: disobedience to laws on a religious, moral, or ethical level. When he speaks of spiritual conflicts, he mentions that these may exist before birth, i.e., other lifetimes. This seems to be a fairly complete picture as to the causes of diseases. (For more details, see *Paracelsus: His Mystical and Medical Philosophy* by Manly P. Hall, Philosophical Research Society, Los Angeles, 1964.)

The first section of this book deals with the roots of disease, cleansing the body and elimination, metabolic types and their dietary needs, and the basics of nutrition like proteins, fats, carbohydrates, vitamins and minerals. Additional nutritional supplements like aloe vera juice, bee pollen, chlorophyll, evening primrose oil, sea vegetables, and protomorphogens are discussed to help us choose appropriate supplements to nurture our bodies. Herbology and homeopathy are introduced as healing modalities that provide us with other tools with which to heal ourselves. Ancient systems of healing like traditional Chinese medicine and Ayurvedic medicine are presented as examples of systems that work with mind-body-spirit.

Once there is a state of balance achieved, it is appropriate to explore various types of exercise and bodywork, mental and spiritual therapies, such as meditation and visualization, as well as vibrational healing techniques like color therapy, music therapy, and crystal and gem therapy. None of this information would be relevant without understanding the various diagnostic tools that are important in determining which systems of the body need particular attention.

In the last section of this book, I have written about 44 different diseases, describing them by the names they are called in Western medicine for the purpose of communication. Recommendations for healing include diet, supplements, herbal medicines and other therapies geared for the physical body. It is my intention and my hope that anyone utilizing these recommendations will explore the psychological and spiritual causes in addition to these suggestions.

This book, then, is a compendium of many healing systems and practices that have proven helpful to individuals and are based on the philosophy of viewing each being as a balanced whole. I hope it will serve the purpose of being a reference book and will lead each of us to explore other methods of natural healing as we become responsible for our own state of health.

THE ROOTS OF DISEASE

How does the physical body become out of balance, and why do conditions of disease begin? What are the underlying causes of the illnesses we refer to as arthritis, heart disease, diabetes, and cancer?

As Paracelsus noted back in the 16th century, our thought patterns and attitudes create our physical states. If our mental thoughts are consistently negative; if we live with anxiety, fear, or worry; if we experience constant stress and tension, our bodies are directly affected.

Emotional states and attitudes are related to corresponding physical conditions. Let's examine the emotion anger. If a person is feeling overwhelmed with anger, or literally "burning up inside," s/he may experience high fevers or conditions like rashes with redness and itchiness over her/his body. If s/he constantly holds back this anger, it affects the bile in the body. (Bile is produced by the liver and stored in the gall bladder.) Her/his skin may begin to turn yellow, and s/he may have difficulty digesting fats and oils.

An example of this is a lady who came to see me for a consultation several years ago. She was dressed in a bright red pants suit with a red purse and shoes; what she was trying to express was obvious. She confessed to envying her son because he could "fly off the handle" so easily—because he was able to release his anger. At the end of the session, she told me that she had had a serious liver disease for several years, that the doctors were keeping her going with heavy medications, and that her skin had been very yellow. As she learned to get in touch with her anger and express it in her daily life, she was able to discontinue the medications and gradually restore her body to its normal functioning.

Paracelsus explained in his writings that violent emotions may cause miscarriages, apoplexies and spasms and result in the malformation of the fetus of an unborn child. Grief can depress a function so that it results in death, whereas great joy and gaiety can stimulate sluggish functions and help to restore bodily health. People with unreasonable dispositions and unpleasant attitudes may have trouble with digestion, assimilation, and elimination.

Other examples of obvious mind/body links are conditions of stiffness and rigidity—a stiff neck, arthritis, bursitis, and many diseases of the bones and joints. These involve attitudes which are inflexible and not amenable to change; therefore, a rigid condition develops within the body. Physical therapies for these diseases work to break up crystallization in the body (such as calcium deposits), but unless new thought patterns and attitudes are created the body reverts to its former state.

How, then, does one go about changing attitudes, thought patterns, and life styles? First, it's necessary to examine all aspects of one's life—job, family situation, relationships. Which areas are atrophied, where is there stagnation, and what thought patterns and activities will bring about new growth and change? Examining childhood patterns and conditioning is one important step as well as seeing where one's life "has not worked," noting the types of negative thoughts one indulges in when this happens. One needs to look at how his/her "buttons have been pushed" and where s/he has placed the guilt and blame. Then s/he can begin to develop a *new way* of handling the situation the next time it reoccurs. This is often referred to as breaking the "conditioned reflex." One has to be strongly motivated to do this work and continue to follow through with it because it takes a long time to break old responses. When one is successful at changing the neurological sequence, the body often becomes very toxic since the old cells die and many new cells are regenerated. This is why physical ailments can be such a positive experience: they provide the body with an opportunity to regenerate and reprogram.

There are many systems of healing that work to eliminate old habits and thought patterns. The *Huna system*, derived from ancient Hawaiian teachings, is one of these. The Hunas use the concept of the three selves—the low self or subconscious, the middle or conscious self, and the high self, that part of us which is related to cosmic or divine energy. These are often referred to as the child, the mother, and the father, and the idea is to bring all three of these into a harmonious balance. By dealing with subconscious thoughts, one brings them to the conscious level, and thus can begin to change the patterns. The subconscious also handles the physical programming, according to this system, and by confronting it one understands why her/his body has taken on various diseased states.

Many other systems of healing also deal with restructuring or repatterning. *Rebirthing* is one such system. Here the traumas of birth are encountered by re-experiencing the birthing process in an effort to clear up negative emotions and programs. *Bioenergetics* is another therapy which deals with breaking up old patterns—in this case, through the body armor. Many unconscious patterns are seen in the muscular shapes and tensions of the body. Bioenergetics attempts to release the physical tensions while dealing with the psychological problems and defense patterns adopted by the body.

The effect of *stress* on the physiological processes of the body have been well documented. Dr. Hans Selye in *The Stress of Life* (McGraw-Hill, 1956) first pointed out, through his experiments with rats, the adaptation in the hormonal system and other biochemical processes when subjected to stressful conditions in one's job or family life. Some of the conclusions Dr. Selye came to follow.

During stress reactions, the kidneys are affected because they regulate the chemical composition of the blood and tissues by selectively eliminating certain chemicals from the body. When one is experiencing a great deal of tension and anxiety, the elimination system does not work correctly and the body may swell up with excess fluid. The kidneys also adjust blood pressure, and this explains why blood pressure may be unusually high during these periods.

The liver is also involved in most of the biochemical adjustments to stress. The liver regulates the concentration of sugar, protein, and other important tissue foods in the blood. When it is not functioning properly, the blood sugar may be too high (hyperglycemia or diabetes) or too low (hypoglycemia). Furthermore, the liver destroys the excess of corticoids when the adrenals make too much. And perhaps most important of all is its role in detoxifying environmental pollutants or poisonous substances that are in the body. Strong allergic reactions may occur when the liver is not able to do its work of detoxifying.

The thyroid gland is also affected during stress reactions. It releases hormones which stimulate the metabolism of every other tissue in the body.

Selye lists many physical symptoms which are related to stress and are often the precursors of serious diseases. Among them are irritability; depression; pounding of the heart (an indicator of high blood pressure); the urge to cry; inability to concentrate; feelings of weakness and dizziness (often associated with hypoglycemia); becoming easily fatigued; trembling and nervous tics; tendency to be easily startled; high-pitched nervous laughter; stuttering and other speech difficulties; insomnia; hyperkinesia (moving about without any reason); sweating; frequent urination; indigestion; queasiness in the stomach; constipation; diarrhea and vomiting; migraine headaches; pre-menstrual tension and missed menstrual cycles; pain in neck and lower back; loss of or excessive appetite; increased smoking; increased use of prescription drugs; alcohol and drug addiction; nightmares; and accident proneness.

Dr. Selye particularly discusses metabolic disease, digestive disorders, rheumatoid disease, infectious diseases, nervous and mental derangements, and cancer.

Fortunately, we now have devices such as *biofeedback machines* which can help us learn how to relax by becoming aware of the parasympathetic nervous system and what the body does when it is extremely tense (fast heartbeat, profuse sweating). By tuning in to these reactions, we can slow down our body processes. We can also learn how to function in the alpha rhythms of the brain (the slower, relaxed rhythms) through various techniques of meditation. Dr. Carl Simonton and his wife Stephanie have been very successful in healing cancer through visualization and meditative techniques (see *Getting Well Again*, Bantam, 1981). The Simontons also work with breaking up old emotional patterns and subsequent changes in the life style to accommodate new ways of thinking.

People who work with visualization often change their life style and gain a higher level and quality of life. Visualization techniques involve the use of *imagery*. Imagery can be used two ways. The first is diagnostic in origin as it is a way for people to express what is *really* going on in their bodies. For example, a cancer patient might draw a picture of two armies attacking each other. What s/he is expressing is the war between the healthy cells and the cancer cells in her/his body. This person experiences her/his illness as a war between two sides. Finding corresponding imagery to heal this division is not difficult. The patient can then visualize the healthy cells overtaking the cancer cells. This visualization would then come under the second type of imagery, that is, imagery designed *to heal.*

Jeanne Achterberg, who, with her husband Frank Lawlis, continued and expanded the work of the Simontons, explains the different purposes of imagery in her book *Imagery in Healing: Shamanism and Modern Medicine* (Shambhala Pubns., 1985). She writes that diagnostic imagery is receptive; it is done in a relaxed state, allowing spontaneous images to appear. Therapeutic imagery, on the other hand, is more programmed and can often involve information from books on anatomy and physiology. In both *Love, Medicine, & Miracles* and *Peace, Love, & Healing* (Harper & Row, 1990), Dr. Bernie Siegel works with the use of imagery and reprogramming negative thought patterns.

Both Achterberg and Siegel, as well as other healers and doctors, speak much of the "placebo effect." The placebo effect is a description for a physiological change that happens without any medical intervention or ingestion of drugs, vitamins, or other medical substances. Since thoughts have substance and affect the body in an electrochemical way, the idea that a certain pill will relieve pain transmits that message to the brain, and the body's pain relief chemicals (the endomorphins and enkephalins) are actually increased. There has been much research and collection of data supporting the placebo effect—in fact, a whole new field of healing has come to be known as *psycho-neuro-immunology* (PNI), which works with mental and emotional states as they affect the immune system.

In Chinese medicine, one of the most ancient systems of healing, various emotional states are, in fact, related to different body organs. The liver and gall bladder are associated with the element Wood, the season spring, and anger. Those with disease of these organs tend to hold back their anger, and often tears as well. In conditions as diabetes and cirrhosis of the liver, as well as among many alcoholics, there is a great deal of suppressed anger.

The small intestine and heart relate to joy and sorrow, the element Fire, and summer. Those who carry much sorrow and sadness within them often have problems with the cardiovascular system.

The spleen and stomach are analogous with sympathy, the

Earth element and late summer. Those with stomach ulcers and those lacking hydrochloric acid seem to have difficulty expressing sympathy and emotions in general. (The acid/alkaline condition of the body is related to the emotional balance. When one lacks sympathy or has difficulty expressing emotions, her/his body may lack acid.)

Lung and large intestine problems correlate with worry and grief; they are related to the element Air and autumn. Those who tend to worry a lot, those who hold a lot of grief within, as well as those who are very mental, experience problems as bronchitis, asthma, pneumonia in addition to digestive problems like colitis, flatulence and indigestion. The fluid mucus is related to these organs, and when one gets in touch with long-standing grief a lot of mucus may get released from the lungs. (Coughing is often an attempt to release this mucus and express the grief.)

The kidney and bladder signify fear, the Water element, and winter. Cystitis, nephritis, and other kidney and bladder problems related to fear often make the body imbalanced in terms of heat and cold (winter relates to cold) as well as acid and alkaline. (The kidneys control the acid/alkaline balance.)

Chinese medicine has integrated within its system the roots of disease and even specifies the organs that are involved with particular emotional and mental attitudes.

MAINTAINING HEALTH AND PREVENTING DISEASE

In order to maintain our total health (physical, emotional, spiritual), we need to become flexible at all times and adapt to the various changes around us. Each day has its particular rhythms in terms of sunrise and sunset. The Sun is related to activity, heat, awareness, and consciousness; the Moon, to passivity, cold, intuition, and the subconscious. The Sun governs the fire and heat in the body; the Moon, water and fluids. Each planet is also related to certain bodily functions and parts of the body. Mars, for example, is the red planet; it rules the blood, the physical energy or vitality, and aggressive tendencies. It also rules the adrenal glands. When the adrenals are depleted through stress or worry, we lack energy. Saturn, the principle of time, governs body structure—the teeth, bones, and body alignment. It is related to calcium metabolism. Psychologically, it refers to holding back or restraint.

In Hindu Ayurvedic medicine, there is a definite relationship between the body humors and the passage of time. *Kapha* (Water and Earth) is predominant from sunrise until 10 A.M. One, therefore, feels energetic and fresh at this time, and a little heavy. At midday, *Pitta* (Fire and Water) increases, which is a time when one feels hungry, light and hot. From 2 P.M. to sunset, *Vata* (Air and Ether) is dominant, and one feels more active, light, and supple. Early evening until 10 P.M. is Kapha time again—cool air, inertia, and low energy. Then 10 P.M. until 2 A.M. are the peak hours of Pitta when food is digested. Before sunrise is Vata time when there is movement and people awake to begin a new day.

In Chinese medicine, different body meridians are active at various times of the day. The *chi* flows though the body in a 24-hour period; it flows through the 12 meridians so that each organ is dominant for a two-hour period. From 5 A.M. to 7 A.M., the large intestine (time of elimination and arising), 7 A.M. to 9 A.M., the stomach (breakfast and digestion), 9 A.M. to 11 A.M., the spleen (heat and warmth), 11 A.M. to 1 P.M., the heart (circulation), 1 P.M. to 3 P.M., the small intestine (digestion and resting), 3 P.M. to 5 P.M., the bladder (cooler time), 5 P.M. to 7 P.M., the kidneys (also cooler and a time of reflection, stressing the water element), 7 P.M. to 9 P.M., the pericardium (time for emotional activity and meditation), 9 P.M. to 11 P.M., triple heater (bedtime, warming and regenerating the body), 11 P.M. to 1 A.M., the gall bladder (quiet time when the bile is being stored and other body processes take place), 1 A.M. to 3 A.M., the liver (also a quiet time), and 3 A.M. to 5 A.M., the lungs (time before awakening and preparing for the first breath of the new day).

We each have our own biological rhythm as well which influences our hormonal cycles and metabolism. In addition, we have our particular routine of work, household responsibilities, and family commitments. To maintain our individual rhythm and *at the same time* flow with the universal rhythms each day is *to walk in balance*. Walking in balance is what we refer to as *health*; to become out of balance is dis-ease. (It is interesting to note that the world *dis-aster* means "separation from the stars" or "away from the stars.")

In order to prevent dis-ease, we need to be aware constantly of the state of our vital energy, the "chi" force that the Chinese refer to, or the *prana* as the Hindus call it. What is the state of our vital force today? How is it flowing to each organ? Where is it blocked and why? Certain days we feel more tired than others; certain days we are more emotionally upset and scattered than others. What tools can be used to find the balance at all times and to keep the "chi" energy from becoming blocked or dammed up?

One of the most important tools is *cleansing*. If we regularly cleanse the body, then it will not only function smoothly, but we will become more sensitized to each part of the body and be able to feel when there are blocks or problems in various areas. Cleansing includes the colon (see chapter 3) through enemas, colonic irrigations, juice fasts; the nose (nasal washes); the skin (sweats, saunas, steam baths); and purification of the blood (through herbs and fasting). In addition to physical cleansing, mental purification is important.

Mental cleansing involves calming the mind. One needs to stop all mental activities and practice some sort of meditative exercise to achieve a more passive state. Physical exercise can often be an excellent adjunct to turning off the mind and becoming more receptive. Yoga and tai chi practices that emphasize the breath help to turn off the mind as well. Dance, walking in the woods, swimming—all of these can be relaxing to the mind and rejuvenating to the body. In addition, it is a good idea to become aware of the dreams and inspirations that come at these quiet times. These act as signs for us to keep in touch with our daily process. If we listen and follow our signs, we can indeed maintain our individual dance and rhythm within the larger cosmos.

Assuming responsibility for the food we put into our bodies is a primary concern—where it is grown, whether it has been sprayed with pesticides, as well as preparation and combination with other foods. Each of us requires particular nutrients at different times. To follow any one diet, such as a Raw Food Diet or Macrobiotic Diet, is to shift responsibility to another human being—the responsibility for tuning in to our own physical vehicles and determining our individual needs, regardless of what is in vogue at the time.

There is a great difference between needs and desires when it comes to food. What we desire may not always be best for our bodies. If we can distinguish between the two, we can balance ourselves accordingly.

There are several ways of determining an individual's nutrition needs. Laboratory blood tests and hair analysis may or may not be helpful in determining vitamin and mineral deficiencies. The *taking of the pulses* in Oriental and Ayurvedic medicine, along with facial diagnosis, studying the tongue, and the iris of the eye, are all excellent ways of diagnosing what is happening in the body.

The type of diet one should follow is best determined through the *metabolic constitution* or the Ayurvedic system of constitutional types, which is a comparable system (see chapter 4 for a full discussion).

Specific methods for testing individual foods include *applied kinesiology* (known as muscle testing or Touch for Health). Applied kinesiology uses simple muscle-testing procedures to assess the energy levels of the life forces which control the body. Through holding the food in one hand and testing out the muscle groups, it is possible to check out various foods and food supplements. Another very successful method is through the science of *radiesthesia*—the use of the pendulum or dowsing rod to test various foods. This is helpful for working with food allergies, and one can also determine doses of herbs, vitamins, and minerals.

In addition to foods, becoming aware of *herbs* that help to balance our bodies is important. Herbs may be used as an adjunct to foods in supplying us with vitamin and mineral needs. They can also be utilized as medicines to correct various conditions of imbalance within our bodies. The most effective way to use herbs is as teas, steeping the leaves or simmering roots and barks.

One of the best ways to maintain health is through some type of regular *bodywork*. Bodywork helps to release tensions and makes us aware of those areas where we tend to block energy. Good bodywork also enables the "chi" energy to circulate through all the meridians and renew each organ. There are many types of bodywork—relaxing massage which works on the muscular system; massage for relieving stress, based on deep tissue work which breaks down body armor and releases pent-up emotions; and techniques which work with the electromagnetic currents to balance the vital energy (polarity therapy, jin shinn, shiatsu, and acupressure). *Acupuncture* is a technique that uses needles at various points on the meridians to enable the "chi" energy to have a more direct, unimpeded flow to each organ. It is an excellent tool for "tuning up" the body, balancing the energy going to each organ, and preventing disease.

Stress-reducing techniques, such as *biofeedback*, and various types of mental exercise that relax the body, like *autogenics* and *hypnosis*, are helpful in controlling diseased states that arise from imbalances in the nervous system. Through the use of a device attached to a person's fingertips, the biofeedback machine is able to help people monitor their inner states and learn to relax, thereby lowering blood pressure and controlling asthma attacks and other physiological processes. Hypnosis and autogenics help to achieve physical relaxation. Once an individual has mastered this, s/he can move into higher meditative states of awareness.

A discussion of preventative tools for maintaining health would not be complete without the mention of *homeopathic medicine*. Homeopathic medicine treats *the person*—not the disease—by finding a specific remedy (called the "constitutional remedy") that vibrates with the individual and helps to increase her/his vital force.

Initially one takes this remedy once or twice, sometimes renewing it every few months. There are also homeopathic remedies for acute conditions such as burns, bee stings, and flu.

Flower remedies and *remedies made from gems* are becoming more frequently used in controlling emotional states that accompany physical imbalances. All disease starts on the higher planes and filters down to our physical bodies. If we can change or transform our emotions, such as grief, depression, and anxiety, we don't need to take on the physical manifestations of these.

◊ 3 ◊

CLEANSING AND ELIMINATION

To keep the body in proper balance and to metabolize and absorb the nutrients from our food, proper elimination is necessary. Whereas the upper portion of the digestive system—mouth, stomach, and small intestine—is designed for absorption, the lower part—the colon or large intestine—is for elimination; it also contains a number of microorganisms, referred to as the intestinal flora, which are essential for proper elimination.

Failure to eliminate waste products from the body causes fermentation and putrefaction, leading to many health problems. When eating several meals a day, it is impossible not to have residues accumulate in the colon in the form of undigested food particles as well as the end products from food which has undergone digestion. Food waste also builds up in the cells and tissues, which become highly toxic if they continue to ferment and putrefy. The purpose of the colon as an organ of elimination is to collect waste material from every part of the body and, through the peristaltic action of the colon's muscles, remove this waste. If it is allowed to accumulate, sickness, disease, and imbalance within the body often occurs.

Constipation is the major condition underlying most health problems.[1] A state of constipation often exists when movements of the bowel *appear to be normal* due to an accumulation of feces somewhere in the colon. Constipation involves not only the retention of feces in the bowel, but also the retention through the first half of the colon (from the cecum to the middle of the transverse colon).

The wall of this section of the colon has nerves and muscles which create wavelike motions known as *peristalsis* to propel the contents of the colon from the cecum to the rectum for eventual evacuation. Besides the formation of these waves, the first half of the colon extracts any nutritional material which the small intestine was unable to collect. This nutritional material is collected by the blood vessels lining the walls of the colon and carried to the liver for processing. If the feces in the colon have fermented, any nutritional elements present pass into the blood stream as polluted products (often referred to as *toxemia*, a condition in which the blood contains poisonous products which are produced by the growth of pathogenic or disease-producing bacteria).

The other important function of the first half of the colon is to gather (from the glands in its walls) the intestinal flora needed to lubricate the colon. Many people believe that colon irrigations and enemas wash out the intestinal flora and deprive the colon of lubrication. This is not the case; when the accumulation of feces in the bowel leads to blockage or incrustation, it is not possible for the lining of the colon to function normally, and the glands cannot produce the necessary lubrication. This incrustation interferes with the necessary intestinal flora for colon lubrication, formation of peristaltic waves for evacuation purposes, and absorption of nutritional elements from the small intestine.

A colon irrigation or colonic is a method of sending water to the colon so that the fecal lining is soaked and saturated in order that its removal may take place gradually and effectively. While the patient lies relaxed on a table which is connected to the colonic equipment, a trained operator (often a nurse, chiropractic doctor or naturopathic doctor) controls the water flow and expulsion going through the colon, massaging the colon as well as helping loosen encrusted fecal material. A colon irrigation requires a period of half an hour to one hour; during that time, 20 or 30 gallons of water (at the rate of about one pint to a quart at a time) are inserted into the colon through the rectum and then expelled. Initially, most people need at least three colonics (about one a week) to break up the old material, and they should continue these treatments every second or third month, depending on the state of the colon. Through cleansing the colon, maximum absorption of food is thus permitted. The proper amount of glucose is transported to all the cells of the body, maintaining the blood sugar at a constant level.

Many diseases and conditions of body imbalance are related to

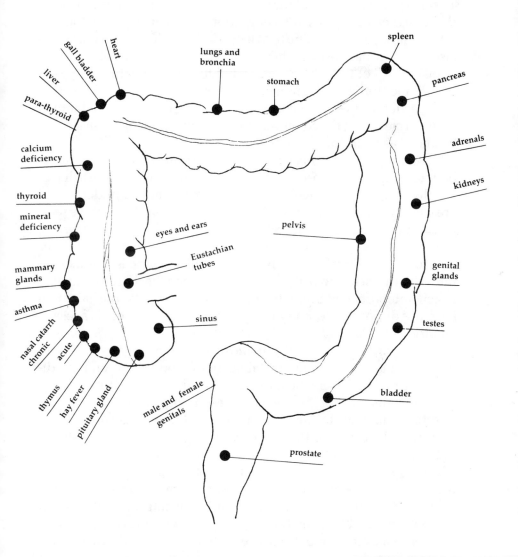

Normal Colon with Anatomical Centers

blockage of fecal material within the colon. One of these is diarrhea—a condition of frequent and fluid evacuation of the bowel. There are several types of diarrhea. The most common is *inflammatory* diarrhea caused by the congestion of mucus in the colon; another type is *pancreatic*, due to a disturbance of the pancreas; there is also *parasitic* diarrhea which is incited by the presence of intestinal parasites. All of these have responded to colonic treatments.

If one studies a diagram of the colon (p. 15), s/he will find that each section of the colon corresponds to another organ within the body. In cleansing the colon, all other organs are being cleansed and balanced as well.

Many people in this country suffer from some type of metabolic condition or disease—hypoglycemia (low blood sugar), diabetes, thyroid imbalance (conditions of overweight and underweight are usually related to the thyroid), and the various diseases we refer to as cancer. The body's metabolism is dependent on the hormone thyroxin for its proper function; *iodine* is the basic ingredient of this hormone. The ability of the thyroid to utilize iodine is commensurate with the lack of toxicity in the colon. When the thyroid is unable to generate sufficient thyroxin, the skin may turn gray, the hair often becomes dry or brittle, body weight increases, and there is a loss of vitality.

The *pancreas* is one of our most important organs; it is intimately connected with the metabolism of blood sugar and the digestive process. Pancreatic juice contains digestive enzymes and is alkaline in its reaction, so it establishes the right conditions for the intestinal enzymes to function in the small intestine. Towards the middle of the pancreas there is a group of glands called the islands of Langerhans, which produce insulin, the hormone responsible for regulating the metabolism of sugar and other carbohydrates. When the body is toxic and there is fermentation in the colon, these glands are unable to produce the needed insulin, causing an intolerance of sugar by the body. When this happens, the volume of sugar is increased in the blood and discharged into the kidneys (known as *diabetes mellitus*).

Working along with the pancreas is the *liver*; it is involved with fat and protein metabolism. It generates bile, which is stored in the gall bladder and helps to break down the fats in the body. It is also a detoxifying agent and a blood reservoir. When the colon is toxic and contains fermented material, toxins build up in the liver as well.

This lowers the immune system, and the body may then develop many allergic conditions and diseased states. Another function of the liver is to break down the hemoglobin of the red cells and to store copper, iron, and other trace minerals.

Congestion of the colon also leads to the *lymphatic system* becoming overloaded with waste material. When the lymph glands are filled to their capacity, lumps often develop in various areas of the body, such as the breasts. *Prostate problems* and other disorders of the reproductive system are also related to blockage in the colon.

In order to aid elimination, there are several foods which should be included in the diet as well as a small amount of fasting, primarily with vegetable juices, broths, and herb teas. Fasting over a long period of time, however, depletes the vitality. Since so many individuals have problems with low blood sugar, one or two days prior to a colonic is sufficient. Fruit juices tend to make the body more acidic and increase the amount of sugar, so very little fruit juice should be used—perhaps one glass of prune or cherry juice in the morning. For the rest, fresh vegetable juices, soup broths made from potatoes and other vegetables (which are alkalinizing to the system), and herb teas will supply the vitamins and minerals the body needs.

Mucilaginous foods and *herbs* are important for lubricating the walls of the colon and aiding elimination. Important mucilaginous foods include flax seeds, chia seeds, and psyllium seeds. These should be ground up and can be added to cereal in the morning, sprinkled on salads and soups, or taken mixed with water or juice. Herbs that are mucilaginous and particularly helpful for the colon are slippery elm and comfrey.

The inclusion of *fermented foods* in the diet is also important as an aid to elimination and to promote growth of healthy intestinal bacteria. Yogurt and kefir are among these foods. If one is particularly sensitive to cow's milk products, goat's milk yogurt is available and can be made from fresh or powdered goat's milk. Seed yogurt and fermented seed cheeses can be made as well from sesame seeds, sunflower seeds, and other seeds. Fermented foods made from soybeans include miso (a soup broth or base) and tamari (soy sauce). One should be careful, however, in the intake of miso and tamari since they are very high in sodium. Therefore, they should not be included in the diet more than once or twice a week. The yellow and white misos are lower in sodium. Other fermented foods include sauerkraut, *kim chee* (an Oriental spicy mixture of cabbage and red peppers), and fermented cheeses like Roquefort.

In addition to cleansing the colon, it is important periodically to remove excess mucus from the nose, throat, and lungs. There are two kinds of mucus—the *lubricating* mucus in the mucosa, which is natural and necessary in every human body—and the *pathogenic* mucus that is the result of eating and drinking certain foods. This pathogenic mucus propagates germs, microbes, and bacteria. Cow's milk and products derived from it are the most prolific source of this type of mucus. Poor food and digestion will also cause an increased mucus flow.[2]

A *nasal wash* is often helpful—pouring warm water in one nostril with a small pitcher (called a "netti pot"), letting it run out the other. There are also various tubes from India which are inserted through each nostril and then pulled out of the throat. This helps to break up mucus in the area of the nose and throat. More complex procedures exist for cleaning the bronchials, stomach, and colon.

The *skin* is another important organ of elimination. Many of the toxins in the body accumulate on the skin, and this accounts for the various body odors we emit. Saunas and steam baths, especially in the winter months when we don't normally perspire, are excellent methods of cleansing the skin. The sweat lodge, used by many Native American tribes, is a fine way of cleansing both mind and body.

NOTES

1. Norman W. Walker, *Colon Health: The Key to a Vibrant Life* (Prescott, AZ: Norwalk Press, 1979), p.11.
2. Ibid., p. 59.

METABOLIC CONSTITUTIONS AND DIET

In our daily observation of people, we experience many physical types—those whose bodies are tall and thin, others who are shorter or heavier, some whose complexions are ruddy, others who are pale or sallow. We also see those who are nervous, tense and underweight as well as those who are more relaxed with a heavier frame. All of these qualities are due to *individual metabolism.*

Metabolism is the function of maintaining life; it is the total exchange of energy with the environment, an exchange involving food, water, air, light, and heat. How each of us uses these raw materials to maintain life differs from one person to another.

In Western medicine and physiology, we speak of metabolic constitutions being determined by the dominance of the sympathetic or parasympathetic nervous systems. *Sympathetic dominance* leads to action-oriented, hyperactive, tense, underweight individuals. They often have problems with constipation; dryness around the mouth, eyes and nose; cold extremities; and adrenal exhaustion. *Parasympathetics* tend to be slower and less active, fall asleep more easily, often have ruddy complexions, and rely more on intuition than reason. Sympathetic dominance is characterized by slow oxidation and digestion because most of the nervous impulses are going to the energy-producing glands. Parasympathetic dominance, on the other hand, has faster oxidation and digestion; these individuals are prone to diarrhea, stomach and intestinal problems, and low blood sugar because they metabolize so fast.

In Ayurvedic medicine, the ancient Hindu system of healing,

19

individuals are categorized by the predominating *dosha* or element—*Vata*, or Air, *Pitta*, or Fire, *Kapha*, or Water. Vata types are very mental, tend to be thin and wiry, and often have problems with constipation and digestion; they are fairly slow oxidizers. Pitta types are fiery, active and energetic, producing a good amount of bile and breaking down foods easily; they are fast oxidizers and are more prone to diarrhea and digestive problems relating to the liver. Kapha types are more emotional, move slowly, and often are heavier due to excess water they carry in their bodies; they are very slow oxidizers.

The various types resulting from sympathetic or parasympathetic dominance have been organized into a system of ten Metabolic Types by Dr. William Donald Kelley, a dentist who cured himself of liver and pancreatic cancer (see *One Answer to Cancer*, The Kelley Foundation, 1974). Kelley found that the diet and supplements that helped him did not work for his wife when she was ill with cancer. In discovering a totally different diet for his wife, Kelley stumbled on an idea that led him to investigate these two branches of the autonomic nervous system.

The autonomic nervous system which regulates metabolism controls involuntary metabolic actions such as heartbeat and digestion. Dr. Kelley found that most people are neurologically influenced more strongly by either the "accelerator" (sympathetic) or "decelerator" (parasympathetic) branch of the autonomic nervous system. Some people may be healthy with "accelerating" or "decelerating" nerve stimulation, while others may be just as healthy with "balanced" stimulation.[1]

The varying degrees of nerve stimulation mean that one's glands and organs function differently. This affects our chemical and hormonal output, which in turn affects personality traits and behavioral patterns as well as physiological characteristics.

Once the metabolic type is determined, the proper nutrients for an individual can be recommended in the form of foods and nutritional supplements. Dr. Kelley identified ten metabolic types ranging from those with pure sympathetic dominance to those with pure parasympathetic dominance. Most people fall in between the two extremes.

Individuals whose sympathetic nervous system is more dominant receive less nerve stimulation in the digestive organs and more in the energy-producing glands. Those dominated by the parasympathetic branch receive more nerve stimulation to the digestive organs and less in the energy-producing glands. Many individuals are balanced; they are neither sympathetically nor parasympathetically dominated.

Individuals dominated by the sympathetic nervous system are often prone to anxiety, nervous strain, and irritability. Parasympathetics tend to have a slow metabolism, indicating that they oxidize blood sugar rapidly and, therefore, have low blood sugar. Those with sympathetic dominance experience food as a heavy feeling in the stomach. Their "fast metabolism" emphasizes the *catabolic* aspect of metabolism which breaks down complex substances into simpler ones. Catabolic processes take place in the absence of oxygen, so the sympathetic oxidizes blood sugar slowly.[2] They have a more acidic body chemistry and do better with alkaline foods such as vegetables. Since the food stays with them so long, they need to eat lightly as they can easily build up waste products in the digestive tract. Parasympathetics and more balanced types can eat more at one sitting. The slow metabolism of the parasympathetics emphasizes the *anabolic* aspect of metabolism, which synthesizes complex substances from simple ones. Anabolic processes are aerobic (take place in the presence of oxygen), so the parasympathetic oxidizes blood sugar rapidly.

How does one determine whether her/his metabolism is dominated more by the sympathetic or parasympathetic system?

SYMPATHETIC	PARASYMPATHETIC
rarely craves sugar	craves sugar frequently
eats small meals often	can eat larger meals
prefers vegetables	often desires meat and heavy proteins
wakes up easily	difficulty getting out of bed
active during the day	often lethargic and sluggish
worries a lot	n.ore relaxed and less anxious
likes exercise	dislikes exercise
makes decisions easily	often has difficulty making decisions
good concentration	poor concentration
acts more on reason	acts more on intuition

These characteristics are the extreme of each type; most of us are combinations of the two, though we often have one system that is more dominant.

ACID/ALKALINE BALANCE

Sympathetic types have a more acid body chemistry, and parasympathetics tend to be more alkaline. Foods are either acid, alkaline, or neutral; this is determined by measuring the *pH* of the ash of the food after it has been burned.

Sympathetics could become too acidic if they overeat proteins. Symptoms of acidosis include dehydration, dry hard stools, rapid heartbeat, muscle cramps, heartburn, and insomnia. Diseases include arthritis, ulcers, hemorrhoids, and hyperactivity. Parasympathetics could become too alkaline from too many fruits and vegetables; symptoms of alkalosis include diarrhea, joint pain, rashes, excessive sweating and teeth sensitivity. Diseases include arrhythmia and edema.

Foods

Alkaline	Neutral	Acid
fruits	milk	fish
meat	butter	poultry
vegetables	cream	lamb
sea vegetables	yogurt, buttermilk	beef
millet	vegetable oils	
seeds	honey	
herbs and spices	sugar	
salt		
soy sauce		
miso		
wine		
tea, coffee		

Citrus fruits contain certain acids which are "buried" by the body forming carbon dioxide and water. The ash that remains has an alkaline reaction in the body tissue. Plums and cranberries contain benzoic acid which is not broken down by the body; they, therefore, cause an acid reaction.

Fruits—Sympathetic dominants like them, but they do not digest them rapidly. Parasympathetics may burn up fruit sugar so quickly that it makes them jittery, just like sugar.

Vegetables—Sympathetics like green leafy vegetables which

are easy to digest and high in potassium. Parasympathetics are more drawn to root vegetables, which are alkalinizing.

Grains—Grains are not so strongly acid; they are more neutral. Parasympathetics convert grains into blood sugar more slowly than fruits, so they are especially recommended in the morning to help stabilize blood sugar throughout the day.

Proteins—Sympathetics need proteins like nuts, seeds, eggs, and yogurt. Parasympathetics can handle proteins such as fish and some meats because they tend to be more lethargic and need more energy. Fish and meat proteins, especially organ meats, contain high purines, one of which, adenine, is a constituent of ATP (adenosine triphosphate), which is an energy carrier at a cellular level.

Acid/alkaline balance is a subtle issue since there are many layers of pH in the body. Stress and emotional factors greatly influence the acid/alkaline balance. Weather and seasonal changes also affect this balance. Food cravings indicate the body is out of balance and that the blood sugar may be low. A varied diet, including different tastes from bitter to sour, sweet, salty, and pungent is helpful.

METABOLIC CONSTITUTIONS AS SEEN
THROUGH AYURVEDIC MEDICINE

In order to compare the differing metabolisms, we need to understand the meaning of each of the three doshas. *Vata* is the principle of *kinetic energy* in the body; it is concerned with the nervous system and controls all body movements. *Kapha* is the principle of *potential energy*, which controls body stability and lubrication. *Pitta* controls the body's *balance* of kinetic and potential energies; the enzyme system and endocrine system are Pitta's territory.[3]

At the cellular level, Vata moves nutrients into and wastes out of cells. Pitta digests nutrients to provide energy for cellular function, and the cell's structure is governed by Kapha. In the digestive tract, Vata assimilates nutrients and expels wastes, and Kapha controls the secretions which lubricate and protect the digestive organs.

Vata is not gas, but increased Vata causes increased gas. Kapha is not mucus, but it is the force which projected in the body causes mucus to arise. Pitta is not bile, but it is the force which causes bile to be produced.[4]

Most people are combinations of these types and are Vata-

Pitta, Pitta-Kapha, or Vata-Kapha.

In terms of food, Vata types have irregular appetites—they often suffer from constipation. Pitta types love to eat; they usually digest well, have loose stools, and are rarely constipated. Kapha types can become attached to food as a means of emotional fulfillment. Vata types do better with three or four small meals a day; they often need to snack in between, but not more than every two hours (the time it takes for food to digest). Pitta types should eat three meals daily with 4-6 hours between them. Kapha types should eat only twice a day with a 6-hour gap between meals.

Vata types require more cooked food than Pitta or Kapha types. Pitta or Pitta-Kapha can handle more raw foods as they have the digestive fire to break them down. Vata people do best on one-pot meals like soups, stews, or casseroles because they are easier to digest than individual foods.

VATA	PITTA	KAPHA
rarely craves sweets	on occasion craves sweets	craves sweets
lots of nervous energy	good physical energy	often lethargic
insomnia and restless	sleeps well	sleeps well
wakes up easily	wakes up easily	difficulty waking
likes exercise	often overdoes exercise	dislikes exercise
logical	logical and intuitive	intuitive
irregular appetite	loves to eat	food emotionally fulfilling

DIET

Diet in the Ayurvedic system is based on six tastes:

1. Sweet is cooling, heavy, and oily. It increases Kapha, decreases Pitta and Vata.

2. Sour is heating, heavy, and oily. It encourages elimination of wastes, lessens spasms and tremors, and improves appetite and digestion.

3. Salty is heating, heavy, and oily. It eliminates wastes, cleans the body, and increases digestive capacity and appetite as well as softening and loosening tissues.

4. Pungent (hot and spicy like chili peppers) is heating, light,

and dry. It flushes all secretions from the body and improves the appetite. It increases Pitta and Vata, decreases Kapha.

5. Bitter is cooling, light, and dry. It purifies and dries all secretions, increases appetite and controls skin disease and fevers. It increases Vata, decreases Pitta and Kapha.

6. Astringent (makes one's mouth pucker) is cooling, light, and dry. It reduces secretions and purifies and constricts part of the body. It increases Vata, decreases Pitta and Kapha.

FOODS FOR VATA CONSTITUTIONS

Sweet, sour, and salty foods are good for Vata constitutions; bitter, pungent and astringent are less desirable because they dry out the system. In terms of grains, well-cooked rice and oats are excellent. Cooked buckwheat, millet, and rye are heating and therefore good. Yeasted bread is not so good because the fermentation fills it full of gas. Freshly cooked grains are better since bread is dried out by baking.

Cooked vegetables are preferable to raw vegetables. Rough, hard vegetables like celery are better digested as juice. Salads of lettuce, parsley, cilantro, or sprouts may be eaten on occasion with a good oily salad dressing like olive oil. Tomatoes are not good raw but infrequently may be used cooked where the skins and seeds are removed.

Most fruits are good, except those which are naturally astringent, such as cranberries and pomegranates, and those which are drying like apples (baked apples or pears are better). All dried fruits are inappropriate unless they are reconstituted with water. Unripe fruits should be avoided, especially unripe bananas because they are astringent. Ripe bananas are good because they are soothing to the intestine and are helpful for constipation.

Vata is the only type who needs animal foods because they need the complete proteins.[5] Too much animal flesh weakens the digestive tract, however. Eggs, fresh fish, chicken, turkey, and venison may be used. Soured-milk products, such as yogurt or kefir, may be used since they aid digestion. Eggs should be scrambled with yogurt or milk or poached; fried eggs are not good.

Legumes are difficult to digest and their metabolic by-product is nitrogen, which is a gas that increases Vata. Mung beans are the lightest to digest. Legumes may be cooked with turmeric, cumin, or coriander seeds to kindle digestive fire. They also may be cooked with ginger or garlic. If legumes are soaked for an hour and the water thrown away, they tend to produce less gas. Splitting peas and lentils makes them more digestible because more of the surface is exposed while cooking.

Almonds are the best nuts, but they should be soaked overnight and their skins peeled. Other seeds and nuts should be made into nut milks or butters so they will not be too concentrated. Overconcentrated foods resist penetration by digestive juices.

All oils are good for Vata types, especially olive, almond, and sesame. Coconut and sesame oils can be used for the hair and skin.

Some sweets reduce Vata; barley malt syrup, rice syrup, molasses or honey may be used. The overuse of sweets increases Vata.

All spices, especially garlic and ginger, can be ingested by Vata types in small amounts. They tend to overuse hot spices to improve digestion so they should be sprinkled with care. Cayenne, cardamom, curry, and turmeric are warming and aid digestion. Fennel, dill, and anise are good for gas.

FOODS FOR PITTA CONSTITUTIONS

Pitta types should avoid sour, salty, and pungent, but should use sweet, bitter, and astringent. Meat, alcohol, and salt should especially be avoided because they increase heat and aggressiveness. Grains, fruit, and vegetables should form the majority of the Pitta diet.

Barley is the best grain for Pitta types because it is cooling and drying and helps reduce excess stomach acid.[6] Rice and oats are also good. Buckwheat, millet, and rye may be too heating, but can be used sometimes. Yeasted bread is not good because of the sourness produced during fermentation, but unyeasted bread is fine.

Most vegetables are beneficial for Pitta types, except sour vegetables such as tomatoes and pungent vegetables such as radishes. Beets, carrots, and daikon radish are good for the liver.

Pitta types should eat sweet fruit and avoid sour fruit like oranges, lemons, limes, pineapples, and pomegranates.

Flesh food is not recommended for Pitta people, but fresh fish as well as turkey, rabbit, or venison on occasion would be okay.

Legumes should be eaten sparingly because of their acidity, but mung beans, tofu, black lentils, split peas and chick peas (red and yellow) are fine. Lentils are too warming.

Nuts and seeds are too hot and oily, except for coconut milk, which is cooling.

Sweet dairy products like milk, ghee, and unsalted cheeses are best. Yogurt may be spiced with cinnamon or coriander if it is eaten.

Sweets can better be handled by Pitta types than other types. However, molasses is heating, and honey can be heating if it is over-used. Only cooling spices such as fennel and dill should be used; cardamom, cinnamon, and turmeric may be used sometimes.

FOODS FOR KAPHA CONSTITUTIONS

Kapha types need to concentrate on bitter, pungent, and astringent foods to invigorate their body and mind and should avoid sweet, sour, and salty tastes. Fat greasy foods and dairy products are the worst foods for these people. They need grains less than the other types, but hot drying grains like buckwheat and millet work best for them. Barley, rice, and corn are also beneficial. Breads are best toasted or dried out.

All vegetables are good for Kapha types, except tomatoes and very sour vegetables. Leafy greens are preferable to root vegetables. Steamed and stir-fried vegetables are easier to digest than raw, though raw may be eaten on occasion.

Very sweet and very sour fruits should be avoided as well as any fruits that are extremely juicy. Dried fruits are good as are fruits such as pomegranates, mangoes, apples, pears, apricots, and peaches.

Kapha people rarely need any flesh foods, but they may eat fresh fish, eggs, broiled poultry or venison. Legumes are better for Kapha types than flesh foods, but they do not need much protein. Heavy legumes like soybeans, kidney beans, and black lentils should be avoided.

Nuts and seeds also should be avoided since they are too oily. The same goes for most oils, except for almond, corn, safflower, or sunflower oils on occasion.

Dairy products are not particularly good, as previously mentioned, though goat's milk products are better than cow's milk.

Sweets should be avoided since they increase Kapha. All spices may be used except salt; ginger and garlic are especially good.

OTHER TYPES

Vata-Pitta types should follow a Vata-controlling diet in fall and winter and a Pitta-controlling diet in spring and summer when Pitta is stronger. They should especially avoid spicy, pungent food.

Pitta-Kapha types should use a Pitta-controlling diet from late spring through early fall and a Kapha-controlling diet from late fall through early spring. Bitter and astringent tastes are best for these types.

Vata-Kaphas should control Vata in summer and fall and Kapha in winter and spring. Since both Vata and Kapha are cold and need heat, they should use sour, salty, and pungent tastes rather than sweet, bitter, and astringent tastes.[7]

These are all general guidelines, and they must be tailored to individual taste and temperament. Though individuals may be typed metabolically, there are many differences within each type.

NOTES

1. *Metabolic Typing—Medicine's Missing Link* pamphlet published by International Health Institute, Winthrop, WA, 1982.
2. Fred Rohe, *The Complete Book of Natural Foods* (Boulder, CO: Shambhala Pubns., 1983), p. 98.
3. Robert Svoboda, *Prakruti: Your Ayurvedic Constitution* (Albuquerque, NM: Geocom Limited, 1988), p. 17.
4. Ibid.
5. Ibid., p. 65.
6. Ibid., p. 67.
7. Ibid., p. 71.

DIETARY REGIMENS

Within the spectrum of natural foods, there are many types of diets. Some diets are strictly vegetarian (elimination of flesh foods, including fish and meat). A lacto-vegetarian diet relies on nuts, seeds, tofu (soybean curd) and other soy products for its proteins. A natural non-vegetarian diet may include fish and organic poultry or other organic meats.

Another distinction in vegetarian diets is those that recommend mostly raw foods and those that use mostly cooked foods. Raw food diets have been popular in warm climates where there is an abundance of fresh fruits and vegetables and body temperature is able to maintain itself without warm, cooked foods. They also are utilized by those who are on a cleansing diet or preparing for a fast, or those who have a serious illness and need to eat a light diet, eliminating protein.

RAW FOODS

Enthusiasts of raw food diets say that enzymes are killed in the cooking process thus making nutrients less available. They do not believe in eating grains because grains form mucus in the system which may reduce the entrance of oxygen into the lungs.[1]

Grains contain a high concentration of starch and mineral salts. When subjected to heat, these minerals are rendered insoluble and may be deposited in body tissues.[2] In addition, unsprouted grains are acid forming in the body. To replace cooked grains, cooked tu-

29

bers or squash are recommended.

Foods should not be eaten cold either. They should be taken out of the refrigerator and allowed to soak in the Sun to absorb solar radiation.[3] Some researchers believe that raw food enzymes continue to work in conjunction with digestive enzymes in the stomach. In the intestines, vegetable enzymes help to detoxify intestinal flora as well as to normalize bacteria in the colon. This reduces the number of disease-producing bacteria.[4]

Dr. Ann Wigmore has become famous for her healing of disease through the use of raw foods and wheat grass juice. She has set up the Hippocrates Health Institute (one in Boston and one in San Diego) where patients learn how to grow sprouts and to juice raw foods. (She has several books out, including *Why Suffer* [Hippocrates Institute, 1964], which delineates the discovery of wheat grass and its effect on health). Many people attribute their ability to heal themselves of cancer and other life-threatening diseases to a raw food diet with lots of vegetable juices.

MACROBIOTICS

The Macrobiotic Diet was developed by the Japanese philosopher George Ohsawa. (*Macro* means "large" or "great," and *bios* means "life.") Ohsawa felt that with a good diet we could experience a deep and fulfilling life. In addition to being a preventive diet to maintain health, Macrobiotics has been used therapeutically for those who are seriously ill.

In Macrobiotics, food is considered not just for its physical effect but for its mental and spiritual effect. Each piece of food is treated as a spiritual manifestation and should not be wasted in the process of preparing and cooking. Before eating, prayers should be offered to nature and the universe which have given us this food. While eating, it is important to chew each particle of food thoroughly in order to spiritualize it and to reflect on the harmony of the universe.[5]

Macrobiotics classifies foods according to *yin* and *yang*.

Yin	Yang
grows in hot climate	grows in cold climate
contains more water	is more dry
fruits and leaves	stems, roots, and seeds
high above the ground	below the ground

Yin
acid reaction in body
hot, aromatic foods

Yang
alkaline reaction in body
salty, sour foods

During the winter, the climate is cold and damp (yin); thus, the energy descends into the roots. Leaves die, the sap goes to the roots, and the vitality of the plant becomes more yang. Plants that grow in late autumn and winter are more dry and have more vitality; they can also be kept a long time without spoiling. Examples are root vegetables such as carrots, turnips, parsnips, and cabbages. The weather becomes more hot and dry (yang). Summer vegetables are more watery and perishable; they need to be stored in a cool place. Fruits ripen in late summer; they are watery and sweet and develop higher above the ground. Foods which grow in hot tropical climates are more yin, whereas foods which grow in northern climates are more yang.

CONSTITUENTS OF THE MACROBIOTIC DIET

1. Grains are the staple of the diet: brown rice, buckwheat, millet, rye, oats, barley, corn and whole wheat form 50-60% of the diet used as whole grains, cereals, and breads.

2. Legumes and seeds form 10-15% of the diet and can be used at every meal in combination with grains.

3. 20-30% of the diet is land and sea vegetables, including soups. About two-thirds of these are cooked, and about one-third is raw as salads. Potatoes (including sweet potatoes and yams), tomatoes, eggplant, avocado and other tropical vegetables are avoided. Seaweeds such as dulse, kombu, wakame, hijiki, arame, and agar-agar are used.

4. Less than 15% animal food is used—primarily white meat fish and seafood.

5. Fruits and nuts are used in small amounts; a fruit dessert is served on occasion if the fruit is growing in the same climatic zone.

6. Fermented food is used in small amounts to provide enzymes and bacteria. These include vegetable-based fermented foods such as miso, tamari, soy sauce, sauerkraut and other pickles.

7. Beverages predominantly made of non-aromatic herbs like bancha twig tea, mu tea, dandelion tea, burdock tea or cereal grains are used. These should be taken as the last part of the meal or separately.

8. Sweets are avoided, except rice syrup, barley malt syrup or other syrups processed from grains. These are used on occasion.

The diet also prescribes a definite order for eating. Whole grains, legumes, and seeds can be eaten throughout the meal. Soups are eaten first, then vegetables, and then vegetable salads or pickles. Fish is often included with the vegetables. Fruit, nuts and beverages are used at the end of the meal and alone. Seasonings include soy sauce, unrefined sea salt, and vegetable oil. Tropical spices and aromatic herbs are avoided.

Some people find the Macrobiotic Diet too heavy because of its emphasis on grains and legumes. Certain body types have difficulty digesting grains and are better off eating grains only once a day, preferably in the morning. In the Ayurvedic system, Vata types, generally thin, airy, and mental people, do not have the enzymes to break down carbohydrates. They do need more protein than other types, however. Kapha types, heavy body types whose bodies seem to be filled with water, may also need a lighter diet since they produce a lot of mucus. They often do better with a light breakfast (vegetables or fruit) rather than a grain breakfast.

The Macrobiotic Diet and certain fasts (combinations of brown rice with vegetables and some fish) have proved very healing for those with many serious ailments. Dr. Anthony Sattilaro, in Philadelphia, who healed himself of cancer through the use of the Macrobiotic Diet and philosophy, is one of its strongest advocates (*Recalled by Life*, Avon, 1982).

OTHER DIETS

More moderate diets than simply raw foods or Macrobiotics work for most people. Whole grains are very grounding and contain most of the B-complex vitamins and other nutrients. Most people do well eating a whole-grain cereal or the whole grains themselves in the morning. This is because the grain is a complex carbohydrate and takes about eight hours to break down in the body. This process of breaking down helps keep the blood sugar up. Whole-grain breads are okay but do not have as many nutrients as the grains themselves. Vegetables may be added to the grain; proteins like eggs, tofu or fish may also be eaten with the grain for a more substantial meal. Those with low blood sugar do well if they have some protein in the morning. As was mentioned previously, certain metabolic types that tend to accumulate mucus function better on a very light breakfast of vegetable juices or cooked vegetables or fruit.

The midday meal should be the largest meal, but this is not always possible for many people who work and bring their food to the office or have to eat at a restaurant. Midday meals should include some vegetables, whether in the form of soups, steamed, or raw in salads. Certain metabolic types and those with low blood sugar benefit from good protein at their midday meal. This may be eggs or fish (if they are eaten) or a soy product like tofu. (Dairy products like cheese tend to form a lot of mucus and are responsible for many allergic conditions. They should be used primarily in the form of soured-milk products like yogurts, kefir, buttermilk, acidophilus cottage cheese, or a small amount of goat milk cheese). Some people need heavier food at midday—a grain or bread, or root vegetables like potatoes or squash.

Dinner depends on what one has eaten for the midday meal. Ideally, dinner should be the lightest meal since one goes to sleep several hours afterwards. Digestive enzymes work best at midday; that is when our fire is at its greatest (the internal fire creates the enzymes that break down food).

Steamed or raw vegetables should be included at dinner with some protein, grain or root vegetable. Heavy carbohydrates such as pasta, beans, and breads should be avoided, as well as heavy proteins and fatty foods like meats and dairy products. Fruits should be eaten separately as snacks in between meals unless it is an all-fruit meal. Fruits can be very acid and are difficult to digest with other foods. Beverages are best after a meal as well, except for vegetable juices which may be drunk before a meal. Herbal teas and grain beverages should be served a short while after eating since the liquids wash away the digestive enzymes.

Alcoholic beverages drunk with meals also have an acidic effect and may interfere with the digestive process. Alcoholic beverages in general are not particularly good for the liver and may interfere with bile production. Certain foods like vinegar, nutritional yeast, cranberries, raw spinach, raw green pepper, and tomatoes are very acidic and should be avoided. (Tomatoes may be used on occasion in a cooked sauce.)

Wheat products form a lot of mucus, and many people are allergic to them. Rye bread, corn bread, and other wheatless breads such as millet bread may be substituted. Rye flour, rice flour, buckwheat flour, and soy flour may be used in baking instead of whole-wheat flour.

A balanced diet includes whole grains at least once a day; vegetables, raw or cooked, twice a day; protein, once or twice a day; and fruit as a snack. If sweets are used, they should be made with honey, barley malt syrup, or rice syrup. Those with low blood sugar do best with the syrups made from grains because they have more complex carbohydrates. There are many cookies and candy bars where these syrups are used; many are also fruit-juice sweetened.

For those who have certain food addictions and cravings, there are ways to balance the body and substitute healthier foods. Many people are used to drinking coffee in the morning and at other times of the day to wake them up. The caffeine in coffee is a stimulant to the nervous system, but it can make one very wired without really increasing vitality or energy. Herbs as gotu-kola or fo-ti which do, in fact, increase adrenal energy, can be used instead. If one likes the taste of coffee, there are grain beverages, such as Roma, Cafix, or Pero, which are coffee substitutes; some of these even come in a package similar to coffee and can be used in drip coffeepots for a comparable taste.

Many people crave sugar, especially mid-afternoon when their energy drops. Usually if they eat a substantial breakfast with a cooked whole-grain product, blood sugar remains higher. Also, a pancreas glandular supplement after meals can help to stabilize the blood sugar. However, it is a good idea to have a mid-afternoon snack like a piece of fresh fruit or some raw vegetables, nuts or seeds. If one wants something sweet, cookies or a candy bar with natural sweetening may be used.

Variety in foods is a good principle to abide by in order to obtain nutrients and to avoid allergies. Eating a different grain every morning is a way to vary breakfasts. Using different vegetables for lunch and dinner and alternating the type of protein is another way to seek variety. The way foods are served may also add nutrition. Foods in combination with certain proteins produce essential amino acids; for example, adding seeds or tofu to a grain dish.

Diet includes much more than the food itself. Diet includes the type of food we buy. Is it organic, or does it have chemical additives? Where was it grown? What kind of store was it bought in? All these factors affect the vibrational quality of the food we eat. How we prepare the food also affects it; if we are feeling angry or upset, it might be better to have a snack and wait until we feel more balanced. In fact, we will take in those angry vibrations with our food; this often is why people get indigestion. It is better to eat meals slowly in a relaxed atmosphere than at one's desk or while driving to and from places. Food eaten in a relaxed atmosphere will be much more healing to our bodies than food, no matter how high the quality, eaten on the run.

Some helpful books on diet include Rudolph Ballantine's *Diet and Nutrition—A Holistic Approach* (Himalayan Intl. Institute, 1978), Gabriel Cousens' *Spiritual Nutrition and the Rainbow Diet* (Cassandra Press, 1986), Fred Rohe's *The Complete Book of Natural Foods* (Shambhala Pubns., 1983), and Frances Moore Lappe's *Diet for a Small Planet* (Ballantine, 1975).

We are what we eat has been a much-overused statement. As spiritual beings, we know we are more than our food intake. Perhaps we could change the statement to "We are *how* we eat." How we eat reflects how we nurture ourselves and each other, and ultimately, how we treat our environment.

NOTES

1. Viktoras Kulvinskas, *Survival into the 21st Century* (Woodstock Valley, CT: O'Mawgo D Press, 1975), p. 41.
2. Ibid.
3. Ibid., p. 46.
4. Ibid., p. 48.
5. Michio Kushi, *The Book of Macrobiotics: The Universal Way of Health and Happiness* (Tokyo: Japan Publications, Inc., 1977), p. 78.

6

CARBOHYDRATES

Carbohydrates make up the bulk of our diet. Through the burning of carbohydrates, energy is produced, and our metabolism is dependent on this energy. We take the carbohydrates, burn them with the oxygen we breathe, and produce carbon dioxide and water. As we do this, we are releasing the energy derived from the Sun that the plants have taken in to produce carbohydrates. By eating these plants, we break them down and utilize their energy.

A *calorie* is a measure of heat produced when a substance is burned or oxidized. One gram of carbohydrate will produce about four calories; a gram of fat will produce nine; a gram of protein, four.[1] If one eats more calories than s/he uses, s/he may convert these to fat and gain weight. Most people, however, do not assimilate much of the food they eat due to the condition of the large intestine, which often serves as a repository of undigested food. Therefore, they can overeat and still remain thin. If carbohydrates are combined with other nutrients, such as protein, fat, vitamins and minerals, one does not have to worry about taking in excess calories. It is only when empty calories are consumed (carbohydrates that have been separated from other components of food) that excess caloric intake occurs.

SUGARS

The carbohydrate molecule contains carbon, hydrogen and oxygen in addition to the Sun's energy. The smallest molecule of carbohydrate produced by a plant is called a *sugar*. Most sugar molecules contain six carbon atoms to which are attached hydrogen or oxygen atoms.[2] The sequence of these makes fructose, the sugar found in fruits, different from, for example, glucose or blood sugar. Fructose plus glucose combine to form sucrose or "table sugar." When purified, white sugar is made from sugar cane; everything is taken out except sucrose. The vitamins, minerals, and other nutrients are removed. Without the proper vitamins and minerals to facilitate the metabolism of the carbohydrate and create the need for exercise, much of the sugar gets stored away as fat, which often leads to obesity. The missing nutrients are then taken from the real food in the diet, from the nutrients in the blood that were intended for other functions, or from the reserves stored in the bones.

A complex carbohydrate (including a sugar made from a grain like rice syrup or barley malt syrup), by contrast, has the accompanying fiber, vitamins, minerals, enzymes, proteins and fat. The sugars of complex carbohydrates are chains of glucose molecules which, when separated by the digestive process, are sent through the walls of the small intestine to the liver for storage as *glycogen*. As we need energy, the liver releases glucose into the blood stream in a smooth, balanced manner.

One of the functions of the liver is to remove excess glucose from the blood. In order to do this, it requires insulin produced in the pancreas. Insulin is the hormone responsible for controlling the metabolism of carbohydrates. The cells that produce insulin receive the signal when we consume a carbohydrate and then send the necessary insulin. Next, the liver converts the glucose into its storage form as glycogen. Later, as glucose is needed for energy other hormones are sent from the adrenals to convert the glycogen back into glucose, which is then released into the blood stream as "blood sugar."[3]

When a simple sugar (as in a candy bar) is consumed, the beta cells which produce the insulin interpret the leap in blood sugar to mean that the liver needs a large amount of insulin to store all that glucose (the same amount it would need if a bowl of rice or a slice of bread were eaten). So the insulin arrives at the liver, waiting for the glucose coming from the small intestine. However, there is no glucose, so the insulin takes the glucose out of the blood (in order for the liver to store it away as glycogen), and the blood sugar plunges way down with the accompanying feelings of tiredness, irritability and depression (or what William Duffy calls *The Sugar Blues* [Warner Books, 1976]). Many people interpret this as a sign for more sugar and, in this way, a sugar addiction is formed. Eventually, diabetes, the failure of the beta cells to produce adequate insulin, may result.

Sugar is also responsible for reducing resistance to disease because it steals the ability of the white blood cells to destroy bacteria. White blood cells are known as *phagocytes*, and phagocyte tests show that a couple of teaspoons of sugar can sap the strength of white blood cells by 25 per cent.[4] Sugar also reacts with saliva to form acids that dissolve the enamel of the teeth, thereby forming an ideal medium for the growth of bacteria.[5] It increases gastric acidity in the stomach, leading to indigestion and possible ulcers; it raises blood pressure and, combined with animal fats in the diet, leads to atherosclerosis.[6]

Sugar takes a transit time of four to five days in the bowel, rather than one and one-half days, and is, therefore, linked with diverticulitis and cancer of the colon.[7] The excretion of calcium in the urine, caused by sugar, is associated with osteoporosis.[8] The fungus *candida albicans*, naturally present in most women, can multiply disproportionately with excessive sugar consumption, leading to infection.[9]

The following are all forms of sucrose, though a few may contain some minor nutrients: raw sugar, light and dark brown sugar, turbinado sugar, maple syrup, corn syrup, invert syrup, cane syrup, sorghum syrup, Barbados molasses, and blackstrap molasses (which does contain more nutrients, but wreaks havoc with the blood sugar as well).

Rice syrup (maltose), barley malt or corn malt syrup (maltose), date sugar (fructose), and honey (glucose and fructose) do not depend on sucrose for their sweetening power. Honey is 98 per cent sugar and 2 per cent enzymes, vitamins and minerals. Although it is a complex carbohydrate compared with sugar, it still enters the blood stream rapidly and causes the same kind of blood sugar rise and strain on the pancreas.[10] So, although honey has many healing properties, including its use as an antiseptic (meaning that bacteria cannot survive in it), it is far better to use the sweeteners made from grain, such as rice syrup, barley malt, or corn syrup. One should also be careful of fructose (fruit sugar) which has been appearing in the form of a sweetener. Much of it being marketed is not pure fructose, and it still remains a simple sugar.[11]

GRAINS AND BREAD

Wheat bread has always been referred to as "the staff of life," and each area of the world is dependent on a different grain for its sustenance. In the United States and much of the Western World, wheat has always been the staple grain. (There is a vast difference, however, between whole-wheat bread and white bread made from refined wheat flour in which most of the nutrients have been removed.) Yet many people are allergic to wheat, and it seems to be the bran in wheat that is the offending substance.

Grains are seeds and are comprised of three parts—the germ, which can be sprouted, the starch or bulk of the grain (called *endosperm*), which nourished the seedling during its early growth, and the bran or outer covering that protects the grain. The germ contains vitamins, oils, and proteins; the endosperm is made up of starch granules packed together, the walls of which contain protein; the bran is composed of several layers and contains fiber, minerals, some protein, and a small amount of vitamins. The gluten in wheat makes up the major part of the protein and can be isolated from the wheat flour to make a meat-like substance that can be sliced into cutlets. The Orientals call this gluten *seitan*. To prepare the gluten, the flour is kneaded until it is stretchy, and then the kneading process is continued under water. The starch or bran falls away and the gluten remains.

Contrary to what many people have thought, it is the bran in wheat and not the gluten that seems to be responsible for allergies. The cellulose comprising the bran contains high amounts of phytic acid. Phytic acid is a phosphorus compound found in large amounts in whole grains, beans, and peas. It has the property of combining with minerals, especially calcium, iron, and zinc, to form insoluble compounds. Therefore, bread with added bran has often caused calcium deficiencies and rickets.[12]

RICE

The staple grain of most of the Far East is rice, and next to wheat it is the grain grown in the largest quantity throughout the world. In the United States, some rice is grown in the southeast, primarily Louisiana and Arkansas. Wild rice is grown in parts of the upper Midwest as Wisconsin and Minnesota. Whole-grain rice, without refining, retains all its nutrients like whole wheat, thus the emphasis on brown rice rather than the polished white rice. The reason that polished rice is used in the Orient seems to be the availability of protein in polished rice compared to unpolished rice.[13] Test subjects maintained a better balance of protein on a polished-rice diet. Polishing, however, removes a large proportion of vitamins and minerals, especially the B vitamins. Beriberi, the thiamine deficiency disease, is found among those who subsist almost exclusively on polished rice.

CORN

Corn was the staple grain of the New World; corn-based diets extended through most of North and South America at the time of the early colonists. The Indians pounded the corn into meal or soaked it until it was soft, and then boiled the whole grain in a solution of ashes. This increased the availability of vitamin B-3 (niacin) and became known as "hominy" among the Southern settlers. The outer edge of the corn grain is hard and requires longer cooking; this part is referred to as "grits."

The growing of corn spread to other countries, but where it was relied on exclusively deficiency diseases like pellagra (lack of niacin) developed.[14] Where green leafy vegetables or beans were added to it for their protein value, these diseases did not develop.

OATS

Next to wheat, rice, and corn, more oats are grown than any other grain. Oats were used by the ancient peoples in Northern Europe. The Scots made oatmeal a national dish around the 17th and 18th centuries. Oats are higher in protein than most other grains[15] and also extremely high in calcium. (Oat straw is used for those suffering from arthritis and rheumatism.) Because oats are soft, the time required to prepare oat cereals is less than that of other grains. Several techniques are used to process oats which make them easier to cook. One is to smash them flat with a roller (rolled oats); another is to cut them with a steel blade into small pieces which cook more rapidly than the whole grain (steel cut oats).

RYE

An advantage of rye is its resistance to cold, so it has been grown widely in Russia, Scandinavia, and the Eastern European countries where a dark rye or pumpernickel bread is produced. It is lower than wheat in gluten but does not make breads which rise as easily. One disadvantage of rye is that it can become afflicted with a fungus that grows on the grains, causing them to swell up and become black. This fungus contains a toxin called *ergot*, which can lead to severe symptoms such as constriction of blood vessels and violent cramps. However, if the grain is watched and harvested correctly, it should not develop this fungus.

BARLEY AND BUCKWHEAT

Barley is grown in colder climates and is useful in cold weather when its warming effects are noticeable. Barley bread is used from Tibet to China and Japan. Sprouted barley has a high content of maltose, a sugar which is the primary ingredient of malt. Malt syrup is used for making beer and as a sweetener. It is preferable to honey because it is a more complex carbohydrate and, therefore, normalizes blood sugar due to its gradual absorption. When barley is milled to remove the outer bran, the process is called *pearling*. Pearled barley is easier to cook, but it is devoid of many of the minerals and proteins. Barley has important medical properties, and barley water has been used for complaints ranging from upset stomach to nervousness.

Buckwheat is technically not a grain; it is not tall and slender like the grasses but grows low with heart-shaped leaves and flowers; the groats are the fruit of the plant. Like rye, it grows well in poor soil and cold climates. It has a warming and drying effect on the body and is cooked whole or cracked like rice.

MILLET

Millet is the staple grain in parts of Africa, India and China. There are three important types of millet among the different species; bulrush millet, which grows on a stalk and is yellow like corn, is the kind we use in the United States. Like buckwheat, millet is a very "yang" grain and is used for its warming and drying qualities.

Sorghum, another species of millet, is grown in South and West Africa, China, and Central and Northern India where it is the principal grain known as *ragil*. Each ear consists of five spikes which rise from a central point like fingers from the palm.

OTHER STARCHES

There are many other sources of starch in the diet in addition to grains and breads. Legumes include various types of beans and peas which are utilized for their protein. Soybeans actually contain more protein than carbohydrate and are, therefore, the source of so many protein derivatives, including tofu or bean curd (made from the curd), and *tempeh* (an Indonesian food made from the soybean that is becoming increasingly popular in this country). Lentils contain twice as much starch by weight as protein, and kidney beans have almost three times as much.

Potatoes, sweet potatoes, yams, and various types of hard or "winter" squashes are also high in starch. The white potato contains a small amount of protein and many vitamins and minerals; yams and squashes are especially high in vitamin A.

NOTES

1. Sue Williams, *Essentials of Nutrition and Diet Therapy*, 2nd ed. (St. Louis, MO: C. V. Mosby Co., 1978), p. 25.
2. Rudolph Ballantine, M.D., *Diet and Nutrition—A Holistic Approach*, (Honesdale, PA: Himalayan International Institute, 1978), p. 52.
3. Paavo Airola, *Hypoglycemia: A Better Approach* (Phoenix, AZ: Health Plus Pubs., 1980), p. 23.
4. Fred Rohe, *The Complete Book of Natural Foods* (Boulder, CO: Shambhala Pubns., 1983), p. 44.
5. Ibid., p. 43.
6. Ibid., p. 48.
7. Ibid.
8 . Ibid.
9. Ibid.
10. Ibid., p. 50.

11. Ibid., p. 51.
12. Ballantine, p. 71.
13. Ibid., p. 76.
14. Ibid.
15. Ibid., p. 81.

PROTEIN

The importance of protein in the diet is emphasized by the fact that protein is a structural material. Calcium and phosphorus are deposited around protein to form bones. Connective tissue is made from collagen, a protein-like substance that creates the fibers that form tendons. An inner framework of protein gives various tissues their shape and is the basis of their organization. Protein molecules are also the largest in the biochemical world. Each protein molecule is a long chain whose links are smaller nitrogen units called *amino acids*. Each amino acid contains at least one atom of nitrogen as well as hydrogen, oxygen, carbon, and sometimes sulphur.

Most of the 22 amino acid molecules can be converted into others or manufactured by the body. However, there are eight which the body cannot synthesize, and these are called the *essential amino acids*. The eight essential amino acids are isoleucine, leucine, lysine, methionine, phenylalanine, threonine, tryptophan, valine, and perhaps histidine.[1] Any amino acids which are not needed for the construction of new protein molecules can be burned as fuel.

The nitrogen fragment of the amino acid molecule and the remains of the other protein substances make up urea and uric acid. When the kidneys are unable to excrete all of the uric acid through the urine, it may accumulate in the tissues and joints and crystallize, promoting protein toxicity and giving rise to symptoms of gout.

PROTEINS IN THE DIET

Important sources of protein include meat, fish, fowl, eggs, dairy products, beans, especially soybeans, nuts, and seeds. Grains contain some protein, and even vegetables have small amounts.

While it is advisable to determine if a protein is complete or incomplete in terms of the essential amino acids it contains, its assimilation potential in the body is also important. NPU, or *net protein utilization*, describes a food's biological value and its relative digestibility. Meat and poultry rank low on this scale; eggs have the highest NPU at 94 per cent, fish, 80 per cent, and milk, 82 per cent. Plant proteins are high in NPU even though they lack some of the essential amino acids.[2] One can, however, work with food complementarily to maintain the correct balance in amino acids. For example, grains are low in isoleucine and lysine, but legumes are high in them. Grains, seeds and nuts are high in tryptophan and methionine.[3]

Though meat has often been regarded as the number one protein food, most meat contains nearly as much fat as protein. Eating too much meat leads to a high blood cholesterol count and eventually may cause arteriosclerosis.[4] In experiments with animals, vegetable protein has been found to protect against arteriosclerosis when compared with animal protein.[5]

Vegetarians or those who eat little meat have less incidence of cancer and heart disease and tend to have lower blood pressure than meat eaters.[6] Eating high-fiber vegetable protein has been correlated with a decrease in diseases such as diverticulosis, arteriosclerosis, and cancer of the colon since vegetable fiber absorbs a variety of environmental pollutants and carries them out of the body.[7] Too much meat may also lead to calcium deficiencies and osteoporosis since meat contains up to 20 times more phosphorus than calcium.[8] Excess animal protein can lead to intestinal sluggishness, overacidity and the formation of ammonia. Ammonia is a carcinogen and a major cause of cancer of the colon.[9] Another important aspect of reducing flesh consumption is to lower ingestion of pesticidal residues. More pesticide residues are found in meat and fish than in grains or legumes.[10] In addition to pesticides, animals are given various hormonal drugs like stilbestrol to fatten them as well as antibiotics.[11]

Eating some meat, however, if it is naturally raised (referred to as "organic"), can be a good way of obtaining the essential amino acids and vitamin B-12, which many vegetarians tend to lack. Organ meats such as liver are very high nutritionally and low in fat as well. Poultry, especially turkey, is high in certain amino acids like tryptophan and methionine.[12]

Fish eating is generally preferable to meat eating because fish has less fat; it is a high source of iodine and other trace minerals from the sea; and it is lower on the food chart than meat and, therefore, may contain less chemical pesticides and residues. However, as some of our waters are badly polluted now, it is important to be discriminating and to determine where the fish came from. Ocean fish should be chosen rather than inland varieties as the degree of contamination is less.[13] It is also important to avoid shellfish since they are scavengers and accumulate a high level of toxic residues. Many come from coastal waters where there have been oil spills and areas have been sprayed for mosquito control with DDT.[14] In and of themselves, shellfish are a cause of many allergies.

EGGS

Eggs are basically an easy-to-assimilate high-protein food *if* fertile eggs are used. Commercial eggs are obtained from hens that are bred in large, factory-like structures with poor ventilation and electric lights. The feed given to the hens has added hormones and antibiotics; water is often withheld from them. The electric lights force the hens to sexual maturity and egg production, and their life span is thus shortened. When the eggs are removed from the hatcheries, they are stored, chilled, and kept for more than a month before incubation.[15]

Tranquilizers also have been used to calm birds and increase egg production. DDT residues have been found, and additives as well as synthetic color are now added since the normal vitamin A content of the yolk is lost.[16] To extend shelf life, commercial eggs are dipped or sprayed with a commercial oil or oil solvent. This makes it impossible, in the absence of refrigeration, for the consumer to distinguish day-old fresh eggs and several-weeks-old oiled eggs.[17]

What is the difference between commercial and fertile eggs? Fertile eggs contain natural growth and reproductive hormones that are beneficial in renewing our glands. They are high in vitamins A and D and methionine, an amino acid low in grains and other plant proteins. They are also a good source of inositol, choline, and lecithin, all involved in balanced cholesterol metabolism.[18]

Frying eggs destroys amino acids and makes their protein difficult to assimilate.[19] The cholesterol content of eggs has made them controversial—some researchers say they raise blood cholesterol; others, that they lower it. The best recommendation here is not to eat eggs in excess of about six a week.

MILK AND DAIRY PRODUCTS

Of all of the available protein sources, perhaps the most problems are caused by cow's milk and products made from it. Milk and cow's milk products are the source of many allergies. This is usually due to a deficiency of *lactase*, the enzyme involved in the digestion of *lactose* (the sugar that supplies the carbohydrate in milk). This milk sugar has to be split by the enzyme lactase into two smaller sugars—galactose and glucose—to be digested. When the enzyme is missing, there is often gas, abdominal pain, and diarrhea. In many ethnic groups where drinking milk has not been traditional, this enzyme disappears about the time of weaning.[20]

In addition to being a source of allergies, cow's milk and cow's milk products form an increased amount of mucus in the throat, nasal passages, and bronchi. This leads to congestion of these areas and increased susceptibility to colds and other allergic reactions. Goat's milk, on the other hand, is less mucus forming; thus, many have switched to goat's milk as well as cheeses and yogurt derived from it.[21] The fat and protein molecules are much smaller in goat's milk so it is easier to digest; it takes 20 minutes in the digestive tract rather than two hours.[22]

Antibiotics, hormones, detergents, viruses, toxins, pesticides, and radioactive isotopes are some of the materials that have been found in regular pasteurized milk.[23] Penicillin has been used since 1945 to treat mastitis in cows, and as many as 28,000 i.u.'s of penicillin per pint have been found in milk from cows treated for this inflammation.[24] One of the processes used to make non-fat milk, drum or roller drying, requires excessively high heat. Milk flows over superheated surfaces and the protein pattern is destroyed. Vitamin C and all other vitamins are reduced. Lysine is almost completely destroyed. Animals fed drum-dried milk deteriorated rapidly.[25] Dry milk is an unbalanced food; the sucrose content is higher than it is in proportion to other elements in fluid milk. This may affect the calcium level in the body. In 1966, the disease organism *salmonella* also turned up in dry-milk products.[26]

Pasteurization of milk is an outmoded solution as it causes loss of vitamin A, 6 per cent of the calcium while the rest is altered into a form more difficult to assimilate, 20 per cent of the iodine, and 40 per cent of the B vitamins, as well as the loss of enzymes that make the milk more digestible, most of the vitamin C, and a reduction of the protein biological value by 17 per cent.[27] Milk partially heated in the pasteurization process tends to coagulate into a tight mass when exposed to stomach acid. It will constipate children; raw milk does not.[28] Since the pasteurization process only heats milk to 145° F (or 62° C), some bacteria still remain. Boiling raw milk, however, will sterilize it without destroying its nutritional advantages.

In addition to goat's milk, other alternatives also exist, and many cultures have long used non-dairy milks. The Chinese and Japanese have used a milk made from ground-up soaked soybeans. Soy milk is now available in this country as well, and there are several companies which produce it. It can be bought with flavors, such as carob or vanilla, added to it. The milk is also curdled and hung in a cheesecloth to form a solid curd called soy cheese or tofu. Tofu is a very assimilable form of protein and can be used in a variety of ways to replace both meat and cheese. There are many such products on the market now—tofu burgers, tofu hotdogs, as well as dips and spreads made from tofu.

Milk can also be made from various nuts and seeds. Sesame milk, made from sesame seeds, is higher in calcium than cow's milk; it is a native drink in the Middle East. Almond milk and cashew milk are both high in amino acids. (They can be made by combining one cup of raw nuts with one cup of water and adding a little malt syrup or honey.) Coconut milk is used in India and West Indian cooking.

Low-fat and non-fat milks have become popular since people are more conscious of fats in their diet. However, the more fat that is removed from milk, the less calcium can be assimilated. Butterfat, found in milk, is an important element in the calcium metabolism of milk and contains vitamins A and D, both fat-soluble vitamins.[29]

In *Nutrition Against Disease* (Bantam, 1973), Dr. Roger Williams says that butterfat protects us against atherosclerosis. Non-fat dry milk fed to rats produced atherosclerosis, but regular milk did not.

CHEESE AND COTTAGE CHEESE

Cheese is coagulated milk with most of the water or whey removed. It is a highly concentrated food and can be difficult to digest except in small amounts. Raw-milk cheese is easier to digest than pasteurized cheese. In addition, most pasteurized cheeses contain additives which give them a yellow or orange color. Traditionally, enzymes and bacterial cultures were added to milk to develop a particular flavor and character in the cheese. Rennet was used to coagulate the casein into a solid mass, which was processed into a hard cheese. It was never subjected to chemical preservatives.

Today, skim milk or milk enriched with a cream may be used instead of rennet. Salt is often added as well as calcium chloride to set the milk in a semi-solid mass.[30] Certain cheese companies in this country use bleaching which adds hydrogen peroxide and catalase (an enzyme) to milk for making cheese.[31] Other companies use benzoyl peroxide or other mold-inhibiting ingredients such as sorbic acid or its salts. In addition to all this, cheese rinds are often coated with wax and vegetable oils which may penetrate the cheese. Often, vegetable dyes in addition to pesticide residues have been found in cheeses.[32] If cheese is included in the diet, it should be raw-milk cheese, aged naturally, without preservatives or chemicals. Again, goat cheese and soy cheese or tofu are good substitutes.

YOGURT AND SOURED-MILK PRODUCTS

The practice of creating soured-milk products like yogurt, buttermilk, and kefir makes milk easier to digest, preserves it, and prevents the growth of undesirable bacteria. The most common method is simply to set the milk aside and allow it to ferment. In the Balkan states, especially Bulgaria, the local bacteria produce a soured milk which is quite delicious. This is called yogurt, and this particular culture is added to milk in the U.S. The milk is boiled before the culture is added; this destroys any bacteria that may be disease-causing and inactivates certain enzymes which would tend to kill the bacteria that are to be added. During the souring process, lactase is broken down to lactic acid; therefore, soured-milk products are more easily handled by those who do not tolerate milk sugar well. The growth of new bacteria in milk during this process of souring may also supply a strain of bacteria which is beneficial to the intestinal tract.[33]

Commercial yogurt has various forms of gelatin and vegetable gums added for thickeners. The fruited yogurts also have sugar and artificial flavoring.

LEGUMES

Beans and dried peas have been used for many centuries throughout the world as a source of protein. Soybeans are popular in the Orient; mung beans and lentils in India (the traditional dish called *dahl* is made from lentils); black beans in Cuba and South America; baked beans in New England; pinto and kidney beans in other parts of the United States and Mexico. When combined with grains, legumes can become a complete protein since legumes are deficient primarily in methionine while grains contain ample amounts of methionine but are deficient in lysine. For grain-legume combinations, the proportion of grain to bean is important—usually about twice as much grain as legumes.

A number of experiments have shown that eating dried beans and peas lowers blood fat and decreases hardening of the arteries.[34] In all races, a high consumption of vegetable protein in the diet was found in those who had the cleanest coronary arteries.[35]

Many people avoid beans because they are difficult to digest. The gas that comes from eating beans is caused primarily by two unusual starches, *stachyose* and *raffinose*.[36] These are short chains of sugar molecules, but they are joined by a special linkage that cannot be broken by any of the enzymes usually found in the intestine. Therefore, they are not absorbed but remain behind in the digestive tract where they are metabolized by certain bacteria that are more common in those who eat meat.[37] These bacteria break down the starches into carbon dioxide and hydrogen, the two main components of gastrointestinal gas.[38] Beans can be de-gassed, however. Soaking overnight helps a little as enzymes in the bean break down the starches into sugars. Boiling for 20 minutes removes a third of these enzymes, and 85 per cent can be removed if soybeans, for example, are boiled five minutes, soaked for a half hour in water, rubbed until the hulls are free, and then cooked for an hour.[39] This may only be necessary, however, for those who are just beginning to eat beans. The cleaner the colon (see chapter 3), the fewer the problems digesting beans and assimilating the protein they contain.

The variety of beans is also important in determining whether they will cause indigestion or gas. Kidney beans and soybeans are harder to digest, while smaller beans, like adukis (traditionally used in Japan; they are very important for the kidneys) and mung beans, are easier. Soybeans can be made into tofu, and all beans can be sprouted, which increases the protein and decreases the starch.[40]

It is important to learn how to cook and prepare legumes since they are an inexpensive source of both protein and starch, are easy to grow in almost any climate, and store well.

NUTS AND SEEDS

Nuts and seeds contain a large amount of high-quality protein and also some of the essential fatty acids. These concentrated fatty acids can make large quantities of nuts difficult to digest, so often they can be ground up and added to various foods or prepared as nut butters and spreads.

Nuts are very delicate because after they have been shelled and allowed to stand for a long time the fats undergo oxidation and become rancid. This rancid flavor is often covered up by oiling, roasting, and salting the nuts.[41] Commercially, cashews may be heated in liquid to make the shells brittle, and English walnuts may be loosened by exposure to ethylene gas. Pecans and English walnuts are often dipped in hot lye and then rinsed in acid, or put into a hot solution of glycerine and sodium carbonate. Pistachios are often dyed red and covered with a layer of salt.[42] Roasting nuts means cooking them in oil and is actually French frying, not roasting. This process kills the vitamin E and 70 to 80 per cent of the thiamine. The oils used are of poor quality and are often reheated or reused, causing carcinogen danger.[43] BHT and BHA are included in most packaged, shelled nutmeats as well as in vacuum-packed tins of nuts. Pesticides also tend to concentrate in oils and fats; nuts often have a concentration of pesticides from spraying of the nut trees.[44] The best way to buy nuts are shelled and from a reputable natural food store. Then, they should be refrigerated.

Although peanuts are not true nuts, they are associated with them. Many peanuts are contaminated with *aspergillus flavus*, an aflatoxin mold found also on wheat, corn, soybeans, rice, cottonseed and other grains stored in a warm, damp place.[45] This toxin can kill ducklings, pigs, and calves. Cows can pass the poison through their milk, and it would be found in dried or pasteurized milk. Investigations uncovered that there is a relationship of aspergillus flavus to human toxicity—it inhibits growth of lung cells and spreads liver disease.[46] This toxin is present in raw and processed peanuts; roasting does not kill it. It is also present in peanut butter, packaged peanuts, candy with peanuts and peanut meal for animal feed.[47] Peanut oil is free from it due to the strong alkali used in processing.

Peanut butter is a very common food in the United States, especially with schoolchildren. To prolong shelf life and prevent oil separation in peanut butter, processors use a hydrogenated vegetable oil. In addition, dextrose or sugar and emulsifiers, such as the monoglycerides and diglycerides, are added. Most processors also degerm the peanut, which lowers the nutritional value. If peanut butter is used, only the old-fashioned natural butter without preservatives should be bought, and it then should be refrigerated.[48]

Seeds such as sesame, sunflower, pumpkin, flax, and chia contain only two or three times as much fat to protein, whereas nuts contain seven times as much.[49] Seeds are often used as a source of cooking oil and make good butters, such as sesame seed and sunflower butter. *Tahini*, a product used in the Middle East, is a paste made from ground, shelled sesame seeds. Sesame seeds are also a very high source of calcium and should be ground up for optimum digestion. They can be added to grains, salads and vegetable dishes to complete the protein. Seeds should be purchased fresh and refrigerated immediately. Roasted sunflower seeds, sold in stores, are often rancid. Roasting fresh sunflower seeds at home, however, makes them more usable and increases their nutritional value.[50]

Flax seeds, chia seeds, and psyllium seeds are mucilaginous foods and help in lubricating the colon. They should be ground up and kept in the refrigerator. A few teaspoons can be cooked with cereal in the morning, or they can be added to salads or juice drinks.

NOTES

1. Vic Sussman, *The Vegetarian Alternative* (Emmaus, PA: Rodale Press, Inc., 1978), p. 83.
2. Ibid., p. 85.

3. Frances Moore Lappe, *Diet for a Small Planet* (New York: Ballantine Books, Inc., 1975), p. 103.
4. Rudolph Ballantine, M.D., *Diet and Nutrition—A Holistic Approach* (Honesdale, PA: Himalayan International Institute, 1978), p. 116.
5. Ibid., p. 117.
6. Ibid.
7. Ibid.
8. Fred Rohe, *The Complete Book of Natural Foods* (Boulder, CO: Shambhala Pubns., 1983), p. 31.
9. Ibid.
10. Lappe, Appendix E, p. 376.
11. Beatrice Trum Hunter, *Consumer Beware!* (New York: Simon and Schuster, Inc., 1971), p. 114.
12. John Yacenda, "Tryptophane: Holiday Friend From Your Pantry and Oven," *Let's Live* (November, 1983).
13. Hunter, p. 197.
14. Ibid., p. 184.
15. Ibid., p. 169.
16. Ibid., p. 172.
17. Ibid., p. 175.
18. Rohe, p. 67.
19. Ibid., p. 68.
20. Ibid., p. 126.
21. Ibid., p. 132.
22. Rohe, p. 63.
23. Hunter, p. 225.
24. Ibid.
25. Ibid.
26. Ibid., p. 234.
27. Rohe, p. 89.
28. Ballantine, pp. 128-29.
29. Ibid., p. 61.
30. Hunter, p. 241.
31. Ibid.
32. Ibid., p. 243.
33. Ballantine, pp. 130-31.
34. Ibid., p. 140.
35. Ibid.
36. J. Rachis, "Soybean Factors Relating to Gas Production by Intestinal Bacteria," *Journal of Food Science* 35 (1970), 634.
37. Ballantine, p. 141.
38. J. Rachis, "Flatulence Problems Associated with Soy Products." Paper presented at First Latin American Soy Protein Conference, Mexico City, 1975.
39. W. Wolf, "Flavor and Oligosaccharides as Limiting Factors in Soy Consumption." Paper presented at First Latin American Soy Protein Conference, Mexico City, 1975.
40. Ballantine, p. 143.

41. Ibid., p. 145.
42. Hunter, p. 198.
43. "Food and Nutrition," Consumer Bulletin Annual, 1962-63, p. 20.
44. Hunter, p. 199.
45. Ibid., p. 200.
46. Ibid.
47. Ibid., p. 201.
48. Ibid., p. 202.
49. Ballantine, p. 145.
50. Ibid., p. 146.

$\Diamond$ **8** $\Diamond$

FATS AND OILS

The subject of fats and oils is perhaps the most controversial topic in the field of nutrition today. Fats and oils are made up of carbon chains. Each carbon atom in the chain may also be attached to two hydrogen atoms. When all the potential hydrogen atom spaces are filled, the fat chain is "saturated"; when there are spaces vacant, it is said to be "unsaturated." Highly saturated fats like animal fats are solid at room temperature while unsaturated vegetable fats are liquid. Animals store their energy in saturated chains; plants store theirs in unsaturated form.

Liquid vegetable oils are unsaturated, and they are often referred to as *poly-* (many) unsaturated since there are a number of unfilled positions on the carbon chain. Polyunsaturated fatty acids are called *essential fatty acids*; they cannot be produced in the body, but are essential for health. They are found in high concentration in grains, beans and seeds, and in lesser concentration in some animal food, especially fish. While polyunsaturated fatty acids are essential, there is no dietary need for saturated fatty acids. The need for polyunsaturates is very small, and two teaspoons of vegetable oil, such as olive, sesame, sunflower, corn, peanut, soy, or safflower, will satisfy this requirement.

Animal fats are mostly made up of saturated fatty acids and are less digestible than unsaturated fats. Polyunsaturated oils are made from vegetable oils and contain high amounts of linoleic acid, the most essential fatty acid. (The other two essential fatty acids are linolenic and arachidonic.) Linoleic acid and the other essential fatty acids are important in strengthening cell and capillary membrane structure, controlling blood clotting, lowering serum cholesterol, and keeping skin and hair lubricated and healthy.[1] Without essential fatty acids, our bodies can't produce lecithin, which, among other things, prevents deposits of cholesterol in the arteries. A deficiency of essential fatty acids may result in stunted growth, dermatitis, and reduced resistance to stress.[2] However, most natural foods contain a high amount of polyunsaturated vegetable oils, so there is small dietary need for additional vegetable oils. Some of the vegetable oils are so highly refined that most of the vitamin E, lecithin, and nutrients are removed. The amount of vitamin E the body needs is directly proportional to the amount of polyunsaturates it consumes; using oils with vitamin E removed creates a vitamin E deficiency.[3]

EXTRACTING VEGETABLE OILS

All vegetable oils come from the seeds of flowering plants. In ancient times, the oil was simply removed by roasting and crushing the seeds, allowing the oil to rise to the top. This wasn't very efficient, so pressing was introduced to extract more oil. High-quality oil made by large producers can be simply pressed, filtered, and bottled. These oils still retain the color, aroma, flavor, and nutrition which natural oils have.

Oils are extracted by two methods—pressure and chemical solvents. Pressing is normally done with an expeller press. In order to remove as much oil as possible, the high pressure used develops excessive heat, which can reach 300° F or more. This high heat can darken the oil and change the all-seed protein. At lower temperatures and lower pressure, the oil loses little of its flavor or nutrition; however, 12-15 per cent of the oil is left in the seed mash.

In solvent extraction, hexane is the most common chemical used. (Hexane is a petroleum derivative and is highly volatile, flammable, and toxic.) Hexane is allowed to flow through the toasted seed meal to dissolve and extract the oil. Removing the solvent also depletes the natural flavors of the oil, so a combination of the press and solvent methods are used. Both press- and solvent-extracted oils are still crude and unrefined; these are merely methods of extraction.

REFINING OILS

The process called refining does remove color, taste, and odor in order to improve shelf life. This process consists of several different operations.

First, the oil is degummed by mixing it with hot water to separate the gummy substance. One of the substances removed is lecithin. (The lecithin in natural oils causes them to smoke at high temperatures.) Next, fatty materials are removed by washing the oil in a high alkaline solution containing lye or sodium carbonate. This extracts the fatty acids and much of the beneficial vitamin E that acts as a natural antioxidant preventing spoilage. It also removes the phosphatides as well as protein and protein fragments.[4] Heated to 140-160° F, this solution neutralizes the free fatty acids to form soaps which are sold to soap manufacturers.[5]

Bleaching follows refining—the oil is treated with bleaching earth, Fuller's earth, or clay. Bleaching removes pigments and any soap left from the refining process; the chlorophyll content is also reduced.[6] Then the mixture is filtered.

After refining and bleaching, vegetable oils have an unpleasant flavor and odor. Therefore, the oil is deodorized at high temperatures. It is stripped with steam distillation and then cooled; this process removes any remaining odor, flavor, or pigments and leaves a bland, unfinished oil that tastes the same no matter what its source. Usually these oils have an antioxidant such as BHA or BHT added.[7]

In general, refining oils removes waxes, resins, stearines, and phosphatides. When these are eliminated, chlorophyll, lecithin, pro-vitamin A, vitamin E, copper, iron, magnesium, calcium, and phosphorus disappear.[8] Dr. Richard Passwater (in his book *SuperNutrition for Healthy Hearts* [Jove Pubns., Inc., 1978]) says that a diet high in *refined* polyunsaturated oils can cause iron deficiency anemia, weight gain, liver disease, intestinal damage, hypertension, gallstones, a raised level of uric acid in the blood, and the promotion of the release of free radicals which accelerate aging and cause cancer mutation.[9]

HYDROGENATION

Many vegetable oils, including margarine, are hydrogenated.

Hydrogenation is the next step after refining in which hydrogen gas is introduced to the liquid oil in the presence of a metallic catalyst, usually nickel or cadmium. Hydrogen ions thus get bonded onto the oil molecules, transforming them from a liquid to a solid. Some margarines do contain small amounts of liquid polyunsaturated oil added to a hydrogenated base, but the bulk of the fat is saturated. In England, a recent statistical analysis of the incidence of heart disease and the consumption of hydrogenated fats has shown a significant correlation. Where margarine and vegetable shortenings were used, the rate of heart attack was always higher.[10] In the Southeastern United States, where margarine consumption is very high, the incidence of heart attacks has also been increasingly high.[11]

A variety of fats and oils are used in the production of commercial margarine, with the selection of the essential ones governed by price. (One year a record amount of lard was used because it was cheaper than vegetable oils.) The remaining non-fat portion may consist of water, milk products, or ground soybeans. The federal standard also permits a variety of chemicals to achieve a butter-like flavor and odor.[12]

Vegetable oil margarines found in natural food stores are made with purer ingredients as well as fewer chemicals, and some of them contain no salt. Since they are made from vegetable oils, they may be better than butter in terms of being easier to digest and forming less mucus in the body, but they are still a hydrogenated product. It would be preferable to use the unrefined oils themselves.

UNREFINED OILS

Unrefined oils are darker in color; sediment accumulates on the bottom of the bottle, and the colors and flavors are strong and distinctive. The most important consideration in choosing an unrefined oil is its stability; it is easy for unrefined oils to become rancid. Olive and sesame are the most stable, and they are the lowest in polyunsaturates.[13] Both these oils have been used throughout the ages, whereas safflower and soy (the two most unstable), corn, sunflower, and peanut oils are fairly recent inventions.

OLIVE OIL

Olive oil is the only oil available that can be considered cold-pressed. Because olive oil comes from the soft, fleshy pulp of the fruit rather than the seed or nut, it doesn't need pre-cooking or high-pressure extraction. Olives are crushed in a mill, which breaks the pulp but not the kernels. The first extraction is a simple pressing that doesn't heat the oil much above room temperature. The oil is then separated from the olive water, either by settling or by centrifuging.

Oil obtained from this first pressing receives no further treatment other than filtering to remove the pulp. This is the only oil that can be labeled "virgin olive oil." Virgin olive oil has three grades: "extra virgin" is oil of perfect flavor and aroma; "fine virgin" has the same flavor as "extra," but a high acidity; "plain virgin" is slightly off flavor and has the highest acidity. This is the grade most often sold in the United States.

Oil labeled "pure" is still 100 per cent olive oil, but not virgin. Pure grades are extracted from the second pressings using higher temperature, pressure, and hot water treatments, or are solvent extracted. These grades are usually blended with virgin oil for better flavor. Pure olive oil has excellent stability and flavor and can sometimes be stored without refrigeration for over a year, but virgin oils degrade more quickly. Most of the unsaturates in olive oil are in the form of mono-unsaturated oleic acid; the lighter polyunsaturated linoleic forms only 15 per cent. This results in a fattier and heavier oil that can be used in soaps and cosmetics.

SESAME OIL

Sesame oil, one of the oldest oils produced, comes in light and dark varieties. The dark oil is made from seeds that have been roasted prior to pressing. This oil has a toasted smoky flavor, whereas the light oil is mild and nutty tasting. Although sesame oil is 87 per cent unsaturated, it contains only 42 per cent linoleic acid. It has excellent stability, resists oxidation, and may be used for salads, sautéing, and deep-frying. Most of the sesame seeds are imported from Central America and pressed in small amounts.

PEANUT OIL

Peanut oil is a by-product of the peanut industry with the poorer nuts being pressed or solvent extracted for oil. Natural peanut oil is fairly high in saturated fat, about 20 per cent, while containing only 30 per cent linoleic acid. This gives it a longer shelf life than safflower oil, so it may be used instead in natural potato chips or corn chips.

CORN OIL

Corn oil is highly saturated (90%) and high in linoleic acid (59%), yet it is very stable due to its relatively high vitamin E content which acts to prevent oxidation. Corn oil is a product of the industry that uses corn as a source of starch for glucose manufacturing, cornstarch, and cereal production. The oil comes mainly from the germ of the corn kernel, which is separated by steaming and mechanical action and then pressed.

SAFFLOWER OIL

Safflower oil is the most popular oil in the natural foods industry. Safflowers grow in arid and semi-arid climates on land not suitable for other crops. In the United States, they are grown in California, Arizona, and other parts of the Southwest. It is the least flavorful of the natural oils, which is one reason it is well liked, especially by those who are used to bland commercial oils. It has the highest percentage (94%) of unsaturated fats of all the oils and is highest in linoleic acid (78%). This gives it an exceptionally short shelf life and makes it too unstable for use in frying.

SUNFLOWER OIL

Sunflower oil is one of the few oils that can be produced in cold climates; it is manufactured in Canada and is of great commercial importance in Russia. In the southern United States, oil-bearing seeds such as sunflower are planted in areas with diminishing cotton yields. Sunflower oil is similar to safflower insofar as it is 92 per cent unsaturated with 72 per cent linoleic acid. Unlike safflower, sunflower oil has good resistance to oxidation and stores better.

SOYBEAN OIL

Soybean oil accounts for over 65 per cent of the oil currently being used commercially. Soybeans have a low oil content, only

16-18 per cent, which makes extraction desirable in commercial products. Natural soy oil is high in linoleic acid (about 50%) and is susceptible to oxidation. Soy oil has the strongest flavor of all the oils, and people often find the unrefined product undesirable. It is used in baking and salad dressings where a strong taste is desired. In commercial use, it is partially hydrogenated besides refined.

RANCIDITY

A rancid oil is one which has been acted on by oxygen. (Oxygen atoms, rather than hydrogen atoms, fill the spaces on the carbon chains.) Oxidation leads to the formation of free radicals. Vitamin E, which is present in unrefined oil, prevents both oxidation and the formation of free radicals.[14] (Free radicals are compounds that hold the oxygen atoms together.)

Unrefined oils should be kept in dark bottles in the refrigerator. The potential for rancidity is related to the amount of unsaturated fat in the oil. Safflower oil, the highest of the oils in polyunsaturates, is also the least desirable because it is the most unstable and the hardest to keep fresh.

Rancid oil tastes bitter and has a bad smell; however, a small degree of rancidity may not be noticed.

CHOLESTEROL

Some fat-like substances in the body are different from the simple carbon chains that make up most oils and animal fat. Cholesterol (*chol* means "bile," and *sterol*, "hormone-like") is a waxy fat-like compound and is the base from which estrogen, cortisone, and testosterone are made by the body.[15] It is also a component of nerve tissue. One end of the molecule can form a "salt" which is soluble in water, while the other end combines with fat. For this reason, cholesterol salts or bile salts promote the mixture of fats in the small intestine with water so they can be broken down and absorbed through the intestinal wall.

Cholesterol is most likely to cause trouble along the walls of blood vessels. As it accumulates, a hardening or plaque develops in the vessel wall. If this process continues, the deposits can become thick and large enough to narrow the space inside the blood vessel.

The blood supply to the area where the vessel leads is reduced. When muscular exertion increases the demand for oxygen, and not enough oxygen is supplied to the tissue, the result is often pain. When people with arteriosclerotic deposits in the blood vessels leading to the legs try to walk, there can be severe leg pain. If the deposits are located in the coronary arteries, the pain is in the chest, and if the arteries are narrow enough, portions of the heart muscle may die because of lack of blood. When the heart wall or myocardium is damaged or destroyed, it is called a myocardial infraction, or coronary. When the arteries that lead to the brain are blocked off, the damage affects the ability to walk, speak, or write; this is called a cerebral vascular accident, or "stroke."

Arteriosclerosis has become more prevalent in the United States and Europe, and heart attacks and strokes have increased. When it was discovered that severe arteriosclerosis is often accompanied by high blood levels of cholesterol and that cholesterol makes up the bulk of the arterial plaques, it was natural to assume that a diet low in cholesterol would help prevent the disease. Therefore, eating eggs, dairy products, and animal fats was discouraged.[16]

As a result of the cholesterol problem, Americans began using more margarine and liquid vegetable oils. Initial research using polyunsaturates first showed an ability to lower cholesterol levels and decrease the number of heart attacks.[17] Further research has thrown doubt on the long-term value of using vegetable oils for this purpose.

Recently, there has been a growing number of reports of increased incidence of cancer in patients who use a high percentage of unsaturated and polyunsaturated oils. Physicians whose patients showed an unusual frequency of malignant melanoma, a form of skin cancer, inquired into their dietary habits and found there had been a switch to vegetable fats and oils.[18] Many writers on nutrition, including Roger Williams in *Nutrition Against Disease* (Bantam, 1973), David Reuben, M.D. in *Everything You Always Wanted To Know About Nutrition* (Avon, 1979), and Dr. Richard Passwater in *Super-Nutrition for Healthy Hearts* (Jove Pubns., Inc., 1978), explain that the increase in American fat consumption, which corresponds to the increase in heart attacks and strokes, is primarily an increase from eating polyunsaturates. From 1950-1970, American polyunsaturated use tripled from 2 per cent to 6 per cent of our diet.[19]

Dr. Robert Atkins in *Nutrition Breakthrough* (Cancer Control Society, 1979) states that polyunsaturates are chock full of free radicals, which may hasten the aging and degeneration process and increase our requirements for vitamin E.[20] Dr. Harry Bieler in *Food is Your Best Medicine* (Random House, 1973) maintains that as long as fats and oils are in their natural state, they do not lead to arterial disease. Eating natural fats, whether they are saturated animal fats or unsaturated vegetable fats, provides the liver with the light, quality raw materials it needs to manufacture good cholesterol. Studies of cultures with diets high in animal fats (Saami, Masai) and high in natural vegetable fats (Greek and Italian peasants) have revealed no arterial disease.

The main trouble arises from ingesting unnatural fats and natural fats which have been overheated. Fats that have been overheated in combination with starch cause much harm. Examples of this would be deep-fried foods and pastries and snacks such as potato chips. As a result of eating this type of food, the liver cannot manufacture good cholesterol, and problems with the arterial cells begin. People who have eaten high-fat diets and have been immune from these problems have taken fats in the form of grains, beans, nuts, seeds, fish, meat, eggs, or milk products.[21]

The question of how much polyunsaturated fats in the diet still remains to be answered. Sticking to natural and unrefined sources as much as possible seems to be a key to maintaining a healthy cardiovascular system and enabling the liver to do its work in the production of cholesterol.

NOTES

1. Dan Seamens and David Wollner, "Shopper's Guide to Natural Foods," *East West Journal*, 31.
2. Ibid.
3. Ibid.
4. Beatrice Trum Hunter, *Consumer Beware!* (New York: Simon and Schuster, Inc., 1971), p. 219.
5. Dan Seamens and David Wollner, p. 32.
6. Hunter, p. 219.

7. Ibid.
8. Fred Rohe, *The Complete Book of Natural Foods* (Boulder, CO: Shambhala Pubns., 1983), p. 74.
9. Ibid.
10. Rudolph Ballantine, M.D., *Diet and Nutrition—A Holistic Approach* (Honesdale, PA: Himalayan International Institute, 1978), p. 96.
11. Ibid.
12. Hunter, p. 215.
13. Rohe, p. 78.
14. Ibid., p. 76.
15. Ballantine, p. 93.
16. Ibid., p. 94.
17. M. Miettinen, "Prevention of Coronary Heart Disease by Cholesterol Lowering Diet," *Postgraduate Medicine* 51 (1975), 47-51, as cited by Ballantine, p. 97.
18. E. Pinckney, "The Potential Toxicity of Excessive Polyunsaturates," *American Heart* 85, 723-25, as cited by Ballantine, p. 97.
19. Rohe, p. 71.
20. Ibid., p. 73.
21. Ibid., p. 72.

NUTRITIONAL SUPPLEMENTS

There are many nutritional supplements available on the market, and it is often difficult to know which supplement performs what functions. Here is a summary of the main supplements available. Each day there are new supplements developed, so it is important to understand what each one does and to be discriminating in the use of these supplements.

ACIDOPHILUS

Lactobacillus acidophilus is a bacterial culture that is in soured-milk products such as yogurt, buttermilk, and kefir. It also may be purchased separately in liquid, powdered, or capsule form. Some new forms of powdered acidophilus are available like Megadophilus and Maxidophilus, which are particularly potent strains of the acidophilus culture.

The function of acidophilus is to reestablish healthy intestinal bacteria and destroy pathogenic organisms in the intestine. Acidophilus is diminished by the foods we eat, the toxins in the environment, antibiotics and other drugs, alcohol and cigarette smoking, food additives and preservatives, and the daily stresses of life. It cannot be replenished without being taken orally or in a good yogurt or kefir product. (Yogurts commonly sold in supermarkets do not qualify; they have the bacteria added before the heating process, which destroys them.)

A potent acidophilus supplement from time to time has been

helpful to those with digestive and excretory disorders, skin problems, chronic illnesses, allergies, an inability to absorb food and vitamins, and a history of antibiotic therapy. Antibiotics destroy acidophilus along with destroying infecting organisms. This often results in diarrhea which continues long after antibiotic use, and, at times, may result in a serious condition known as *candida* of the intestinal tract.[1] Candida is a fungus usually kept under control by acidophilus.

In recent research it was shown that some strains of lactobacillus acidophilus may lower cholesterol.[2] Pigs were fed 1,000 mg of pure crystalline cholesterol. One group received lactobacillus acidophilus in their milk, while another group did not. The animals that were fed acidophilus registered a smaller gain in serum cholesterol concentration. A reduction in cholesterol level in infants fed a formula of lactobacillus acidophilus was also found.

Lactobacillus supplies an enzyme missing in many who cannot digest lactose in milk. Since this enzyme changes the lactose to lactic acid, they can drink acidophilus milk, yogurt, buttermilk, and kefir. Acidophilus reduces the risk of colon cancer by producing metabolites that inhibit the growth of a variety of bacteria in the intestines that are capable of producing carcinogens.

Another area in which lactobacillus acidophilus is helpful is in controlling flatulence. Flatulence is generally caused by colon bacteria acting on fats. Acidophilus alters the composition of colon bacteria and creates a situation where there is less fermentation or gas.

ALOE VERA PRODUCTS

The products from the aloe vera plant—aloe vera juice, salve, and gel—have proved remarkable healing agents for a variety of health problems. This plant, known for its healing properties since Biblical times, is rich in *saponins*, a chemical known to block the inflammatory enzymes in the body and remove mucus; it is also high in *anthraquinone*, which are natural antibiotics with antifungal and antiviral properties. In addition, aloe contains a protein with the 18 amino acids, wound-healing hormones, growth stimulators, vitamins, and minerals.

Externally, aloe has been used to treat burns (including those from x-ray and radiation), acne, and other skin conditions. The ointment in the aloe regenerates the skin tissue. Complete healing of skin ulcerations caused by beta radiation was accomplished within two months of treatment, while the untreated ulcerations were not healed for more than four months.[3]

Internally, aloe has healed many digestive complaints as well as conditions of constipation and diarrhea. It has the highest concentration of a certain glycoside known as *barbaloin*, which exhibits cathartic properties and is able to transport the glycoside to the large intestine.[4] For those suffering from food poisoning and other conditions causing diarrhea, it has been effective immediately.

Individuals with arthritis have reported a lessening of pain after drinking aloe juice.[5] Rubbing the gel on the skin has also relieved aching joints and muscles. At the Moscow Somatological Institute, scientists showed that the aloe extract regenerated nerve fibers. They found it effective in treating hearing impairments (applying the extract to the remaining nerve fibers.)[6] Soviet research also showed the efficacy of aloe in patients with pulmonary tuberculosis. They coughed less, chest pain ceased, appetite improved, and x-rays showed a decrease in lung congestion.

Other cases of "miraculous" cures involve periodontosis, a disease of the bone holding the teeth. Three to four injections of aloe extract reduced bleeding of gums as well as the itching.[7] Peptic ulcers were also healed by drinking aloe juice regularly,[8] and those with nasal congestion had their symptoms cleared by extracts and injections of aloe.[9] Bed wetting in children disappeared after 7-10 injections of aloe, and their poor appetite and irritability cleared up.[10]

Drinking aloe juice twice a week is a good preventative measure against digestive problems, constipation, ulcers, colitis, and allergens. Regular users of the plant have more energy and better digestion. Their bodies are also able to handle harmful toxins and pollutants in the environment since the aloe serves to detoxify the liver and cleanse the colon.

BEE POLLEN AND PROPOLIS

Bee pollen, taken from the hives of bees, has been known for many years to have a number of healing properties. It has been used for colds and allergies since it contains vitamin C and the bioflavonoids (vitamin P) which enhance the effectiveness of vitamin C.

More recently, propolis, a resinous substance lining bee hives and collected by the bees from buds, stalks, and twigs, has proved to be a strong healing agent for its antibiotic *and* antiviral properties. Propolis is chestnut or greenish brown in color and has a pleasant aroma of poplar buds, honey, and vanilla. It is used to seal the cracks in the hive as well as to protect the bees from infection. When other insects enter the hive and are killed, they are encased in propolis and wrapped with beeswax. They thus remain embalmed without decay or decomposition. Scientists are using this same principle to immobilize infectious bacteria and viruses.

Since propolis is high in bioflavonoids, it is effective in healing sore throats, respiratory disorders, high blood pressure, hemorrhage, and female disorders. The bioflavonoids in propolis inhibit the enzymes that produce the prostaglandin that causes pain and fever. Thus, it acts like a natural aspirin. The bioflavonoids also stimulate the white blood cells to produce *interferon*, a natural protein substance that fights many diseases. Furthermore, propolis is a strong source of histamine and serotonin, which are needed to help cope with allergens.

Propolis has been effective in periodontal problems or the erosion of gums and tissues. The bioflavonoids block the formation of the prostaglandin which causes decomposition. This diminishes bleeding. The bioflavonoids also stimulate enzyme formation to fortify the walls of the blood vessels in the gums.

At the Institute of Radiology in Yugoslavia, patients suffering from irradiation diseases with serious liver damage were given propolis in a double-blind test, and the radiation problems lessened or disappeared.[11] In China, propolis was given to patients with hyperlipidemia, or high blood fat, and after four weeks there was a lowering of blood fat.[12] In Austria, Dr. Franz Feeks used propolis effectively in the treatment of ulcers and in healing internal sores and wounds. He also used it locally, applied with a brush, to treat herpes zoster.[13] The pain disappeared in 48 hours. At the Crimean Medical Institute, doctors applied a solution of propolis as a salve for women who had erosion of the neck of the uterus, an irritated cervix, and vaginal problems. In four to five days some healing was noted. Propolis has also been used successfully for women with dysmenorrhea.

According to research, propolis activates the thymus gland and, therefore, the immune system. The thymus gland is in the root of the neck and consists of developing lymphocytes, the white blood cells needed to provide immunity against illness and infection. Other uses for propolis have been to clear up skin diseases and blemishes, nasal congestion, respiratory problems, flu, and viruses.

BLUE-GREEN ALGAE

Blue-green algae is a single-cell algae that grows in only one place, Klamath Lake in Oregon. This algae grows and reproduces itself by photosynthesizing nitrates from the air. It is one of the oldest foods on the planet and is harvested for human consumption through freeze-drying.

Blue-green algae is rich in chlorophyll, the eight essential amino acids, B vitamins including B-12, and beta-carotene (the vitamin A precursor). It contains 60 per cent pure protein (glyco-proteins as opposed to lipo-proteins found in vegetable matter and beef). In glyco-proteins, the glucose molecule is attached to the amino acid molecule so that the process of converting protein to glucose has already begun.

Blue-green algae can help rejuvenate the thymus gland (the central factor in the immune system), stimulate the spleen, and help to correct imbalance of the pituitary and pineal glands.

Some people are greatly affected by the algae and notice an increase in mental alertness and stamina, clarity, memory, intuitive perception, and creativity. For many, it helps to balance moods, counteract chronic fatigue, and create a greater sense of centeredness and well-being. These efforts seem due to its content of "essential neuropeptides," short chains of amino acids which help the brain initiate certain functions. Neuropeptides function as either neurotransmitters or hormones in the human body. They are capable of activating the neurotransmitters in the brain. Blue-green algae seems to promote a more even flow of nerve impulses throughout the body. It also stimulates the cellular memory or genetic code (DNA), which helps to promote extra cell regeneration essential to the healing process.

In addition, blue-green algae is a powerful detoxifier, affecting the liver. It seems to remove heavy deposits of lead and mercury. It has also been successful in treating allergies.

The most interesting piece of research about this algae is that its cellular structure remains stable at radiation levels that are harmful to human beings. It only mutates when exposed to 100 times the amount of this radiation, and, after two generations of reproducing itself in mutated form, it continues to reproduce itself normally. This suggests a high level of life force.

EVENING PRIMROSE OIL

Evening primrose is an herb that grows throughout North America and Europe. It has many names, including rock rose, coffee plant, and night willow. Generally two to five feet tall, it has large flowers with a light green vein running down the center of each petal. The flowers last one night and wither to a pinkish color.

The Pilgrims learned of the evening primrose from the Indians who used extracts externally to heal wounds and soothe skin inflammations and eruptions. Internally, they used it to control coughs and infections. A cough syrup can be made from the root that is effective against whooping cough as well as coughs from asthma and tuberculosis.

In recent times, scientists have found that the oil of the evening primrose seed is rich in a rare nutrient, GLA, or *gamma linolenic acid*, which alleviates many health problems , including heart disease, arthritis, and skin disorders. Gamma linolenic acid is not the common form of linolenic acid, known as *alpha linolenic acid*, or ALA. GLA is needed for the body to make a family of hormone-like compounds called prostaglandins (PG's). A deficiency of GLA results in a deficiency of PG's. Previously it was thought that GLA could be made from linoleic acid, one of the essential fatty acids. Now we're discovering that due to deficiencies in overconsumption of saturated fats, alcohol, cholesterol, exposure to radiation, and chemical carcinogens, GLA, and subsequently PG, production is not complete.

PG's are not stored in the body; every tissue makes PG's as needed. They can be quickly inactivated by enzymes in certain organs. In the 1930s, two doctors working independently, one in England and one in Sweden, found that a certain substance reduced blood pressure in lab animals. Since this material was found in high concentration in the prostate gland, it was named *prostaglandin*. Years later, research revealed that prostaglandin was actually a family of compounds closely related to EFA's (essential fatty acids). Many disease states were found to have an excess or deficiency of PG's in the body. PG's are named similarly to vitamins with the main classes being E, F, A, B, C, and D. These classes are determined by chemical constituents.

Other than in mother's milk, the only substantial source of GLA is the seed oil of evening primrose.

Studies with evening primrose oil have shown dramatic results when administered to patients with various heart diseases. It has been found to be effective in lowering cholesterol levels, in inhibiting the formation of clots, and in lowering blood pressure in those with mild to moderate hypertension.[14] The effects on clotting are rapid (1-4 hours), while the effects on cholesterol and blood pressure take three to four weeks. Experiments indicate that GLA, which is converted into PGE (prostaglandin E), can be used as a direct dietary supplement in patients to lessen the risk of heart attack.

Diseases involving the inflammatory system and immune system have been greatly helped by evening primrose oil. These include rheumatoid arthritis, eczema, inflammatory bowel disease, and multiple sclerosis. These diseases share two common features: improper functioning of certain lymph cells (T-suppressor lymphocytes) and excessive production of class 2 prostaglandin. T-suppressor lymphocytes are cells which keep other parts of the immune system under control. They help ensure that the immune system attacks only foreign bodies and not the body's own tissues. When these cells are defective, damage by the immune system attacking body cells occurs. This phenomenon of the body attacking itself is a major component in rheumatoid arthritis, ulcerative colitis, and multiple sclerosis. In the case of rheumatoid arthritis, evening primrose oil was effective in 4-12 weeks, with the course of the disease arrested in some cases.[15]

Eczema-like skin disorders are also due to a deficiency of EFA's. Evening primrose oil rubbed on the skin of infants with eczema produced complete healing. Eczema often develops when the infant switches from mother's milk to cow's milk (which contains less GLA, and many infants are allergic to it).

Lab tests for MS patients became normal after using evening primrose oil.[16]

The Hyperactive Children's Support Group in England conducted research with children who were hyperactive using evening primrose oil. These children were found to have deficiencies of EFA's, especially GLA. With some of the children, results were better when the oil was rubbed onto the skin instead of taken orally.[17]

Prostaglandin E has been found to be a strong determinant of mood, and low levels of PGE were found in alcoholics, especially in the case of hangovers since the alcohol itself temporarily elevates the level of PGE. Evening primrose oil has been used successfully in the treatment of alcoholism.[18]

Evening primrose oil was also found to relieve premenstrual symptoms in women: bloating, breast pain, irritability, depression and other symptoms.[19] By taking evening primrose oil along with vitamins B-6 and E, women were able to get rid of all PMS symptoms. This oil was also helpful to women with heavy and prolonged bleeding during menstruation. In cystic mastitis (benign breast disease) where there are tender and painful lumps prior to the menstrual flow, this oil helped the cystitis to soften or disappear.[20]

In the case of cancer, PGE was found to be one of the most potent natural agents to induce cancer cell reversal. In addition to measures to strengthen the immune system, reversal of cancer cells through the use of evening primrose oil and vitamin C is now being researched at various centers in England.[21]

Other conditions in which evening primrose oil has been found helpful are weight loss and brittle nails. Evening primrose oil capsules were taken over a period of six to eight weeks; subjects felt less hungry, and some of them even lost weight.[22] Those who wished to soften their nails reported the effects after three to four weeks of using the oil. Brittle nails are a sign of EFA deficiency.

LINSEED OIL

Linseed oil, or flax seed oil, is an edible polyunsaturated vegetable oil used in many parts of the world. It is very rich in linoleic and linolenic acids. When correctly processed (not heated, filtered, or refined), it consists of 58 per cent of the essential fatty acids which are converted in the body to prostaglandins.[23]

Without essential fatty acids, prostaglandin biosynthesis cannot take place. Prostaglandins are chemically active substances which affect the cardiovascular system and are present in the prostate gland, menstrual fluid, brain, lungs, kidneys, thymus gland, seminal fluid, and pancreas.[24] There are more than a dozen prostaglandins which are derived from essential fatty acids. (See Evening Primrose Oil.)

Flax seeds and flax seed oil have been used throughout the centuries in many healing traditions. Herbologists use the seeds as an internal demulcent. They are mucilaginous and soften the intestinal lining; they are also used in poultices for rheumatism, gout, and carbuncles. The oil is used as an enema to treat impacted feces. When it is mixed with limewater, the oil is applied topically to promote the healing of skin lesions and to soothe the itching of eczema.

Linseed oil is used in many parts of Europe for the prevention and treatment of cancer, arteriosclerosis, arthritis, stroke, irregular heartbeat, fatty degeneration of the liver, bronchial spasms in the lungs, regulation of intestinal activity, the normalization of stomach ulcers, and for all auto-immune diseases.[25]

CHLOROPHYLL

Chlorophyll is the basis of all plant life; it absorbs energy from the Sun, using it for the manufacture of sugar, starch, and proteins. Chlorophyll has the same chemical structure as hemoglobin, but in hemoglobin the metallic atom consists of iron; in chlorophyll, the atom is magnesium.

Chlorophyll aids in rebuilding the blood stream. In studies of various animals, the red cell count was returned to normal within four to five days after the use of chlorophyll.[26] Laboratory investigation has shown that tissue cell activity and its regrowth is increased by the administration of chlorophyll.[27] It also produces an unfavorable environment for bacterial growth; therefore, it has been used effectively in treating infected and ulcerated wounds. Chlorophyll helps to counteract toxins which have been ingested; it is an aid in purifying the liver and improves blood sugar problems.

Chlorophyll can be obtained in large amounts by juicing certain green plants. Chief among these is wheat grass. Wheat grass juice has been successful in helping to remove toxic minerals, such as lead, cadmium, mercury, aluminum, and copper, from the body.[28]

WHEAT GRASS JUICE

Wheat grass juice is a good blood purifier. It aids in proper digestion since it is high in enzymes. It also helps to prevent tooth decay and has been used successfully in cases of pyorrhea. For skin problems, such as eczema and psoriasis, wheat grass has been extremely effectual, and it is also an excellent skin cleanser when used externally in a bath.

In cases of anemia, wheat grass has been very effective.[29] It reduces high blood pressure by removing toxins from the body and by providing more iron in the blood. It is excellent in cases of constipation and has also been used as an implant in enemas for healing and detoxifying the colon walls. Implants also heal and cleanse the liver, pancreas, and other organs. (After an enema, wait about 20 minutes and follow with another enema made with four ounces of wheat grass juice, which should be retained for 20 minutes.)

In cases of radiation, tests have been made which show that wheat grass and other vegetables high in chlorophyll affect the survival of experimental animals undergoing lethal doses of radiation.[30] Wheat grass is rich in laetrile (B-17), which destroys cancer cells but has little effect on normal cells. A wheat grass plant in front of the TV will absorb radiation from the TV.

Wheat grass is an excellent source of vitamins A and C as well as calcium, magnesium, potassium, and phosphorus. It is grown from wheat berries. The berries need to be soaked for a day and then allowed to sprout for another day or two. When they have sprouted, fill a tray with soil (about one inch mixed with 50 per cent peat moss). Spread the seeds over the tray, and cover with a dark plastic bag for three days. Then place the tray in the sunlight. Wheat grass will grow to seven inches high and can then be harvested and juiced.

BARLEY GREEN

Another strong source of chlorophyll is barley green. Barley green is the juice from the leaves of young green barley plants. Dr. Yoshida Hagiwara, a pharmacist and medical doctor in Japan, was searching for a super-nutritious food to offset many of the commercially processed foods in the Japanese diet. He found the leaves of the barley plant especially high in chlorophyll and enzymes.

One of the enzymes in barley green, SOD, *superoxide dismutase*, is found in all body cells and acts as a cellular antioxidant, protecting against radiation and chemical-free radicals, as well as an anti-inflammatory agent which prevents cellular damage following heart attacks.[31] Another enzyme, *nitrogen reductase*, transforms nitrogen dioxide, a major pollutant, into nitrogen hydroside, a harmless compound. Seventy per cent of known carcinogens are nitric compounds, and the enzymes in green barley juice that detoxify these are important in preventing cancer.[32] Barley green was found to deactivate the carcinogenic effects of 3.4 benzopyrene found in charcoal-broiled meats and fish. (Japan has a high rate of stomach cancer due to this.) Barley green also contains a factor called P4D1, which protects reproductive cells against known carcinogens. P4D1 also has been found to have an anti-inflammatory effect, suppressing pancreatitis, stomatitis, dermatitis, ulcers, and colitis.[33]

SPIRULINA

The use of spirulina as a food supplement has become a very controversial issue. Spirulina is a micro algae that grows naturally in alkaline lakes in Mexico and Africa. It is 60-70 per cent protein, which is almost all digestible, and also contains B-complex vitamins and minerals such as calcium, phosphorous, magnesium, and zinc.[34]

Spirulina has no vitamin B-6, C, or D, as well as no carbohydrates, fat, or fiber, so it is not a complete food. It may be useful as a food supplement to boost certain nutritional requirements.[35]

Many of those who have worked with and researched spirulina feel unsure about its source. They feel that some of the lakes it originates from are polluted and would like some kind of quality control before harvesting.

LECITHIN

The body produces lecithin in the liver, utilizing it to form bile. Lecithin is manufactured from choline that comes both from the diet and the body's own manufacturing process. The concentration of choline in the body and the blood depends on dietary choline intake. Liver, eggs, and soybeans are high sources of choline and lecithin. Once the dietary lecithin is taken in, it is broken down in the intestinal tract to substances which are absorbed into the blood and made into lecithin in the liver.

There are a number of tissues that use the blood levels of choline in the manufacturing of specific substances like lecithin or acetylcholine. (Acetylcholine helps transport messages across the nerve junctions so that the nervous system functions properly.) These tissues include the brain, kidney, liver, and spleen. The tissues which synthesize choline are the liver, testes, and heart.

Newborn babies have extremely high choline content in their blood. Deficiencies of choline may produce abnormalities in the nervous system. Mother's milk is much higher in lecithin than cow's milk and is important in providing high levels of choline for the nervous system of the infant.

Therapeutically, choline and lecithin have been used in many ways. About 9-12 grams of choline chloride per day have been given to treat Tardive Dyskinesia, a neurological condition resulting as a side effect from anti-schizophrenic medicine which creates a deficiency of acetylcholine in certain neurons of the brain.[36] Lecithin and choline remove the symptoms of motor shaking, slurred speech, and palsy-like reactions.[37]

Another effect of increasing choline and lecithin in the diet has been improved memory. Alzheimer's disease is a condition associated with memory loss. It is related to excessive aluminum exposure and concentration of aluminum in the brain.[38]

Using lecithin, along with lithium, has been very effective in treating manic-depressives. Lecithin reduces the need for lithium and improves the level of acetylcholine. Seventy-five per cent of patients taken off choline and kept only on lithium had symptoms of their manic-depression worsen.[39]

Clinical trials have not confirmed lecithin to be useful in reducing blood cholesterol levels.[40] However, the emulsifying factors of lecithin help to make cholesterol more soluble and to prevent cholesterol gallstones.[41]

The success of using lecithin as a dietary supplement is dependent upon the quality of lecithin as it relates to its phosphatidylcholine content. The lecithin must be at least 30 per cent phosphatidylcholine. Many commercially available lecithins are heavily diluted with other oils. Also, lecithin should be taken in the liquid form; granular lecithin is not very potent, and the capsules are difficult to digest and contain very small amounts of lecithin.

SEA VEGETABLES

Sea vegetables are the most important of all the nutritional supplements. If sea vegetables were used generously in the American diet, there would be less need for mineral and vitamin supplements. Sea vegetables are used in the cuisine of coastal and island peoples and as medicines for many types of ailments. Kelp ointments and liniments are used for cuts, stings, sprains, and bruises. These alginates increase the rate of healing without inducing a toxic reaction or antigen response in the body. Sea plants are used for a variety of skin ointments as a component in skin cream and shampoo.

An abundance of minerals, which comprise 5 per cent of our body weight, is found in sea vegetables. Iodine has been sought as a goiter preventative in all cultures. It also functions as an antiseptic and is prophylactic in bacterial and viral diseases. High amounts of calcium, phosphorus, magnesium, zinc, and iron are also contained in these plants from the ocean. By maintaining balanced thyroid function and promoting fluid balance in body cells, algae work to counteract obesity (since upsets in fluid balance bring about water retention).

Physicians have prescribed seaweeds for prostate and ovarian dysfunctions, including sterility in males, due to the high presence of zinc.[42] Since zinc is a constituent of insulin, it also contributes to the health of the pancreas and is important in treating hypoglycemia and diabetes. Recent research has found zinc to be one of the most important factors in the health of the immune system as well.

Alginates from kelp were proven to inhibit the body's absorption of radioactive strontium and cadmium up to 7/8 of the radioactive dosage received.[43] Research in this area has been done at McGill University, Montreal, where strontium 90 which was absorbed into the tissue has been removed.

In addition to minerals, sea vegetables also contain one to nine per cent fats, present as the fat-soluble vitamins A, D, E, and K; essential fatty acids; lecithin; and certain sterols such as cholesterol and ergosterol, which in the presence of sunlight are converted by the body into vitamin D. The Japanese have used sea vegetables to reduce cholesterol in blood plasma.[44]

Seaweeds contain strong amounts of B-12, which is impossible to obtain in a vegetarian diet, and vitamin C. They are 20-30 per cent protein, which is completely digestible. Whereas minerals in soil are constantly being leached out and carried back to the sea, they are absorbed there by the algae. Algae do not absorb pollutants along with other elements. When the level of pollution is high, they fail to grow, as seen by Japan's polluted sea waters where the nori crop has been reduced.[45]

Doctors have begun to prescribe kelp and other sea vegetables for a wide range of mineral-related diseases including arthritis, rheumatism, obesity, high blood pressure, and thyroid problems.[46]

KOMBU AND THE KELPS

The brown seaweeds known as kelps have over 890 known species—kombu and rockweeds and serpent kelp—all of which are harvested industrially and processed to procure algin. In some cases they are powdered or pressed into mineral tablets.

Many people throughout the world use kelp for its medicinal power. Peruvians living in the Andes carry a bag containing kelp "to guard the heart." The Tibetan *sherpas* also carry kelp at high altitudes to aid breathing and restore leg muscles. Dr. D. C. Jarvis, author of *Folk Medicine* (Fawcett, 1978), has treated patients for heart pain, rheumatic fever, and arthritis with kelp.[47] The Japanese use kombu to prevent high blood pressure. Kelp also aids digestion, helps to loosen toxins from the colon lining, aids kidneys and the urinary tract, relieves anemia, and helps to normalize reproductive organs.[48]

DULSE

Dulse, the dark red sea vegetable, has the highest concentration of both iron and iodine of any food source. It is also rich in potassium, which is important for body fluid balance as well as adrenal, kidney, and muscle function, and magnesium, an aid to the nervous system and a muscle strengthener. A recent medical use of dulse is as a combatant of the herpesvirus.[49]

NORI

Next to the kelps and rockweeds, the most popular and widely consumed seaweed is nori. Porphyra, the purple greenish variety of nori (called "laver" in England), is used in several dishes in England and Wales. The Japanese use it in combination with fried foods as it decreases cholesterol and aids digestion.[50] Nori provides B and C vitamins as well as calcium, potassium, magnesium, and phosphorus.

WAKAME

Wakame accounts for about 15 per cent of the total Japanese seaweed harvest. It is closely related to kombu and used in soups and salads.

In North America, *alaria* is similar to wakame and contains vitamins B and C as well as calcium, magnesium, phosphorus, and potassium.

ARAME

Arame is a social plant which grows in association with another brown seaweed, ecklonia, and sometimes with hijiki. Japan is the only country that harvests arame commercially. It has been used along with kombu and hijiki for high blood pressure.[51] It is also used as an emergency food in times of famine since it maintains its taste, dried for two to three years. A substitute for soy sauce has been developed from arame and ecklonia.

HIJIKI

Hijiki is used along with arame and wakame for hair loss.[52] It is very high in calcium; a portion of 100 grams provides 1400 micrograms of calcium, 14 times the amount in a glass of cow's milk.[53] It is also high in vitamins A, B, B-2, niacin, and C. Hijiki has been used as a food for dieters since the dried plant expands, making it a filling meal.

AGAR-AGAR AND IRISH MOSS

Agar is a Malay word which means "jelly." It is a complex polysaccharide starch related to cellulose and found in the cell walls of certain species of red algae. Agar is used to make kanten bars (which when broken yield a gelatinous substance). It has generous quantities of calcium, iodine, phosphorus, and vitamins A, B-1, B-6, B-12, biotin, C, D, and E. It aids intestinal action and also bonds with radioactive wastes, carrying them out of the body.[54]

Irish moss, like agar, has been valued for its gelling properties. It has many medicinal uses as well. It is recommended for scrofulous complaints, dysentery, diarrhea, and disorders of the kidneys and bladder.[55] The extract carrageenan is used in prescription medication for peptic and duodenal ulcers.[56] Calcium chloride, a mineral compound found in Irish moss, acts as a heart tonic and maintains glandular balance.[57]

WHEAT GERM AND OCTACOSANOL

Wheat germ has been one of the most popular food supplements. The germ, which contains all the vitamin E from the wheat, is removed in the process of refining. Wheat germ oil has an even greater concentration of vitamin E. However, much of the available wheat germ is rancid. Rancidity occurs because most wheat germ is rolled into flakes, which breaks open the sac containing the wheat germ. When it is exposed to air, oxygen begins to work on the oil. If, however, the flakes are vacuum-packed the day they are rolled, they will have a sweet smell (rather than an acrid odor) and will not be rancid. After opening, they should be stored in the refrigerator.

Octacosanol is the active ingredient in wheat germ responsible for its ability to increase stamina and endurance.[58] Studies with individuals using octacosanol showed a decrease of blood cholesterol.[59] There was also improved muscle-glycogen storage, stability of the basal metabolic rate under stress, improved reaction time, and reduced oxygen debt.[60] Octacosanol has also been used to prevent muscle pain after exercise and for neuromuscular disorders and muscular dystrophy.[61]

NUTRITIONAL YEAST

Nutritional yeasts are excellent sources of B-vitamin proteins. However, since many people are allergic to yeast, and since it produces a very acidic reaction in the body, it is not particularly desirable as a food supplement. Most people need to be careful as well in using B vitamins because they are made from a yeast base. There are, however, hypo-allergenic vitamins which do not use yeast.

AMINO ACIDS

Amino acids are being used individually and in combination to achieve many beneficial effects within the body and to alleviate many diseases and ailments.

The essential amino acids that must be obtained from foods are histidine, isoleucine, leucine, lysine, methionine, phenylalanine, threonine, tryptophan, and valine. Two other amino acids are derived from these—cysteine, which is made from methionine, and tyrosine, which is made from phenylalanine.

Amino acids that our bodies can manufacture include alanine, aspartic acid, asparagine, glutamic acid (glutamine), glycine, proline, and serine.

The nature of any given protein is determined by the sequence in which these amino acids are linked and the amounts of each amino acid present. Amino acids rarely act alone; many other co-factors, such as vitamins and minerals, are necessary to manufacture the final chemical from the particular amino acid. If any of these co-factors are missing, increasing the amino acid by supplementation will not alter the manufacturing process. Amino acids compete with other amino acids for transportation into the body and at other sites along the way. Therefore, the use of any single amino acid may be impaired by the presence of other amino acids. Excessive use of any one can inhibit the availability of certain others.

An *L* before the name of an amino acid signifies that the structure of the amino acid is wholly natural since it appears in food and in our bodies. A *DL* indicates that it was constructed in the laboratory; it contains the same amounts of carbon, hydrogen, oxygen, and nitrogen, but these elements are arranged in a different pattern.

PHENYLALANINE

Phenylalanine is used by the brain to manufacture *norepinephrine*. One of the functions of norepinephrine is as a neurotransmitter, allowing certain brain cells to communicate with each other. It is stored in "pouches" at the end of neurons located in the brain. When it transmits impulses to another cell, it is released from these pouches. Drugs such as amphetamines block norepinephrine from re-entering these pouches. These drugs stimulate memory and improve learning, but once the stored norepinephrine is released, the decreased stimulation is often accompanied by depression. Norepinephrine requires tyrosine for its synthesis, which comes from phenylalanine.

Certain types of depression have responded favorably to

phenylalanine, and attention span and learning have improved.[62] In studies at the University of Chicago, significant pain relief was experienced four to five weeks after beginning the treatment.[63] In addition to pain relief, phenylalanine has anti-inflammatory effects in arthritis.[64] Doctors at the University of Chicago believe that the reduced swelling and inflammation may be due to an increase in endorphins (the body's own painkiller compounds) that phenylalanine stimulates. It has also been effective in treating gout, ankylosing spondylitis, lupus, and bursitis.[65]

TRYPTOPHAN

Tryptophan is related to the neurotransmitter in the brain called *serotonin*. Serotonin requires a number of compounds for its synthesis in our bodies—oxygen, iron, B-6, and tryptophan. Researchers have used tryptophan supplements to manipulate serotonin levels in the treatment of depression and sleep disorders. Many studies have been conducted correlating levels of tryptophan in the blood with mood and depression. These include studies with post-menopausal women and women during the postpartum period. Tryptophan was compared with several anti-depressants—Tofranil, Elavil, and Endep. Groups to whom tryptophan was administered held up better during a six-month period; the drug-treated group had a greater tendency to relapse.[66]

Since the neurotransmitter serotonin plays a major role in inducing sleep, tryptophan was used to induce sleep and decrease the time needed to fall asleep. It also increased the duration and the quality of sleep.[67] Tryptophan has been used as well in treating migraine sufferers who have a below-normal level of serotonin, especially during migraine attacks.[68] It is also being used to defend the immune system since it helps to form antibodies in the blood which protect the body against foreign substances.[69]

The recent problem with tryptophan, which started in the summer of 1989, concerns the side effects that many have been suffering from using this amino acid. A painful blood disorder, known as eosinophilia-myalgia syndrome, induces an abnormally high number of white blood cells and causes severe muscle pain. The disease was reported in 43 states by the Center for Disease Control. As of April 1990, federal researchers were able to trace the cause of the blood disorder to a specific company and a contaminant in its product. The particular company is Showa Denko, one of Japan's largest chemical manufacturers. Though all of their products have been recalled, federal health officials are urging all Americans to stop using tryptophan.[70]

GLUTAMINE

Glutamine or glutamic acid is the most prominent amino acid in wheat protein. Dr. Roger Williams (author of *Biochemical Individuality* [Univ. of Texas Press, 1956]) has been doing research for years with glutamine at the Clayton Foundation for Research, University of Texas. This research has shown that glutamine decreases the craving for alcohol consumption in alcoholics as well as the desire for sweets in hypoglycemic patients.[71] Glutamic acid serves as a fuel for the brain, which is something that only one other compound, glucose (blood sugar), can do. Glutamic acid restores hypoglycemic patients in insulin coma to consciousness at a lower blood sugar level than when glucose alone is used. Since the brain can store only a small reserve of glucose, it is dependent on the immediate supply of blood sugar. This explains the dizziness and other nervous symptoms in hypoglycemics. Glutamic acid is the only other compound used by the brain for energy. The gray matter in the brain contains a special enzyme to convert glutamic acid to a compound that regulates brain-cell activity.[72]

Dr. Lorene Rogers reported that glutamine improved the IQ's of mentally deficient children. Dr. William Shive found that glutamine shortened the healing time for ulcers. Glutamine has also been used to fight fatigue, depression, and impotence. Dr. Abram Hoffer has successfully used it with other nutrients against schizophrenia, senility, and mental retardation.[73]

SULFUR-CONTAINING AMINO ACIDS

Methionine, cysteine, cystine, and taurine contain high amounts of sulfur. Every body cell contains sulfur, with the greatest concentration in the cells of the skin, hair, and joints. Keratin, one of the layers of skin, has a high concentration of sulfur, as do the fingernails, toenails, and hair. These amino acids function as antioxidants, free radical deactivators, neutralizers of toxins, and aids to protein synthesis. Sulfur also protects against radiation and pollution.

A property of these amino acids that helps eliminate free radicals is their ability to chelate or grab onto certain metallic elements such as copper. This ability to chelate heavy metals helps to eliminate the build-up of toxic minerals, such as lead, mercury, and cadmium.

Since we cannot use elemental sulfur to make these amino acids, we need to get our sulfur from our diet. One egg, for example, supplies 60 mg of sulfur. When vitamin C is converted in the body, it is a form that requires sulfur. Large doses of C may place demands on the sulfur reserves, and extra amounts of the sulfur-containing amino acids may be needed. These amino acids also play a role as natural carriers of the trace element selenium (which is a prominent anti-aging nutrient and anti-cancer supplement).

METHIONINE

Methionine is a member of the lipotropics, which include choline, inositol, and betaine. Its primary function as a lipotropic is to prevent excess accumulation of fat in the liver. By increasing the liver's production of lecithin, methionine helps prevent cholesterol build-up.[74]

The other amino acids that provide sulfur—cysteine, cystine, and taurine—can be made in the body as long as we consume adequate amounts of the essential amino acid methionine. Many vegetables and legumes are low in methionine and must be combined with grains, seeds, or nuts to provide this amino acid. One way to conserve methionine is to provide a dietary source of choline so that methionine is not needed for choline synthesis. The best source of choline is lecithin.

TAURINE

Taurine, made from methionine, helps stabilize the excitability of membranes which are important in epileptic seizures. Research is underway to determine if taurine is better in controlling epilepsy than drugs such as Dilantin and Phenobarbital.[75] Dr. André Barbeau, a Montreal physician, was able to reduce seizures in 12 epileptics by using taurine and zinc. The seizures were eventually eliminated, although the patients are still taking their regular drugs.[76]

In 1974, a fatal hereditary disease which caused severe mental depression and other mental and nervous symptoms was discovered in a British Columbia family. Six members died of the disease over three successive generations. Canadian doctors found that they all had below-normal levels of the amino acid taurine in their blood. No other defects were found except for malabsorption in the intestines and increased amounts of fat in the stools. This suggests that lack of taurine may be related to diseases in which foods are not absorbed normally.[77]

CYSTEINE AND CYSTINE

The amino acid cysteine is unstable and is readily converted to cystine. As an antioxidant, cystine works closely with vitamin E and selenium. Cystine has been used along with pantothenic acid in the treatment of arthritis (both osteo and rheumatoid) by Dr. Eustace Barton Wright in London.[78] Cystine is also necessary for vitamin B-6 utilization, according to Dr. William Philpott. He recommends that patients who have the B-6 utilization problem take cystine three times a day for a month and then reduce the amount to twice daily.

TYROSINE

If the diet is deficient in tyrosine, the requirement for phenylalanine goes up since tyrosine can be synthesized from phenylalanine. Tyrosine plays a role in the synthesis of the neurotransmitter *norepinephrine*, according to Dr. Alan J. Gelenberg of the Department of Psychiatry. This amino acid is important in controlling anxiety and depression. A lack of tyrosine results in a deficiency of the neurotransmitter norepinephrine at a specific site in the brain. Dr. Gelenberg reported a considerable improvement in two patients whose depressions were not responsive to conventional drug therapy.[79]

Tyrosine can also trigger migraine headaches since it breaks down into a product called *tyramine* in foods such as beer, wine, aged cheese, yeast and pickled herring. Eliminating these foods often helps in eliminating migraines.[80]

Dr. Jeffrey S. Rosecan reported decreased use of cocaine in addicts who were given tryptophan and tyrosine along with an antidepressant drug. Fourteen of 25 patients he treated with this combination stopped using cocaine entirely, and six decreased their use.[81]

LYSINE

An important function of lysine is to aid adequate absorption of calcium. It also serves to form collagen. (Collagen is the protein that makes up the matrix of bone, cartilage, and connective tissue.) Before lysine can be utilized in the formation of collagen, it must be converted to another configuration; this conversion process is regulated by vitamin C. Without vitamin C or adequate protein to supply lysine, wounds would not heal properly and we would become more susceptible to infection.

The new use of lysine is in the treatment of herpes simplex. Doctors Chris Kagan and R.W. Tinkersley, working in a lab at a Los Angeles hospital, noted that the amino acid arginine was always added to the solution used to grow tissue cells infected with the herpes virus. When lysine was added to the growth media, the virus did not grow.[82] It was then suggested to use lysine clinically as a therapy for herpes. The doctors found that it suppressed symptoms of herpes in 90 per cent of the 45 patients tested.[83] Inactive herpes can be helped with lysine supplementation if the individual works on balancing his acid/alkali intake through diet.

LEUCINE, ISOLEUCINE, AND VALINE

Leucine, isoleucine, and valine cannot be manufactured by the body and must be supplied in the diet. They are found in adequate amounts in liver, fish, chicken, beef, eggs, dairy products, some nuts, and some legumes. Most vegetables and grains do not have high amounts and need to be balanced with legumes and nuts.

Normally, these three amino acids are metabolized into simple acids. However, in the disease known as "maple syrup urine," these amino acids are not completely broken down and end up in the urine. (The urine has the odor of maple syrup, and this is a clue to the disease.) Infants with this disease have difficulty sucking and swallowing a few days after birth. They may have seizures and mental retardation.[84] Restrictive diets have helped, but they will not gain weight without some supply of these amino acids.

Another metabolic disease that involves the amino acid leucine is leucine-induced hypoglycemia. At about four months old, the infant may start to have convulsions, slowed growth, delayed mental development, and symptoms like Cushing's syndrome, including obesity, acne, osteoporosis, and facial hair growth.[85] It is impossible to treat these infants with a diet that has leucine removed without extracting all protein from the diet, but by careful work with food intake the child may be able to tolerate a normal diet by five or six years of age, when the disease has run its course.[86]

HISTIDINE

Histidine is necessary for growth in children and is fairly essential for adults since it can't be manufactured. It is the amino acid from which the biochemical substance histamine is derived. Both histidine and histamine can chelate or grab onto trace minerals, such as copper and zinc. In certain forms of arthritis, there is an overload of copper and other metals. Because of the chelating properties of histidine, it is used in the treatment of arthritis to remove these metals.[87]

THREONINE

Threonine is readily available from most protein foods, including soybeans and other legumes. Along with other amino acids, it is an important constituent of collagen, elastin, and enamel protein. When choline, one of the lipotropics, is deficient in the diet, threonine takes on the role of a lipotropic to prevent fatty build-up in the liver.

PROTOMORPHOGENS

Protomorphogens are animal glands and organs used in human nutrition. The use of protomorphogens is known as *glandular therapy*. The most ancient histories of healing from the Egyptians, the early Hindus, and the Greeks refer to the use of animal glands for the treatment of human glandular deficiencies.[88]

In the 1930s, Dr. Paul Niehans of Switzerland was the first to treat problems of the immune system with organ tissue extracts from the endocrine glands. Niehans found that the time involved in achieving a therapeutic effect from his organ therapy varied according to the organ involved; some took five to eight weeks while others took months. He found that underfunctioning of an endocrine gland was best treated by material from the same gland, while over-functioning required material from an antagonistic gland.[89] In Germany, medical research has shown, using radioactive isotope tracing, that nutritional factors from glandular tissues are absorbed from the blood stream by the corresponding glands of the patient.[90] An example of glandular therapy in curing diabetes would be regenerating the cells of the islands of Langerhans of the pancreas rather than giving insulin shots.

Animal glands seem to work best when used raw, and the raw organs and glands are often freeze-dried and pressed into tablets. More recently, however, sublingual glandular supplements have been developed, which have an advantage in assimilation over the tablets. Absorption from tablets can be slow or erratic because it may occur anywhere in the alimentary canal. (The higher up it occurs, the more rapid its action.) Mingling substances with food in the stomach also delays absorption since foods are antagonistic to some substances and may destroy them. In sublingual absorption, the results are more rapid and more potent. Drainage from the mouth is direct to the right side of the heart, bypassing dilution in the stomach and liver.[91]

CO-ENZYME Q (CoQ 10)

Co-Enzyme Q is a nutrient that plays a part in the production of energy in the cells of the body and in the oxygenation process. It has been used in Japan since 1974 and is available there in 252 different preparations.[92]

Co-Enzyme Q is produced by the body and can be obtained in the diet, but research has shown low amounts of CoQ 10 in tissues which have become diseased. Many co-enzymes in human energy systems are vitamins, and researchers are debating whether CoQ 10 is among them.

CoQ 10 is important therapeutically in various conditions, especially in heart disease and hypertension. Karl Folkers of the University of Texas at Austin (the American pioneer in CoQ 10 research) found evidence of CoQ 10 deficiency in heart disease in 1970.[93] Significant improvement has been found in angina, cardiac failure, and other heart disease following long-term therapy with oral CoQ 10. Conclusions were that CoQ 10 improves cardiac function and relieves symptoms in patients with heart problems. Studies have shown a decrease in blood pressure in hypertensive individuals following treatment with CoQ 10.

In 1974, research was conducted on CoQ 10 and muscular dystrophy. Older children and teenagers were treated and were monitored. It was found that some forms of muscular dystrophy responded to therapy with CoQ 10 as it reduced abnormal levels of serum enzymes.

Another area in which CoQ 10 is extremely effective is in periodontal disease. CoQ 10 is deficient in cases of pyorrhea. Seventy per cent of cases of patients with pyorrhea responded well to treatment with CoQ 10.[94]

CoQ 10 becomes scarcer as we get older because the breakdown of cellular membrane occurs at an accelerated rate. Less is made available from the diet as the efficiency of the digestive system diminishes. CoQ 10 helps to prevent degeneration of tissue and is, therefore, a good remedy for aging.

CoQ 10 is also helpful in alleviating fatigue that accompanies low thyroid output; in weight loss since it increases the body's ability to burn stored fat as heat; in maintaining blood sugar levels; and in restoring muscle efficiency where a lack of energy results in muscular weakness.

CoQ 10 can be taken daily or on alternate days. It comes in several different potencies and in capsule or tablet form.

NOTES

1. Frank Murray, "Acidophilus May Improve Your Digestion," *Better Nutrition* (December 1984), 11, 41-42, 44.
2. *Science News* (August 25, 1984).
3. Laurie Taylor-Donald, "Aloe Vera—Nature's Miracle," *Bestways* (June 1981).
4. Ibid.
5. Ibid.
6. Ibid.
7. Ibid.
8. Ibid.
9. Ibid.

10. Ibid.
11. Carlson Wade, *Propolis: Nature's Energizer* (New Canaan, CT: Keats Publishing, Inc., 1983), p. 10.
12. Ibid.
13. Ibid., p. 11.
14. Alan Donald, "The Powerful Healing Magic of the Evening Primrose," *Bestways* (June 1981).
15. Ibid.
16. Ibid.
17. Ibid.
18. Ibid.
19. Richard A. Passwater, *Evening Primrose Oil* (New Canaan, CT: Keats Publishing Inc., 1981), p. 21.
20. Ibid., p. 22.
21. Ibid., p. 19.
22. Donald, op. cit.
23. William L. Fischer, *How to Fight Cancer and Win* (Fischer Publications, 1987), chapter VI.
24. Ibid.
25. Ibid.
26. Betsy Russell-Manning, *Wheatgrass Juice: Gift of Nature* (Calistoga, CA: Betsy Russell, 1979), p. 6.
27. Ibid.
28. Ibid., p. 15.
29. Ibid., p. 9.
30. Ibid., p. 20.
31. Robert Picker, "Barley Green: Guardian Against Cancer," *Lifestyle* (April 1983), 10.
32. Ibid.
33. Ibid.
34. John O'Rourke, "Spirulina: New Food from the Ancients," *Let's Live* (March 1984), 42-44.
35. Fred Rohe, *The Complete Book of Natural Foods* (Boulder, CO: Shambhala Pubns., 1983), p. 167.
36. Jeffrey Bland, Ph.D. *Choline, Lecithin, Inositol and Other "Accessory" Nutrients* (New Canaan, CT: Keats Publishing Inc., 1982), p. 9.
37. Ibid., p. 10.
38. Ibid., p. 11.
39. Ibid., p. 10.
40. Ibid., p. 11.
41. Ibid.
42. Sharon Rhoads, *Cooking with Sea Vegetables* (Brookline, MA: Autumn Press, 1978), p. 25.
43. Ibid., p. 26.
44. Ibid., p. 25.
45. Ibid., p. 26.
46. Ibid.

47. Ibid., p. 41.
48. Ibid., p. 42.
49. Ibid.
50. Rhoads, p. 76.
51. Ibid., p. 54.
52. Ibid., p. 91.
53. Ibid., p. 92.
54. Ibid., p. 41.
55. Rhoads, p. 114.
56. Ibid.
57. Ibid.
58. Jeffrey Bland, Ph.D. *Octacosanol, Carnitine and Other "Accessory" Nutrients* (New Canaan, CT: Keats Publishing Inc., 1982), p. 2.
59. Ibid., p. 3.
60. Ibid., p. 4.
61. Ibid.
62. Robert Garrison, Jr., *Lysine, Tryptophan and Other Amino Acids* (New Canaan, CT: Keats Publishing Inc., 1982), p. 2.
63. Ruth Adams, "Phenylalanine May Stop Your Pain," *Better Nutrition* (July 1984), 29-32.
64. Ibid.
65. Ibid.
66. Garrison, p. 11.
67. Ibid., p. 12.
68. Ibid., p. 13.
69. Ibid.
70. "Researchers Trace L-Tryptophan Poison," *San Francisco Chronicle,* April 26, 1990.
71. Ibid., p. 14.
72. Richard Passwater, Ph.D., "L-Glutamine, the Surprising Brain Fuel," the newsletter of Super-Natural Foods, Corte Madera, CA.
73. Ibid.
74. Ibid., p. 15.
75. Ibid., p. 16.
76. Ruth Adams, "Can the Amino Acids Improve Your Health?," *Better Nutrition* (July 1984), 11, 46, 48.
77. Ibid.
78. Garrison, p. 17.
79. Ibid., p. 19.
80. Ibid.
81. Adams, p. 46.
82. Garrison, p. 21.
83. Ibid.
84. Ibid., p. 22.
85. Ibid.
86. Ibid.
87. Ibid., p. 23.

88. Gene Birkeland, "Sub-linguals: A New Way of Taking Glandulars," *Your Nutritional Consultant* (November 1984), 11.
89. Ibid.
90. Rohe, p. 467.
91. Birkeland, p. 48.
92. Karl Folkers and Y. Yamamura, editors, *Biochemical and Clinical Aspects of CoQ 10* (New York: Elsevier/North-Holland Bio-medical Press). Vol. 1, 1977. Vol. 1, 1980. Vol. 3, 1981. This reference is from Vol. 3.
93. Ibid.
94. Ibid., Vol. 1, p. 294.

10

VITAMINS

Vitamins are substances found in living organic matter, plants, and animal cells. With a few exceptions, vitamins cannot be synthesized by the body; therefore, they must be supplied through food or food supplements. Vitamins have no energy value or calories but are constituents of enzymes, which function as catalysts in metabolic reactions. They serve to regulate the metabolism, help convert fat and carbohydrates into energy, and assist in forming bone and tissue.

Vitamins in food and herbs and in liquid and powdered supplements are absorbed better than capsules or tablets, which have a low absorption value. There are two major reasons for this. The intestinal surface is large and the absorption of swallowed material may occur anywhere en route, all the way to the rectum. The higher up in the alimentary tract absorption occurs, the more rapid its action. Also, mingling substances with food in the stomach will delay absorption. Slow acting substances in the stomach with slow emptying time may be inactivated and destroyed. Some foods are antagonistic to certain substances and thus eliminate them. The gastric tract has a variable pH level which can wipe out some liquids or precipitate them too rapidly.

Certain vitamins are now being processed sublingually, which means they are absorbed under the tongue. The drainage from the mouth is direct to the right side of the heart, bypassing dilution in the stomach and the liver.

When vitamin supplements are used in tablet and capsule form, amounts taken in excess of what is needed for the metabolic processes will be excreted in the urine in the case of water-soluble vitamins, or stored in the body for fat-soluble vitamins. Excessive ingestion of fat-soluble vitamins (A, D, E, F, and K) may result in toxicity, so it is important to be careful when using these. The water-soluble vitamins (C, B complex, and P) are measured in milligrams. The fat-soluble vitamins are measured in international units.

VITAMIN A

Vitamin A is essential in the formation of visual purple, a substance in the eye which is necessary for proper night vision. It is also important in treating infections and in resistance to infection. When a group of mice were given four consecutive daily injections of 3,000 i.u.'s of vitamin A, and then injected with different stains of virulent bacteria and fungus, 90 per cent of the vitamin A-treated mice survived, while only 35 per cent of those unprotected lived.[1] A correlation between vitamin A deficiency and increased frequency of respiratory and gastrointestinal infections in humans has recently been discovered.[2] Many infections that respond dramatically to vitamin A occur in the protective covering of the body, the lining or mucous membranes that line the respiratory passages, the gastrointestinal tract, the urinary passages, and the eyes, ears, and nose.

Recent studies show a definite relationship between vitamin A and the synthesis of RNA. RNA (ribonucleic acid) is a nucleic acid that transmits instructions to the cells of the body. Using laboratory animals, researchers found that vitamin A facilitated the absorption of RNA in the liver and in the nucleus of the individual cells in other parts of the body.[3] An association between vitamin A and cancer of the lungs and cervix has also been noted. Lung cancer arises in the epithelial linings of the respiratory tract by a process similar to that which results in cancer of the cervix.[4]

Vitamin A is found in two forms: preformed vitamin A or retinol, which is present in large amounts in animal and fish livers, and beta-carotene, one of the carotene pigments found in green and yellow vegetables and fruits. Green leafy vegetables are even richer in usable carotene than carrots; this is because carotene has a particular preference for chlorophyll.[5]

Vitamin A toxicity can occur if too much is taken. This often happens as a result of preformed A taken in fish liver oil capsules; very little toxicity has occurred from beta-carotene.[6] Symptoms of vitamin A toxicity include nausea, vomiting, diarrhea, dry skin, hair loss, headaches, sore lips, and flaky, itchy skin.[7]

Factors interfering with vitamin A absorption include excessive consumption of alcohol, too much iron, the use of cortisone and other drugs, gastrointestinal and liver disorders, and any obstructions of the bile duct. Cooking, puréeing, and mashing of vegetables rupture cell membranes and make the carotene more available for absorption.[8]

Deficiencies of vitamin A include night blindness, an inability of the eyes to adjust to darkness, other eye diseases, and rough, dry, or prematurely aged skin. Severe conditions include corneal ulcers and softening of the bones and teeth since a deficiency of vitamin A leads to loss of vitamin C.[9]

The highest source of vitamin A is hot red pepper. Other sources are green leafy vegetables, orange vegetables, and fruits such as carrots, apricots, sweet potatoes, and winter squashes. Although vitamin A is found in high amounts in fish liver, this is not a recommended source at this time due to the high level of toxic residues in the liver and other organs of fish.

VITAMIN B COMPLEX

B-complex vitamins are water-soluble substances that can be cultivated from bacteria, yeasts, fungi, or molds. Known B-complex vitamins include B-1 (thiamine), B-2 (riboflavin), B-3 (niacin), B-6 (pyridoxine), B-12 (cyanocobalamin), B-13 (orotic acid), B-15 (pangamic acid), biotin, choline, folic acid, inositol, PABA (para-aminobenzoic acid), and B-17 (laetrile or amygdalin). All of these vitamins are grouped together because they are found in the same foods, have a close relationship in vegetable and animal tissues, and work together in maintaining certain body functions.

The B vitamins are necessary for the normal functioning of the nervous system. They provide the body with energy by converting carbohydrates into glucose, which is then burned by the body. They also are important in maintaining muscle tone in the gastrointestinal tract and in the health of the skin, hair, eyes, mouth, and liver.[10]

Since B vitamins are not stored in the body, their excess amounts are secreted, and they need to be continually replaced.

Sugar and alcohol destroy B vitamins; sulfa drugs, sleeping pills, insecticides, and estrogen create a condition in the intestinal tract which can destroy the B vitamins.[11]

Deficiencies of the B complex result in malfunctions of the nervous system, such as insomnia, irritability, nervousness, depression, defects in memory, dizziness, and headaches. Other deficiencies may manifest as anemia, baldness, gray hair, acne and other skin problems, constipation, and a high cholesterol level. Lack of B vitamins can show up in a sore mouth with cracks at the sides, a burning sensation inside the mouth, and an enlarged tongue which is swollen, shiny, and bright red or purple.

The B vitamins have been used successfully in the treatment of alcoholic psychoses, barbiturate overdose, and drug-induced delirium. Massive doses have been used to cure polio, to improve cases of shingles, and to control migraines and Meniere's disease.[12] Menstrual difficulties are relieved with a small dose as are post-operative nausea and vomiting resulting from anesthesia. [13]

The richest sources of B complex are the germ and bran of seeds like cereals, nuts, beans, and peas. Liver is especially rich in B complex, particularly B-12; however, only organic liver should be eaten because of the liver's tendency to concentrate contaminants and pollutants. Nutritional yeast is a strong source of B-complex vitamins and has been recommended by many nutritional experts. However, many individuals tend to be allergic to yeast; for those who are not allergic to it, it still has a strong acidic effect on the body. It has been shown that uric acid levels were elevated after using three tablespoons of yeast a day.[14] This could lead to problems such as gout. Most B-complex vitamins are also yeast based and, therefore, much discrimination and reading of labels should be exercised before taking a B-complex supplement. Supplements of the individual B vitamins are often made from other substances.

VITAMIN B-1 (THIAMINE)

Thiamine combines with pyruvic acid to form a substance necessary for the breakdown of carbohydrates into glucose. Thiamine is a component of the germ and bran of wheat, the husk of rice, and that portion of grains which is commercially milled away to give the grain a lighter color and texture. Beriberi, the deficiency disease that results from lack of thiamine, has been found both in the Orient among those who eat polished rice and in the West among wheat eaters who eat white bread.

Low intake of thiamine with experimental groups led to symptoms of irritability, depression, lack of cooperation, and fearfulness. The subjects also became inefficient and lost manual dexterity. Their hands and feet became numb as well.[15] Many ailments have been aided by the administration of thiamine. Thiamine is essential in the manufacture of hydrochloric acid, which aids in digestion. Thiamine helps improve muscle tone in the stomach and intestines so that constipation is relieved. Herpes zoster, a clustering of blisters behind the ear, has been successfully treated with thiamine.[16] Nutrients such as thiamine and niacin have been used together to treat multiple sclerosis patients with success. [17]

A deficiency of thiamine makes it difficult for a person to digest carbohydrates and also leaves too much pyruvic acid in the blood. This causes an oxygen deficiency that results in loss of mental alertness, labored breathing, and cardiac damage. First signs of this deficiency include fatigue, loss of appetite, irritability, and emotional instability. Confusion, loss of memory, abdominal pain and gastric distress may follow. A thiamine deficiency also affects the cardiovascular system and the gastrointestinal system with symptoms such as indigestion, severe constipation, and loss of appetite.[18]

Foods high in thiamine include rice bran, wheat germ, rice polish, sunflower seeds, pinyon nuts, peanuts, other nuts and seeds, and whole grains.

VITAMIN B-2 (RIBOFLAVIN)

Riboflavin is part of a group of enzymes that are involved in the breakdown and utilization of carbohydrates, fats, and proteins. It works with enzymes in the utilization of cell oxygen. Along with vitamin A, it is necessary for good vision, and it plays an important role in the prevention of cataracts. Riboflavin has also brought relief to children suffering from eczema.[19]

Riboflavin deficiency is the most common vitamin deficiency in the United States.[20] It may result from poor diets and from restricted diets for digestive problems such as ulcers or from diabetes and blood sugar problems. Symptoms of B-2 deficiency are cracks and sores in the corner of the mouth and lower lip; a red, sore tongue; eye fatigue; burning of the eyes; dilation of the pupil; and sensitivity to light. A strong deficiency can cause some type of cataracts as well.[21]

High natural sources of B-2 include liver, tongue and other organ meats, wheat germ, mushrooms, whole grains, and green leafy vegetables.

VITAMIN B-3 (NIACIN)

Niacin is an important vitamin for the proper activity of the nervous system and is effective in improving circulation and reducing the cholesterol level in the blood.[22] Niacin also assists enzymes in the breakdown and utilization of proteins, fats, and carbohydrates.

Large doses of niacin have been used successfully with psychiatric patients and in disorders such as elevated blood cholesterol and cholesterol deposits in the skin.[23] Large doses have also prolonged blood coagulation time, which may be helpful in treating heart attacks and strokes.[24] Niacin has been used in treating Meniere's disease (vertigo) and in some cases of deafness.[25] Acne has also been treated successfully with B-3.

Symptoms of niacin deficiency begin with muscle weakness, fatigue, loss of appetite, indigestion, skin eruptions, irritability, tension, and depression. Severe niacin deficiency results in pellagra, which is characterized by diarrhea, digestive disorders, skin lesions and canker sores, redness of the skin, rough, dry skin (the Italian name *pellagra* means "skin that is rough"), as well as anxiety, tremors, and other nervous disorders.

Pellagra has occurred in the southeastern United States and other countries where corn is eaten as the principal grain. Corn is not all that low in niacin, but it is the way that the corn is prepared that is important. The American Indians prepared the corn by soaking it in water that had been mixed with ashes. This ash water would soften the coating and make the niacin available for intestinal absorption. Sometimes the grain was pounded into a meal and then the ash water added; this not only liberated the niacin but also added minerals from the ash.[26] A similar custom exists in Mexico where limewater is added to soften the corn and make it into a dough.[27]

There are three synthetic forms of niacin—niacinamide, nicotinic acid, and nicotinamide. Niacinamide is sometimes used as a supplement since it does not cause the flushing of the skin that niacin does. Care should be taken, however, in using either of these forms as excess niacin has been known to cause deep depression and liver damage.[28]

Small amounts of pure niacin are contained in foods, but many foods contain tryptophan, an amino acid that can be converted into niacin by the body. Rice bran, rice polish, wheat germ, peanuts, lean meats, poultry, fish, and whole grains are rich in both niacin and tryptophan.

VITAMIN B-6 (PYRIDOXINE)

B-6 is required for the proper absorption of B-12 and for the production of hydrochloric acid and magnesium. The release of glycogen for energy from the liver and muscles is facilitated by B-6. It also aids in the conversion of tryptophan to niacin and helps maintain the balance of sodium and potassium in the body.

Pyridoxine is related to hormonal balance in women. Prior to the onset of menstruation, women seem to need additional doses of B-6; this helps to control irritability, nervousness, and outbreaks of acne. "Morning sickness" in early pregnancy is also the result of a B-6 and magnesium deficiency.[29] The use of B-6 has reduced the incidence of pre-eclampsia and toxemia which may occur during pregnancy.[30] Disorders of the nervous system like epilepsy have responded well to B-6 supplementation.[31] This is because these disorders are related to magnesium deficiency as well, and B-6 helps the absorption of magnesium.

B-6 is involved in fat metabolism, and a diet high in animal fat may cause cholesterol plaque when B-6 is low. Arteriosclerotic conditions have been produced in animals by putting them on pyridoxine-deficient diets.[32] Cases of Parkinson's disease have responded to B-6 injections in combination with magnesium.[33] Vitamin B-6 has also been used to help treat a form of anemia in which red blood cells are too small.[34]

Deficiencies of pyridoxine may appear similar to those seen in niacin and riboflavin deficiencies, which includes muscular weakness, nervousness, irritability, depression, and dermatitis. In cases of B-6 deficiency, there is also low blood sugar and low glucose tolerance, resulting in a sensitivity to insulin.[35] Deficiency may also cause numbness and cramps in arms and legs, tingling hands, and forms of neuritis and arthritis.

Foods high in B-6 include rice bran, rice polishings, organ meats, and whole grains.

VITAMIN B-12 (COBALAMIN)

Vitamin B-12 is the only vitamin that contains essential mineral elements, primarily cobalt. It cannot be made synthetically but must be grown in bacteria or molds. Animal protein is the only source in which B-12 occurs naturally in substantial amounts. In a culture where food is grown organically and not highly processed, there are rarely deficiencies of B-12, even when meat, eggs, or milk are not in the diet. This may be because organic foods contain traces of bacteria from the soil or tiny bits of insects which are difficult to remove completely. These may contain the little amount of B-12 necessary.[36]

B-12 can be absorbed from the gastrointestinal tract if a certain mucoprotein enzyme is present. It needs to be combined with calcium during absorption to benefit the body properly. The presence of hydrochloric acid also aids in the absorption of B-12. Age, iron, calcium, and B-6 deficiencies decrease B-12 absorption. The use of laxatives depletes the storage of B-12.[37]

Cobalamin is necessary for the metabolism of nerve tissue and is involved in protein, fat, and carbohydrate metabolism. It helps iron function better in the body and prevents the disease known as "pernicious anemia." B-12 helps red blood cells to mature up to a certain point, and then protein, iron, vitamin C, and folic acid help to finish the development of the cells. It has been used successfully in treating osteoarthritis, a degenerative joint disease, and osteoporosis, a softening of the bones.[38] B-12 has also proved helpful in the condition known as "tobacco amblyopia," a dimness of vision due to poisoning by tobacco.[39] It has provided relief in conditions of insomnia, mental depression, an inability to concentrate, lack of balance, as well as bursitis and asthma.[40]

Symptoms of B-12 deficiency may take five or six years to appear after the body's supply from natural sources has been restricted.[41] A deficiency is usually due to an absorption problem caused by a lack of the mucoprotein enzyme known as the "intrinsic factor." A deficiency starts with the nervous system—soreness in arms and legs; loss of balance; a red, raw, ulcerated tongue; and mental symptoms such as confusion and loss of memory. In extreme deficiencies, permanent mental deterioration, paralysis, and a type of brain damage resembling schizophrenia may occur.[42]

Food sources high in B-12 include the organ meats, fish, aged cheeses such as Roquefort, brewer's yeast, eggs, milk and dairy products, raw wheat germ, comfrey leaves, kelp and sea vegetables.

FOLIC ACID

Folic acid was first isolated from spinach, and it was successful in curing anemia that resulted during pregnancy. When it was tried as a cure for pernicious anemia, the red blood cells improved, but the neurological symptoms did not. Research showed that the biochemic role of B-12 and folic acid overlapped to some extent. They both involve the synthesis of DNA, the protein chain which is the basic substance of chromosomes and carries the genetic coding that governs the cell's metabolism. When either B-12 or folic acid is missing or deficient, the duplication of chromosomes cannot occur at the normal rate and the reproduction of cells is slowed. During pregnancy, cells are multiplying quickly and new tissue is being formed, so large amounts of folic acid are needed.[43] Deficiencies of folic acid have been seen in women who have taken birth-control pills.[44]

Deficiency of folic acid results in poor growth, graying of the hair, tongue inflammation, gastrointestinal disturbances, and metabolic disturbances. A deficiency can also lead to anemia which cannot be corrected by supplementary iron.[45] A number of studies have shown folic acid deficiencies to be a contributing factor in mental illness; psychiatric patients were found to have low levels of folic acid.[46] Interference with the metabolism of folic acid in the fetus can lead to deformities such as cleft palate, brain damage, and poor learning ability in children.[47]

Folic acid is found in liver, mushrooms, green leafy vegetables, broccoli, and asparagus.

PABA (PARA-AMINOBENZOIC ACID)

PABA stimulates the intestinal bacteria, enabling them to produce folic acid, which aids in the synthesis of pantothenic acid. It is an important vitamin in the health of the skin and in helping respiratory disorders. Used in ointments, it is soothing for burns and sunburn. It is also helpful in eczema, lupus, and skin changes due to aging. PABA has been used in combination with pantothenic acid, choline, and folic acid in the treatment of gray hair with some success.[48] It is also used in treating some parasitic diseases, including Rocky Mountain Spotted Fever.[49]

A deficiency of PABA may result from the use of sulfa drugs, which reduce the capacity of PABA to function properly in the intestines. Symptoms include fatigue, irritability, nervousness, constipation, and other digestive disorders.

Sources rich in PABA include liver, blackstrap molasses, yogurt and soured-milk products, and whole grains.

PANTOTHENIC ACID

Pantothenic acid is another of the B vitamins which is synthesized in the body by the bacteria in the intestines. There is a close correlation between pantothenic acid and the functioning of the adrenal cortex. Pantothenic acid stimulates the adrenal glands and increases production of cortisone and other adrenal hormones. Pantothenic acid, therefore, helps in withstanding stressful conditions. When pantothenic acid was eliminated from the diet in experiments, subjects complained of tiredness, difficulty sleeping, and tingling sensations in the hands and feet.[50] Other symptoms of pantothenic acid deficiency are graying and loss of hair, mental depression, and an increased tendency to infections and allergies.[51] Deficiencies may also lead to low blood sugar, insufficient amounts of HCL in the stomach, and disturbances of the motor nerves.

Although pantothenic acid is found in most foods, 50 per cent of it is lost in the processing of whole grains, and 33 per cent in the cooking of meat.[52] Taking pantothenic acid in tablet form may increase the need for B-1 and other B vitamins, so it is best to obtain it from food sources. Foods high in this nutrient include liver and organ meats, blackstrap molasses, whole grains, egg yolks, and green leafy vegetables.

CHOLINE

The most important function of choline is its collaboration with inositol as part of lecithin. Lecithin helps to absorb and transport fats and the fat-soluble vitamins A, D, E, and K in the blood.

Choline is important in minimizing deposits of fat and cholesterol in the liver and arteries. It also regulates the liver and gall bladder function, helps prevent gallstones, and is necessary for manufacturing a substance in the blood known as phospholipids. Along with inositol, it nourishes the myelin sheaths of nerve fibers.

A deficiency of choline may lead to high blood pressure, cirrhosis and degeneration of the liver, atherosclerosis and hardening of the arteries. Good sources of choline are liquid or granular lecithin, liver, blackstrap molasses, egg yolks, green leafy vegetables, and whole grains.

INOSITOL

Inositol is closely associated with choline and biotin. It is effective in aiding the body's production of lecithin. Fats are moved from the liver to the cells with the aid of lecithin; inositol thereby helps in the metabolism of fats and in reducing blood cholesterol. It prevents the hardening of the arteries and protects the liver, kidneys, and heart. It also prevents thinning hair and baldness and has been found to be helpful in brain-cell nutrition and in the treatment of schizophrenia.[53]

Caffeine may create an inositol shortage in the body.[54] A deficiency of inositol may cause constipation, eczema, and abnormalities of the eyes. It also contributes to hair loss and high blood cholesterol level, which may result in heart and artery disease. Inositol is found in liquid and granular lecithin, liver, blackstrap molasses, egg yolks, green leafy vegetables, and whole grains.

BIOTIN

Biotin assists in the making of fatty acids and in the oxidation of fatty acids and carbohydrates. Without biotin, the body's fat production would be impaired. Biotin also aids in the utilization of protein and some of the B vitamins.

Raw egg white contains the protein *avidin*, which binds with biotin in the intestine, preventing its absorption by the body. Since eggs are usually eaten in cooked form, there is no real danger of a biotin deficiency. Experimental animals who were fed uncooked egg whites developed fatigue, depression, nausea, pain, and lack of appetite.[55]

A biotin deficiency may cause hair loss, eczema, dandruff, seborrhea, and other skin disorders. A severe deficiency may interfere with the body's fat metabolism. High food sources of biotin include unpolished rice, liver, kidney and organ meats, whole grains, soybeans, and green leafy vegetables.

B-13 (OROTIC ACID)

Vitamin B-13 is not yet available in the United States, but it has been synthesized in Europe and is used to treat multiple sclerosis. It is important for the restoration of cells and is utilized by the body in the metabolism of folic acid and vitamin B-12.[56] Deficiency symptoms are not known, but it is believed that a deficiency may lead to liver disorders, cell degeneration, and premature aging.[57] Orotic acid is found in the whey portion of milk and particularly in souredmilk products.

B-15 (PANGAMIC ACID)

Pangamic acid is a water-soluble nutrient that was originally isolated in extracted apricot kernels and later obtained in crystalline form from rice bran, rice polish, whole-grain cereals, brewer's yeast, and horse liver. It promotes oxidation processes and cell respiration and stimulates glucose oxidation. Its chief function is its ability to eliminate *hypoxia*, an insufficient supply of oxygen in living tissue (especially in the cardiac and other muscles).[58] It is essential in promoting protein metabolism; it also regulates fat and sugar metabolism and is, therefore, useful in cases of atherosclerosis and diabetes. It is helpful in treating high blood cholesterol levels and impaired circulation and can protect against carbon-monoxide poisoning.[59]

A deficiency of B-15 may cause diminished oxygenation of cells, heart disease, and glandular and nervous disorders. Food sources include apricot kernels, seeds and nuts, and whole grains.

B-17 LAETRILE (AMYGDALIN, NITRILOSIDES)

Laetrile is a natural substance made from apricot kernels which has a specific function in preventing and treating cancer. It has been legalized in several states in this country; however, many doctors reject its use on the grounds that it may be poisonous because of its cyanide content. It is manufactured and used legally in over 17 countries, including Mexico, Germany, Italy, Belgium, and the Philippines.[60]

Natural cyanide is locked in a sugar molecule. It is found in over 200 known unrefined foods and grains. A concentrate of two to three per cent laetrile is found in the whole kernels of most fruits, including apricots, apples, cherries, peaches, plums, and nectarines.

According to those who have experimented with laetrile, it attacks only cancerous cells. When laetrile is heated and absorbed by normal cells, an enzyme called *rhodanese* detoxifies the cyanide, which is then excreted through the urine. Because cancer cells are deficient in rhodanese and are surrounded by another enzyme, *beta-glucosidase*, which releases the bound cyanide from the laetrile at the site of malignancy, laetrile is believed to attack only the malignant areas.

A prolonged deficiency of B-17 may lead to diminished resistance to malignancies. Dosages of 0.25 to 1.0 grams may be taken with meals, but not more than one gram at a time. Dosages as high as 20 grams daily of combined oral and intravenous administration have been used on patients whose detoxification and elimination levels of laetrile were adequate.[61]

VITAMIN C (ASCORBIC ACID)

Vitamin C has had such dramatic effects on various body conditions and disease states that too much of it tends to be used, especially in its acidic forms, thus creating an acid/alkaline imbalance in the body. When vitamin C is used, it should be utilized in its ascorbate form as calcium, potassium, or magnesium ascorbate (not sodium ascorbate; we already have plenty of sodium in the body). Vitamin C should also be used in conjunction with the bioflavonoids, or vitamin P, alternating between vitamin C one day and bioflavonoids the following day since they help vitamin C assimilate in the body.

One of the primary functions of vitamin C is maintaining collagen, a protein necessary for connective tissue in skin, ligaments, and bones. Vitamin C is used for healing wounds and burns because it facilitates the formation of connective tissue in the scar. In addition, it fights bacterial infections and reduces the effects on the body of certain allergy-producing substances. It also helps in forming red blood cells and preventing hemorrhaging.[62]

When cultures of human cells were bathed in a solution containing vitamin C, they were able to produce large quantities of a substance known as *interferon*, which "interferes" with the ability of viruses to invade cells.[63] There is also evidence that vitamin C exerts some detoxifying effect in those who have been exposed to heavy metals like lead and cadmium.[64] High doses also seem to have a protective effect against pesticides and food additives.[65]

One should be careful in taking large doses of vitamin C because it can disrupt calcium absorption. Vitamin C is sometimes converted to calcium oxalate in the urine, which can result in the formation of kidney stones.[66] In some animals, large doses produced demineralization of the bones.

A deficiency of vitamin C results in swollen or painful joints, a tendency to bruise easily, bleeding gums, pyorrhea, tooth decay, nosebleeds, lowered resistance to infections, and slow healing of wounds and fractures. A severe deficiency results in scurvy. Smoking lowers the blood level of vitamin C.[67]

Ascorbic acid is found in most fruits and vegetables, especially leafy green and yellow vegetables, green peppers, citrus fruits, rose hips, acerola berries, and tomatoes. However, it is recommended that green and yellow vegetables be used as primary sources since many people are allergic to citrus (particularly oranges) and tend to overalkalinize their bodies through the use of too much citrus fruit. (Although citrus fruit is acid, it turns to alkali in the body.) In addition to green and yellow vegetables, sprouts made from the seeds of grains and beans, such as alfalfa, red clover, sunflower, buckwheat, lentil, and mung bean, are exceptionally high in vitamin C.

VITAMIN D

The strongest source of vitamin D is sunlight, although certain foods also contain this vitamin. The Sun's ultraviolet rays activate substances in the skin which are related to cholesterol; these substances are transformed to vitamin D. Vitamin D regulates calcium metabolism along with the parathyroid hormone. It aids the absorption of calcium from the intestinal tract and the assimilation of phosphorus, which is required for bone formation. If there is not enough calcium in the intestinal tract, it absorbs it from the bones themselves. This vitamin is essential in maintaining a healthy nervous system, normal heart action, and normal blood clotting since all these functions are related to the body's utilization of calcium and phosphorus.

Vitamin D is best utilized when taken with vitamin A; a high natural source of both of these vitamins is found in fish liver.

Since vitamin D is a fat-soluble vitamin, it does not dissolve in water; therefore, it is not easily excreted in the urine. If it is taken in large quantities, it tends to accumulate, and there may be difficulty getting rid of excesses. When too much vitamin D is taken, so much calcium can be absorbed and removed from the bones that it begins to form deposits which damage the tissues of the heart, blood vessels, and lungs. Other symptoms of vitamin D toxicity are nausea, vomiting, diarrhea, dizziness, and weakness.

For those individuals who live in northern climates, vitamin D can be obtained through diet since it is found in large amounts in fish liver oil. (This is because fish eat plankton which thrives near the surface of the sea and is exposed to sunlight.) Milk contains another form of vitamin D—D-2, or *ergocalciferol*. This synthetic form is made by taking a substance produced by yeast called ergosterol and exposing it to ultraviolet radiation. The ergosterol is then separated, purified, and added to milk.[68]

Symptoms of vitamin D deficiency are inadequate absorption of calcium from the intestinal tract and retention of phosphorus in the kidney, leading to faulty mineralization of bone structures. Rickets, a bone disorder in children, is a result of vitamin D deficiency. Signs of rickets are softening of the skull and bones with bowing of the legs and spinal curvatures, enlargement of wrist, knee, and ankle joints, poorly developed muscle, and nervous irritability.[69] Adult rickets, known as osteomalacia, may also occur.[70] Vitamin D deficiency may cause tetany, a condition characterized by muscle weakness, tingling, and spasm. This is because vitamin D and parathyroid hormones work together to regulate the transport of calcium.

Foods high in vitamin D include fish liver, calves' liver, chicken liver, beef liver, egg yolks, yogurt and soured-milk products.

VITAMIN E

Vitamin E is a fat-soluble vitamin composed of a group of compounds called *tocopherols*. *Alpha tocopherol* is the most potent form of vitamin E and has the greatest nutritional and biological value. Tocopherols occur in the highest concentrations in cold-pressed vegetable oils, raw seeds and nuts, and soybeans. Vitamin E was first obtained from wheat germ.

Vitamin E is an antioxidant; it opposes oxidation of substances in the body. It prevents saturated fatty acids and vitamin A from breaking down and combining with other substances in the body. Fats and oils containing vitamin E are less susceptible to rancidity than those devoid of it. Vitamin E can unite with oxygen and prevent it from being converted into toxic peroxides; this leaves the red blood cells more fully supplied with pure oxygen that the blood carries to the heart and other organs.

In areas where there is high air pollution, vitamin E has proved very helpful. Rats exposed to ozone concentrations in the air similar to what occurs in air pollution were given doses of vitamin E. When their lungs were examined for damage, it was found that the greatest injury occurred in those who had been given the least vitamin E.[71] Air which is polluted with combinations of ozone and oxides of metals like nitrogen, cadmium, and lead requires us to need increasing amounts of protective antioxidants like vitamin E. These oxidating reactions (called peroxidation) also enter the body through food. The principal source of reactive oxygenation in food are vegetable oils which have become rancid.[72] When peroxidation occurs, it produces a pigment that accumulates, causing discoloration in the tissues. These deposits show up in the fatty tissue and the skin of those who are advanced in age.[73] Rats exposed to high concentrations of oxygen were fed large amounts of wheat germ oil, and they lived their normal life span.[74] Therefore, vitamin E could have an effect on the aging process, especially in industrial areas where smog and pollution lead to peroxidation damage. This could also be true for individuals who consume large amounts of unsaturated vegetable oils in their diet.[75]

Vitamin E plays an important role in heart disease since it makes it possible for the cardiac muscle to function with less oxygen, thereby increasing endurance and stamina. It also causes dilation of the blood vessels, permitting a fuller flow of blood to the heart. In coronary thrombosis, a heart attack in which the vessels are blocked by blood clots and the heart is deprived of its blood supply, vitamin E causes arterial blood clots to disintegrate. Angina pectoris, a chest pain resulting from an insufficient supply of blood to the heart tissue, has also been treated successfully with alpha tocopherol.[76]

Furthermore, vitamin E is also helpful in the functioning of the reproductive organs (*tocopherol* means "bringing forth normal births"). Rats on a diet in which vitamin E was absent failed to reproduce.[77] It has been used to regulate flow during menstruation and as a treatment for "hot flashes" and headaches during menopause.[78] Applied as an ointment, vitamin E aids in healing burns and skin ulcers, and dissolves scar tissue.

A vitamin E deficiency is not responsible for any deficiency diseases, but its lack may lead to many other conditions. The first sign of vitamin E depletion is the rupture of red blood cells, which results from their increased fragility. A deficiency may result in abnormal fat deposits in the muscles and an increased demand for oxygen. Iron absorption and hemoglobin formation are also impaired. A severe deficiency can cause damage to the kidneys and nephritis. This occurs when kidney tubules plug up with dead cells so that urine is unable to pass. Vitamin E deficiency makes red blood cells more susceptible to damage from medication and environmental stresses.[79]

Thus, the amount of vitamin E given should be carefully watched, especially in those with high blood pressure and those with rheumatic heart disease. People taking digitalis need to be careful of vitamin E since it magnifies the effect of the drug and could cause arrythmia.[80] Iron metabolism can also be impaired by too much E, and if iron supplements are being taken, they should be used at a different time of day. It is very important that vitamin E (like A and D) be taken in its dry form—not as an oil-based capsule, but in a dry capsule or a chewable tablet.

Food sources where vitamin E is found in high concentration include vegetable oils, seeds, nuts, and soybeans.

VITAMIN F

Vitamin F is a fat-soluble vitamin consisting of the three essential fatty acids—linoleic, linolenic, and arachidonic. The body cannot manufacture these EFA's (essential fatty acids), so they must be obtained in the form of food. EFA's make it easier for oxygen to be transported to all the cells, tissues, and organs; they help lubricate the cells, regulate the rate of blood coagulation, and break up cholesterol deposited on arterial walls.[81] These unsaturated fatty acids work with vitamin D in making calcium available to the tissues, assisting in the assimilation of phosphorus, and stimulating the conversion of carotene into vitamin A.

A balance of twice as much unsaturated fatty acids to saturated ones is beneficial for heart and arterial health. A higher consumption of food such as butter, cream, cheese, milk, and carbohydrates increases the need for unsaturated fatty acids. When there is sufficient linoleic acid in the diet, the other two essential fatty acids can be synthesized from it. In order to get the full benefit of vitamin F, the proper amounts of vitamin E need to be included.

Vitamin F deficiencies may be responsible for dry and brittle hair, dandruff, eczema, acne, dry skin, as well as diseases of the heart, circulatory system and kidneys associated with faulty fat metabolism.[82] Vitamin F has been used in preventing heart disease; it keeps cholesterol soft and prevents it from forming any hard deposits in the blood vessels or under the skin.[83]

Natural sources of vitamin F include lecithin, vegetable oils such as safflower, soy and corn, wheat germ, seeds and fish liver oils.

VITAMIN K

Vitamin K is found in three forms: K-1 and K-2, which are fat-soluble and can be manufactured in the intestinal tract in the presence of certain intestinal bacteria, and K-3, which is produced synthetically for those who are unable to utilize naturally occurring vitamin K due to lack of bile (necessary for the absorption of fat-soluble vitamins). If yogurt, kefir, and other soured-milk products are included in the diet, the body should be capable of manufacturing sufficient amounts of K.

Prothrombin, a chemical involved in blood clotting, needs vitamin K for its formation. Vitamin K is also involved in a body process called *phosphorylation* in which phosphate in combination with glucose is passed through the cell membranes and converted into glycogen, a form in which carbohydrates are stored in the body.[84] It is also important for normal liver functioning.

Vitamin K is absorbed in the upper intestinal tract with the aid of bile and is transported to the liver where it synthesizes prothrombin and other proteins involved in blood clotting. Excessive use of antibotics can destroy the intestinal flora needed to synthesize K.[85]

Deficiencies of vitamin K result from inadequate absorption or the body's inability to utilize vitamin K in the liver. Vitamin K deficiency is common in diseases such as celiac disease (intestinal malabsorption); colitis, which affects the lining of the small intestine and causes a loss of intestinal contents; and hypothrombinemia, where blood clotting time is prolonged.[86] Vitamin K is useful in reducing the blood flow during prolonged menstruation; it has also been used with vitamin C in the prevention of hemorrhage.[87]

Natural sources of vitamin K are yogurt, kefir, and soured-milk products, sea vegetables, alfalfa, leafy green vegetables, blackstrap molasses, fish liver oils, and other polyunsaturated oils.

VITAMIN P (BIOFLAVONOIDS)

Bioflavonoids are composed of a group of substances that appear in fruits and vegetables in conjunction with vitamin C. The components of bioflavonoids are citrin, hesperidin, rutin, flavones, and flavonals. Bioflavonoids were discovered in the white segments of citrus fruits.

One of their uses is in the absorption of vitamin C. They help vitamin C by keeping collagen, the intracellular cement, in healthy condition. They increase the strength of the capillaries, help prevent hemorrhage in the capillaries and connective tissues, and build a protective barrier against infections. Along with vitamin C, they are helpful in treating bleeding gums, eczema, rheumatism, and rheumatic fever.[88]

Bioflavonoids are also important in treating allergies and asthma. Vitamin P is beneficial in the treatment of muscular dystrophy because it helps lower blood pressure. Studies have been conducted on the use of bioflavonoids with rheumatoid arthritis, where much improvement took place.[89] Thirty-six patients with bleeding duodenal ulcers were also treated with bioflavonoids along with an orange juice/milk/gelatin mixture. Bleeding stopped within four days, and in most of the cases there was no recurrence of bleeding.[90] Rutin, one of the bioflavonoids, is important in treating ailments of the kidneys.

The bioflavonoids are absorbed from the gastrointestinal tract into the blood stream. Excess amounts are excreted through urination and perspiration. Deficiency symptoms are related to vitamin C deficiencies—the increased tendency to hemorrhage and bruise easily.

Vitamin P is found in buckwheat, buckwheat sprouts, rose hips, lemons, blackberries, black currants, grapes, cherries, grapefruits, oranges, and herbs like St. John's wort.

NOTES

1. Rudolph Ballantine, M.D., *Diet and Nutrition—A Holistic Approach* (Honesdale, PA: Himalayan International Institute, 1978), p. 163.
2. Ibid.
3. John D. Kirschmann, *Nutrition Almanac* (New York: McGraw-Hill, 1979), p. 14.
4. Ballantine, p. 166.
5. Ibid., p. 167.
6. Ibid.
7. Kirschmann, p. 15.
8. Ibid., p. 14.
9. Ibid., p. 15.
10. Ibid., p. 18.
11. Ibid.
12. Ibid., p. 19.
13. Ibid.
14. Ballantine, p. 170.
15. Ibid., p. 173.
16. Kirschmann, p. 22.
17. Ibid.
18. Ibid.
19. Ibid., p. 25.
20. Ibid., p. 24.
21. Ibid.
22. Ibid., p. 36.
23. Ballantine, p. 181.
24. Ibid.
25. Kirschmann, p. 36.
26. Ballantine, p. 180.
27. Ibid., pp. 37-38.
28. Ibid., p. 182.
29. Ibid., p. 183.
30. Ibid.
31. Ibid.

32. Ibid., p. 184.
33. Paavo Airola, *How To Get Well* (Phoenix, AZ: Health Plus, 1974), p. 262.
34. Kirschmann, page 26.
35. Ibid., p. 25.
36. Ballantine, p. 185.
37. Kirschmann, p. 26.
38. Ibid., p. 28.
39. Ibid.
40. Ibid.
41. Ibid., p. 27.
42. Ibid., p. 28.
43. Ballantine, p. 188.
44. Ibid., p. 189.
45. Kirschmann, p. 32.
46. Ballantine, p. 189.
47. Kirschmann, p. 32.
48. Airola, p. 264.
49. Kirschmann, p. 38.
50. Ballantine, p. 191.
51. Airola, p. 265.
52. Ballantine, p. 191.
53. Airola, p. 266.
54. Ibid.
55. Ballantine, p. 193.
56. Kirschmann, p. 29.
57. Ibid.
58. Ibid., p. 39.
59. Ibid.
60. Ibid., p. 35.
61. Ibid.
62. Ibid., p. 43.
63. Ballantine, p. 98.
64. Ibid., p. 201.
65. Ibid., pp. 109-10.
66. Ibid., p. 201.
67. Kirschmann, p. 44.
68. Ballantine, p. 208.
69. Kirschmann, p. 48.
70. Ibid.
71. Ibid., p. 50.
72. Ballantine, p. 214.
73. Ibid., p. 215.
74. Ibid.
75. Ibid., p. 216.
76. Ibid.
77. Kirschmann, p. 50.
78. Ballantine, p. 210.
79. Kirschmann, p. 56.

80. Ibid., p. 52.
81. Ballantine, p. 212.
82. Kirschmann, p. 56.
83. Ibid., p. 51.
84. Ibid.
85. Ibid., p. 58.
86. Ibid.
87. Ibid., p. 59.
88. Ibid., p. 60.
89. Ibid.
90. Ibid.

11

MINERALS

Mineral salts are found in the Earth. When rocks and stones break down into fragments, they accumulate in the soil. From the soil, they are passed on to plants, and from plants they are available to nurture both animal and human. When plant or animal tissue is burned, the nitrogen, hydrogen, sulfur and carbon that make up fats, carbohydrates and proteins are released as gases and the minerals alone remain as "ash." The minerals found in the body are primarily sodium, potassium, calcium, phosphorus, magnesium, sulfur and chlorine. These are known as the *macro-minerals* because they are found in large amounts in the body. However, there are a number of other minerals like iron, zinc, iodine, manganese, and copper that are found in small amounts, and these are referred to as *trace minerals*.

Although only four to five per cent of body weight is mineral matter, minerals are vital to mental and physical health. They are constituents of the bones, teeth, soft tissue, muscle, blood, and nerve cells. They are catalysts for many biological reactions within the human body, including muscle response, transmission of messages through the nervous system, digestion, metabolism of foods, and production of hormones. Minerals help to maintain the water balance essential to the proper functioning of mental and physical processes. They keep blood and tissue fluids from becoming too acid or alkaline and permit other nutrients to pass into the blood stream.[1] All of the minerals needed in the body must be supplied by the food and herbs we ingest.

CALCIUM

Calcium is the most abundant mineral in the body. About 99 per cent is deposited in the bones and teeth, and the remainder is in the soft tissue. To function properly, calcium needs magnesium, phosphorus and vitamins A, C and D.

Calcium's major role in combination with phosphorus is to build and maintain bones and teeth. It is also essential for the contraction of muscles. If a muscle doesn't have enough calcium, its fibers are motionless and do not slide together and mesh. Therefore, the muscle cannot contract, or once it has contracted, it will not relax, causing a "cramp." Calcium is also important, along with magnesium, in maintaining a healthy nervous system. This mineral assists in the process of blood clotting and helps prevent the accumulation of too much acid or alkali in the blood. Furthermore, it aids in the body's utilization of iron, helps activate several enzymes, and regulates the passage of nutrients in and out of the cell walls.[2]

Calcium absorption is inefficient; usually only 20-50 per cent of ingested calcium is absorbed. Absorption takes place in the duodenum and ceases in the lower part of the intestinal tract when the food content becomes alkaline.[3] Calcium absorption depends on the presence of adequate amounts of vitamin D, which works with the parathyroid hormone to regulate the amount of calcium in the blood. Phosphorous, vitamin A and vitamin C are also needed.

Certain substances interfere with the absorption of calcium. When excessive amounts of fat combine with calcium, an insoluble compound is formed which cannot be absorbed. Oxalic acid, found in chocolate, spinach, and rhubarb, makes an insoluble compound and may form into kidney or gall bladder stones. Large amounts of phytic acid, present in the bran of grains, may also tie up calcium absorption.[4] The amount of protein taken is significant. Too little protein will result in reduced absorption, while a high intake of animal protein can depress calcium retention. Studies show that vegetarians often have stronger bones.[5]

When one is inactive and at rest, calcium tends to be pulled out of the bones to be used for other purposes. This is especially true of older people who exercise less. After the hormonal shifts of menopause, women seem to be more susceptible to the action of the parathyroid hormone which promotes the removal of calcium from the bones. The result is a gradual demineralizing of the bones with increasing age and a growing incidence of fractures.[6] (See Osteoporosis in chapter 21.)

Large amounts of calcium are found in sesame seeds, sea vegetables, green leafy vegetables like kale, turnip greens, mustard greens, collard greens and dandelion greens, and some nuts like almonds and filberts. Herbs as comfrey root and leaf also contain strong amounts of calcium.

MAGNESIUM

Nearly 70 per cent of the body's magnesium is located in the bones along with calcium and phosphorus, while 30 per cent is found in the soft tissues and body fluids. Magnesium is important in activating the enzymes necessary for the metabolism of carbohydrates and amino acids. It balances the effect of calcium, thereby playing an important role in neuromuscular contractions.[7] It helps regulate the acid/alkaline balance in the body and promotes absorption of other minerals, such as calcium, phosphorus, sodium, and potassium. Magnesium enables one to utilize the B-complex vitamins and C and E. It is important for the proper function of the nerves and muscles, especially the heart muscle.

The balance between calcium and magnesium is critical. If calcium consumption is high, magnesium needs to be high also. The amounts of protein, phosphorus, and vitamin D also influence the magnesium requirement. The need for magnesium is increased when blood cholesterol levels are high and when consumption of protein is high.[8]

Magnesium is important in controlling the manner in which electrical charges are utilized by the body to induce the passage of nutrients in and out of cells.[9] It is vital in preventing heart attacks and coronary thrombosis.[10] It has also proved beneficial in the treatment of neuromuscular disorders, nervousness, tantrums, and hand tremors.[11] It it has been used to control convulsions in epileptic patients. Magnesium, rather than calcium, forms the kind of hard tooth enamel that resists decay. No matter how much calcium is ingested, only a soft enamel will be found unless magnesium is present.[12] It also helps to protect the accumulation of calcium deposits in the urinary tract by making calcium and phosphorus soluble in the urine and preventing them from turning into stones.[13]

Symptoms of magnesium deficiency include anxiety, confusion, muscle twitches, tremors, cramps, and spasms. A magnesium deficiency is also related to coronary heart disease. An inadequate supply may result in the formation of clots in the heart and brain and may contribute to calcium deposits in the kidneys, blood vessels, and heart. One of the first steps in treating magnesium deficiencies, among children especially, is to eliminate milk from the diet. Milk contains high amounts of *calciferol*, a synthetic vitamin D, which binds with magnesium and carries it out of the body.[14]

Magnesium is found in very high amounts in green leafy vegetables since it is an essential component of chlorophyll. (It has the same relationship to chlorophyll that iron has to hemoglobin.) It is also found in oil-rich seeds and nuts, especially filberts, almonds, and cashews. Herbs such as alfalfa, borage and red raspberry leaf contain significant amounts of magnesium.

POTASSIUM

Potassium and sodium are alkalis; they have a single electrical charge instead of the two charges on many other minerals. Therefore, they move readily through solutions, especially water. Potassium tends to be concentrated inside the cell, whereas sodium is high in the fluid surrounding the cell. Sodium is found in the waters on the Earth's surface, whereas potassium is concentrated inside plants.

Potassium and sodium help regulate the water balance within the body; they check the distribution of fluids on either side of cell walls.[15] Potassium is necessary to preserve the proper alkalinity of body fluids. It assists the conversion of glucose and glycogen (the form in which glucose is stored in the liver). It stimulates the kidneys to eliminate body toxins and wastes. Potassium is also important in maintaining the skin. With sodium, it normalizes the heartbeat and nourishes the muscular system. It also unites with phosphorus to send oxygen to the brain and works with calcium in the regulation of neuromuscular activity.[16]

Potassium is absorbed from the small intestine. It is excreted through urination and perspiration. Aldosterone, an adrenal hormone, stimulates potassium excretion. Excessive use of salt drains the body's conservation of potassium. Potassium can also be depleted by prolonged diarrhea, vomiting, excessive sweating and fluid loss. Contrary to the theory of losing sodium through excessive sweating and replacing it with salt tablets, it is actually potassium that is lost.[17] I tested several individuals who had undergone many days of sweating in Native American Sweat Lodges, and the only nutrient they were deficient in was potassium. Both alcohol and coffee increase the excretion of potassium; a high intake of sugar also increases potassium elimination. A low blood sugar level is a stressful condition that strains the adrenal glands, causing additional potassium to be lost in the urine while water and salt are held in the tissues. An adequate supply of magnesium is needed to retain the storage of potassium in the cells.

Potassium has been used to treat cases of high blood pressure which were caused by excess sodium intake. Injections of potassium chloride have been used to treat colic in infants.[18] Potassium chloride is also effective in treating allergies. Giving potassium to diabetic patients has reduced blood pressure and blood sugar levels.[19]

Symptoms of potassium deficiency may include nervous disorders, insomnia, constipation, slow and irregular heartbeat and muscle damage, and acne and dry skin conditions. When a deficiency of potassium impairs glucose metabolism, energy is no longer available to the muscles, and they may become paralyzed. Infants who have diarrhea may have a potassium deficiency because the passage of the intestinal contents is so rapid that there is decreased absorption of potassium. Diabetic patients are often deficient in potassium as are those taking hormone drugs, such as cortisone and aldosterone, which cause the retention of sodium.

Food sources high in potassium include potatoes, bananas, peanuts, and leafy green vegetables. Herbs such as plantain and alfalfa are also rich in potassium.

SODIUM

Sodium is found predominantly in the body's extracellular fluids. The remaining amount is found in the bones. Along with potassium, sodium equalizes the acid/alkaline factor in the blood and helps regulate water balance within the body. Sodium and potassium are also involved in muscle contraction and expansion and in nerve stimulation.

Sodium keeps the other blood minerals soluble so they will not build up as deposits in the blood stream. It works with chlorine to improve blood and lymph health and is necessary for hydrochloric-acid production in the stomach. Sodium is absorbed in the small intestine and stomach and then filtered out and carried by the blood to the kidneys. The excess is excreted in the urine. The adrenal hormone aldosterone regulates sodium metabolism.

Excesses of sodium are found much more readily than deficiencies. Excess may cause abnormal fluid retention accompanied by dizziness and swelling of ankles, legs, and face. Excess also contributes to high blood pressure. Low sodium diets are important, particularly eliminating table salt and substituting herb seasonings with no salt (for example, Bio-salt, the herbal blend from Switzerland that has various potassium compounds; Dr. Bonner's mineral seasoning; Veg-It, the low-sodium vegetable seasoning; and Wachter's Sea-Land Seasoning, a delicious seasoning with garlic, green pepper, various vegetables and spices, but no salt). Soy sauce, tamari (naturally fermented soy sauce), and miso soup are high in sodium.

If a sodium deficiency occurs, it can cause intestinal gas, weight loss, vomiting, and muscle shrinkage. The conversion of carbohydrates into fat for digestion is impaired when sodium is absent.[20]

Balanced foods high in sodium include sea vegetables, such as dulse, hijiki, arame, nori, wakame, kombu, and kelp, and seafoods.

IRON

The major function of iron is to combine with protein and copper in making *hemoglobin*. Hemoglobin transports oxygen in the blood from the lungs to the tissues. Iron is also necessary for the formation of *myoglobin*, which is found in the muscle tissue. Myoglobin supplies oxygen to the muscle cells to enable the muscles to contract.

The balance of calcium, iron, and phosphorus is important. Excess phosphorus hinders iron absorption. In addition, the lack of hydrochloric acid, the taking of alkalis, and a high intake of coffee and tea all interfere with iron absorption.[21] Protein promotes iron absorption since certain amino acids tend to chelate the iron and help carry it into the system. The absorption of chelated forms of iron is greater than that of the free ionic form. Chelated iron supplements have, therefore, been used in treating iron-deficient anemia.[22] Iron is also more efficiently absorbed from animal products than from vegetable foods.[23] However, it is becoming a common mineral deficiency in plants due to worn-out soils. Plants which are iron deficient have bleached-out yellowish leaves.[24]

In addition to iron, copper is also necessary for building blood, as is manganese and adequate levels of protein, calcium, vitamin E, vitamin C, and several of the B vitamins, particularly B-12 and B-6.

The most common deficiency of iron is iron-deficient anemia in which the amount of hemoglobin in the red blood cells is reduced and the cells become smaller. Symptoms of anemia are fatigue, pale skin, difficulty breathing, and decreased resistance to disease.

Foods high in iron include organ meats, beef, lamb, fish, sea vegetables (especially dulse), wheat grass juice, blackstrap molasses, eggs, beets, red cabbage and other dark red vegetables such as red chard, cherries, black mission figs, prunes, and green leafy vegetables. Herbs such as nettle leaf, yellow dock, and burdock root are especially high in iron. These can be made into teas.

ZINC

Zinc is found in the body in larger amounts than any other trace mineral except iron. Zinc is essential for the growth and development of the reproductive organs and for normal functioning of the prostate gland. It is important for nourishing the immune system and in preventing colds, flus, and other diseases. Zinc is found in high concentrations in the prostate gland and semen, and zinc supplements have been used to treat prostate problems as well as retarded development of the genital organs.[25] It is beneficial in healing wounds and burns since it is involved in certain enzymes which produce new cells and form keratin, a substance present in hair and nails as well as the skin.[26] It has also become an effective treatment for acne. Veterinarians found that animals whose feed contained inadequate amounts of zinc developed red and cracked skin with loss of hair or wool.[27] Zinc helps eliminate cholesterol deposits and has been used successfully in the treatment of atherosclerosis.[28] It has also been utilized in treating cirrhosis of the liver and alcoholism. For diabetics, it regulates the effect of insulin in the blood. It has also been administered to those suffering from Hodgkin's disease and leukemia.[29]

Phytic acid present in bran can tie up zinc and interfere with its absorption, carrying it through the intestinal tract in a way similar to what occurs with calcium. Fermenting bread with yeast to make it rise increases the availability of zinc by providing enzymes that destroy some of the phytic acid.[30] Zinc also has an important relationship to cadmium, a toxic mineral which is heavier than zinc that tends to replace it. The presence of a small amount of cadmium in food increases the need for adequate zinc.[31]

Signs of zinc deficiency are stretch marks on the skin and white spots on the fingernails. Other symptoms are abnormal fatigue, poor appetite, a loss of taste sensitivity, and retarded growth. Zinc deficiency makes one more susceptible to infection and to prolonged healing of wounds.

Recent studies show that a prolonged zinc deficiency causes sterility and dwarfism in humans. It leads to changes in the size and structure of the prostate gland. Low zinc levels in the blood were found in those suffering from alcoholism, cirrhosis, liver diseases, ulcers, diabetes, heart attacks, mongolism, and cystic fibrosis. Women taking oral contraceptives also had low levels of zinc in their blood.[32]

Foods high in zinc include oysters, pumpkin seeds, sea vegetables, and fish.

IODINE

Iodine is one of the most important trace minerals since it is essential in the functioning of the thyroid gland and is an integral part of thyroxin, the principal hormone produced by the thyroid gland. Iodine helps regulate energy production, promotes growth and development, and stimulates the rate of metabolism, helping the body to burn excess fat. When thyroxin production is normal, the synthesis of cholesterol is stimulated, carotene is converted to vitamin A, and the absorption of carbohydrates from the intestine work more efficiently.

Care should be taken in prescribing iodine as a drug because an overdose can become serious. Large doses of iodine may impair the synthesis of thyroid hormones.

An iodine deficiency can result in goiter characterized by thyroid enlargement or hypothyroidism (low rate of secretion of thyroid hormones). Such a deficiency may also lead to hardening of the arteries, obesity, sluggish metabolism, slow mental reaction, rapid pulse, and heart palpitation. A severe iodine deficiency may result in cretinism (a congenital condition characterized by physical and mental retardation in children born to mothers who have had low iodine intake).[33] Iodine therapy has been used successfully in treating goiter, children suffering from cretinism, and arteriosclerosis. Enough dietary iodine will also reduce the danger of radioactive iodine collecting in the thyroid gland.[34]

Iodine is found in all sea vegetables, particularly dulse, fish and seafood, and mushrooms, especially if the soil they are grown in is rich in iodine.

COPPER

Copper assists in the formation of hemoglobin and red blood cells by facilitating iron absorption. It is required for the synthesis of phospholipids and helps the body to oxidize vitamin C, working with it in the formation of elastin.

Copper and zinc have an inverse relation to each other. When copper levels are high, zinc levels are low. In schizophrenic patients, a substance called *cryptopyrole* has been found in the urine. This combines with zinc and pulls it out of the body, permitting the elevation of copper levels. Zinc, therefore, is helpful to schizophrenics in producing an anti-anxiety effect.[35]

Too much copper tends to produce epileptic-type seizures. Copper levels are usually elevated in women before their menstrual cycle begins, especially if they have used birth-control pills.[36] Too little copper may predispose to cardiovascular disease. In experimental animals, deficiencies of copper produced disease of the heart and blood vessels similar to strokes and heart attacks.[37] Deficiencies have also produced iron-deficient anemia and edema in children.

Foods high in copper include liver, sea vegetables, fish, and some green leafy vegetables.

MANGANESE

Manganese is a trace mineral which is extremely important in nourishing the brain and the nervous system. It also aids in the use of choline and activates enzymes that are necessary in utilizing biotin, thiamine, and ascorbic acid.[38] It is related to the connective tissue which provides the framework for the bones. In experimental animals, manganese deficiencies produced bone deformities which were not due to a lack of calcium but to a failure of the bone to stretch out to its normal length and shape.[39]

Manganese is beneficial in the treatment of diabetics; several diabetics who were unresponsive to insulin were able to control their symptoms by drinking alfalfa tea, which contains large amounts of manganese.[40]

Manganese has been helpful in treating schizophrenia, Parkinson's disease, and myasthenia gravis (failure of muscular coordination and loss of muscle strength).[41] Patients with a tendency to extreme allergies respond well to manganese supplements. In schizophrenic patients, manganese helps to restore balance when histamine, the substance that is released during allergic reactions, is either too high or too low in the blood.[42]

High calcium and phosphorus intake increase the need for manganese. Industrial workers exposed to manganese dust sometimes absorb enough of the metal in the respiratory tract to develop toxic symptoms. Motor difficulties and psychological imbalance are a result of manganese toxicity.[43]

A deficiency of manganese can affect glucose tolerance, resulting in the inability to remove excess sugar from the blood by oxidation or storage.[44] Ataxia, the failure of muscular coordination, has been linked with an inadequate intake of manganese. Deficiencies may also lead to paralysis and concussions in infants and dizziness, ear noises, and loss of hearing in adults.[45]

Manganese is found in high amounts in blueberries, boysenberries, and other dark blue berries such as olallie berries, alfalfa tea, and alfalfa sprouts. It is also found in whole grains and leafy green vegetables.

CHROMIUM

Chromium, an essential trace mineral, is important in producing an enzyme-like substance called *GTF*, or Glucose Tolerance Factor. This substance is necessary in proper production and utilization of insulin. When deficient, elevated blood sugar levels may exist, creating the condition known as *diabetes mellitus*. Experimental animals given a diet free of chromium developed all the symptoms of diabetes with sugar in their urine.[46] When chromium was replaced, the symptoms cleared up. Animals placed on chromium-free diets also developed arteriosclerosis with plaques in the arteries.[47]

Americans seem to be deficient in chromium as compared with other nationalities. This may relate to chromium deficiencies in the soil and a large percentage of lead poisoning, which depletes the chromium as well as the use of refined carbohydrates.[48]

Deficiencies of chromium may upset the functions of insulin and result in depressed growth rates and glucose intolerance in diabetics. Chromium and insulin may also be related to amino acid metabolism. Chromium may inhibit the formation of aortic plaque, and a deficiency could contribute to atherosclerosis.[49]

Chromium is found primarily in yeast and is also in whole grains.

SELENIUM

Selenium is a trace mineral that works closely with vitamin E in its metabolic actions and in the promotion of normal body growth and fertility. Selenium supplements have been helpful to women during menopause and at other time periods when they are undergoing hormonal change. As a natural antioxidant, selenium helps preserve the elasticity of tissues by delaying the oxidation of polyunsaturated fatty acids.[50]

Demonstrations with mice showed that selenium increased resistance to disease by increasing the number of antibodies that neutralize toxins. In the *Archives of Environmental Health* (Sept.-Oct. 1976), it was reported that areas with soil levels high in selenium reported lower male cancer death rates.[51] A deficiency of selenium may lead to hormonal imbalances and premature aging.

High natural sources of selenium are green leafy vegetables such as kale, Swiss chard, mustard greens, turnip greens, dandelion greens, chicory, cabbage, broccoli, and asparagus. Rice polishings and the bran and germ of whole grains also contain this mineral.

SULFUR

Sulfur makes up 25 per cent of body weight. It has an important relationship with protein as it is contained in the amino acids methionine, cystine, and cysteine and is necessary for collagen synthesis. It is found in keratin, a protein substance necessary for the maintenance of skin, hair, and nails.[52]

Sulfur works with thiamine, pantothenic acid, biotin, and

lipoic acid, all of which are necessary for metabolism and strong nerve health. It is important in tissue respiration where oxygen and other substances are used to build cells and release energy. Sulfur is helpful in treating arthritis; the level of cystine, a sulfur-containing amino acid, in arthritic patients is lower than normal. It is also used topically in the form of an ointment in treating skin disorders. There are no known deficiency effects from a lack of sulfur.

Sulfur is found in large amounts in certain vegetables, such as cabbage, broccoli, Brussels sprouts and cauliflower, eggs, fish, and meat.

PHOSPHORUS

Phosphorus is the second most abundant mineral in the body. It works along with calcium in maintaining the proper calcium/ phosphorus balance in the body. Phosphorus plays a part in almost every chemical reaction in the body since it is present in every cell. It helps in the utilization of carbohydrates, fats, and protein for the repair of cells and production of energy. It stimulates muscle contractions, including the contraction of the heart muscle. Phosphorus is an essential part of nucleoproteins, which are responsible for cell division and reproduction and transference of hereditary traits. It is also necessary for proper skeletal growth, tooth development, and kidney functioning.

Phosphorus speeds up the healing process in bone fractures and has reduced the loss of calcium; it has been used successfully in the treatment of osteomalacia and osteoporosis. It is helpful in treating arthritic conditions and disorders of the teeth and gums.

An insufficient amount of phosphorus may result in stunted growth, poor quality of bones and teeth, and other bone disorders. A deficiency in the calcium/phosphorus balance can cause diseases such as arthritis, pyorrhea, rickets, and tooth decay. Phosphorus absorption depends on the presence of vitamin D and calcium. Absorption can be interfered with by excessive amounts of iron, magnesium, and aluminum, which tend to form insoluble phosphates.[53] The use of refined sugar also disturbs the calcium/phosphorus balance.

Phosphorus is found in whole grains, seeds, nuts, eggs, fish, poultry, and meat.

CHLORINE

Chlorine is an essential mineral occurring in compound form with sodium or potassium. Chlorine helps regulate the acid/alkaline balance in the blood, stimulates production of hydrochloride, an enzyme needed in the stomach for digestion, and stimulates the liver to function as a filter for wastes. It is sometimes added to water for purification purposes because it destroys water-borne diseases such as typhoid and hepatitis. There has been much controversy over adding chlorine to drinking water because it is a reactive chemical and may join with inorganic minerals and other chemicals to form harmful substances. It destroys vitamin E and many of the intestinal flora that help in the digestion of food.[54]

A deficiency of chlorine can cause hair and tooth loss, poor muscular contraction, and impaired digestion. Chlorine is found in sea vegetables such as dulse, wakame, kelp, arame, and hijiki.

COBALT

Cobalt is an essential mineral which is an integral part of vitamin B-12, or cobalamin. Cobalt is necessary for the functioning and maintenance of red blood cells as well as other body cells. It also activates a number of enzymes in the body.

A deficiency may cause symptoms of pernicious anemia and a slow rate of growth. It may also lead to nervous disorders.[55] The body does not have the ability to synthesize cobalt so must depend on outside sources for obtaining it.

The best food sources of cobalt are liver and organ meats, seafood and sea vegetables. Cobalt is lacking in almost all land foods.

FLUORINE

Fluorine is an essential trace mineral found primarily in the skeleton and teeth. Fluorine occurs in the body in compounds called *fluorides*. There are two types of fluorides—sodium fluoride, which is added to drinking water, and calcium fluoride, which is found in nature.

Fluorine increases calcium deposits and, therefore, strengthens the bones. It helps reduce the formation of acid in the mouth caused by carbohydrates through reducing tooth decay.[56]

Traces of fluorine are beneficial to the body, but excessive amounts can be harmful. Fluorine can destroy the enzyme phosphatase, which is important to many body processes, including the metabolism of vitamins. High levels of fluorine can also depress growth, cause calcification of the ligaments and tendons, and bring about degenerative changes in the kidneys, liver, adrenal glands, heart, central nervous system, and reproductive organs.[57] Calcium is an antidote for fluorine poisoning.

Toxic levels occur in water when the content exceeds two parts per million.[58] In areas where the fluorine levels are high, tooth mottling (enamel discoloration) is epidemic; where fluorine is not added to the water, dental decay is higher.[59]

Fluorine is found in sea vegetables and seafood. The fluorine in plant food varies according to environmental conditions; for example, the type of soil used.

MOLYBDENUM

Molybdenum is an essential part of two enzymes—xanthine oxidase, which aids in the mobilization of iron from the liver, and aldehyde oxidase, which is necessary for the oxidation of fats.

Molybdenum is absorbed from the gastrointestinal tract. It may play a role in the prevention of anemia. There's no known deficiency effect. High intake can result in copper deficiency, and toxic symptoms include diarrhea and depressed growth rate.[60]

Molybdenum is found in dark green leafy vegetables, but the amount varies with the soil content.

TOXIC MINERALS

LEAD

Lead is a highly toxic trace mineral. Lead may enter the body via inhalation through the skin and the gastrointestinal tract. The lead that is absorbed enters the blood and is stored in the bones and soft tissues, including the liver. Sources of lead poisoning include drinking water, food from lead-lined containers, lead-based paint, lead in water pipes, cosmetics, cigarette smoking, and motor vehicle exhausts. Thirty to fifty per cent of the lead in inhaled air is absorbed into the body.

Lead poisoning attacks the central nervous system and can cause hyperactivity, irritability, fearfulness, crying, and listlessness in children. Acute lead toxicity is also manifested in abdominal colic, encephalopathy (dysfunction of the brain), myelopathy (any pathological condition of the spinal cord) and anemia.

The most effective way to prevent lead poisoning is to include a small amount of algin in the diet. Algin is a non-nutritive substance found in kelp which is used in the preparation of food. It attaches itself to any lead that is present and carries it out of the system.

Treatment for lead poisoning includes the use of chelation therapy, where a chelating agent (a large molecule that locks around the mineral and holds it) is put into the body carrying a calcium ion. The lead displaces the calcium and both are excreted in the urine. Injections of calcium chloride solution and administration of vitamin D help prevent lead from being leached out of the bones into the circulatory system.

ALUMINUM

Aluminum is a toxic trace mineral which can be dangerous if excess amounts are found in the body. Aluminum weakens the tissue of the alimentary canal, the digestive tube from the mouth to the anus. Many of its harmful effects result from its destruction of vitamins. Foods cooked in aluminum utensils may absorb small quantities of the mineral; it is also an ingredient in some baking powders and white flour.

Symptoms of aluminum poisoning include constipation, colic, loss of appetite, nausea, skin ailments, excessive perspiration, and loss of energy. There may be motor paralysis and areas of numbness with fatty degeneration of the kidney and liver.

CADMIUM

Cadmium is a toxic trace mineral with many structural similarities to zinc. Its toxic effects are kept under control in the body by the presence of zinc. Refining processes disturb the cadmium/zinc balance. Cadmium is found primarily in refined foods such as flour, rice, and white sugar. Coffee and tea also contain high amounts of cadmium. It is present in the air as an industrial contaminant, and soft water usually contains higher levels of cadmium than hard water.

Cadmium seems to be related to high blood pressure and hypertension. High blood pressure was produced in rats by putting cadmium in their drinking water. Treatment with a chelating agent to remove the cadmium reversed the high blood pressure. In humans, the urine of hypertensive patients contains up to 40 per cent more cadmium than does the urine of healthy persons. A correlation was also found between the cadmium content and the air in different parts of North America and the incidence of death from high blood pressure and other cardiovascular disease. Emphysema also seems to be related to the high cadmium inhaled by cigarette smokers.

Cadmium is associated with testicular tissue, perhaps because it replaces zinc. Industrial workers exposed to cadmium often were found to have cancer of the prostate. An injection of cadmium produced hemorrhage and destruction in rat testes as well.

Zinc and selenium can help prevent cadmium toxicity. Selenium is important because of its antioxidant effects along with vitamin E. However, selenium supplements should be taken with care as too much selenium can be toxic.

MERCURY

Mercury is another toxic mineral which has no function in the human body. Fish from certain inland waters are known to be polluted by toxic mercury dumping. Mercury's damage to the body consists of being exposed to certain compounds rather than organic forms Methyl mercury and ethyl mercury are two highly toxic forms. Methyl mercury is found in pesticides, fungicides, in the chemical by-products of chlorine, and in a form of mercury vapor from smokestacks. These are retained in the body for long periods and can affect the central nervous system. Symptoms of mercury poisoning may be diarrhea or neurological symptoms such as Parkinsonian tremors, vertigo, irritability and depression.

Cleansing the body regularly through colonics for the digestive tract and saunas for the skin helps remove toxic minerals. In addition, a balanced natural-foods diet with sufficient amounts of trace minerals (especially zinc), vitamin C, bioflavonoids, and vitamin E are important. An RNA/DNA tablet is also helpful.

NOTES

1. John D. Kirschmann, *Nutrition Almanac* (New York: McGraw-Hill, 1979), p. 12.
2. Ibid., p. 163.
3. Ibid.
4. Ibid., p. 164.
5. Rudolph Ballantine, M.D., *Diet and Nutrition—A Holistic Approach.* (Honesdale, PA: Himalayan International Institute, 1978), p. 228.
6. Ballantine, p. 226.
7. Kirschmann, p. 73.
8. Ibid., p. 74.
9. Ibid.
10. Ibid.
11. Ibid.
12. Ibid.
13. Ibid.
14. Ibid.
15. Ibid., p. 78.
16. Ibid., p. 79.
17. Ballantine, p. 261.
18. Kirschmann, p. 79.
19. Ibid., p. 82.
20. Ibid.
21. Ibid., p. 71.
22. Ballantine, p. 251.
23. Ibid.
24. Ibid., p. 256.
25. Ibid., p. 248.
26. Ibid., p. 247.
27. Ibid.
28. Kirschmann, p. 84.
29. Ibid.
30. Ballantine, p. 251.
31. Ibid.
32. Kirschmann, p. 54.
33. Ibid., p. 70.
34. Ibid.

35. Ballantine, p. 243.
36. Ibid., p. 246.
37. Ibid.
38. Kirschmann, p. 75.
39. Ballantine, p. 241.
40. Ibid., p. 240.
41. Kirschmann, p. 76.
42. Ballantine, p. 42.
43. Kirschmann, p. 95.
44. Ibid., p. 76.
45. Ibid.
46. Ballantine, p. 238.
47. Ibid.
48. Ibid.
49. Kirschmann, p. 67.
50. *Complete Book of Minerals for Health* (Emmaus, PA: Rodale Press, Inc., 1981), p. 235.
51. Kirschmann, p. 80.
52. Ibid., p. 82.
53. Ibid.
54. Ibid., p. 66.
55. *Complete Book of Minerals for Health*, p. 187.
56. Kirschmann, p. 68.
57. Ibid., p. 69.
58. Ibid.
59. Ibid.
60. Ibid., p. 77.

HERBOLOGY

The simplest and most natural form of medicine is herbal medicine. From earliest times we have been surrounded with plants, and by observing where these plants grow and experimenting with the different parts of them—the flowers, roots, leaves—we have been able to heal ourselves of many conditions.

Utilizing plant medicine is such a strong form of healing because it connects us with our environment, with Gaia, with the living Earth. Plants were placed in our environment so that we might *relate* to them; this relationship includes touching, smelling, and utilizing them for their medicinal properties in teas, tinctures, poultices, salves, etc. Plants are our healers and our teachers; by observing them and ingesting them when appropriate, we may become attuned to many spiritual and metaphysical truths.

Herbs can be used both internally in the form of teas, tinctures and capsules and externally as salves, ointments, and poultices. The first pharmacies made their medicines exclusively from herbs. Many of these are still around as cough syrups and cough drops from horehound and wild cherry bark and liniments from wintergreen and eucalyptus. Many medications used in treating serious disease conditions also derive from herbs; an example would be digitalis, used for heart conditions, which comes from the herb foxglove.

Internally, herbs are used in three major ways: to *eliminate toxins* from the body and cleanse it (this would include "blood purifiers," diuretics, and laxatives) to *build* or *maintain* the body (herbs that enable the body to heal itself); and to *tone* the body (herbs that tone the organs).[1] Certain herbs have a toning effect on specific organs or systems in the body. Dandelion root tones the liver and pancreas; comfrey root, the lungs and large intestine.

Herbs have many properties which combine to make them strong medicines. First is their *smell* or scent—the aroma of an herb can produce an effect before it is even ingested. The smell of peppermint, for example, begins to soothe and stimulate the digestive tract before the tea is drunk. *Aromatherapy* is a branch of herbology where the herbs are used specifically for their scents. The *taste* of herbs is another factor: sour tastes work on detoxifying; salty tastes influence the water balance; sweet tastes are nutritive; bitter tastes fight inflammation and cleanse the liver; pungent tastes open the respiratory tract and skin.

There are a number of herbal therapies that are used to treat different types of disease. In the course of a disease, several of these therapies might be appropriate, depending on the energy level of the individual and the changes occurring in her/his body at that time.

DETOXIFYING OR CLEANSING

Detoxifying includes sweating, vomiting, and purging. *Sweating* is used to treat diseases such as cold, flu, and fevers. Stimulating diaphoretic (herbs used to induce sweating) teas provide heat and increase circulation; they treat weaknesses in the internal organs. (Stomach and bowels should be emptied before ingesting through fasting, an enema, or a colonic irrigation.) Teas made from ginger, cayenne, Chinese cinnamon (cassia bark), and peppermint fall in this category. Relaxing diaphoretic teas such as catnip, spearmint, skullcap, or lemon balm treat ailments where the pores of the skin are closed and the energy has retreated from the surface. In addition, a hot bath or sauna should be taken after which one covers up with warm blankets to promote sweating.

Emetic herbs induce *vomiting* and are used after eating poor combinations of foods or to alleviate food poisoning. Ipecac is an herbal syrup which is a useful emetic. Other herbs may also be used, but caution should be exercised in using emetics since overuse tends to weaken the individual and deplete the vitality.

Purging through herbal laxatives may be helpful in treating excess toxins or constipation. One should be extremely careful, however, in using herbal laxatives as they often force food through the intestinal canal too quickly. They also deplete energy. Dietary changes and the addition of mucilaginous foods and herbs should be used to improve elimination. Colonic irrigations and enemas help cleansing and detoxifying.

Mild herbs like slippery elm, marshmallow root and comfrey are soothing to the intestinal mucus and may be readily used. Aloe vera juice may also be utilized; it is beneficial to the mucous linings and helps to cleanse the colon. Ground psyllium seed, flaxseed, and chia seed may be added to grains or other foods. These are bulk laxatives which increase bulk in the intestinal tract, thus aiding peristalsis. Other herbs stimulate bile secretions which also have a laxative effect. Herbs in this category include Oregon grape root, wild yam, and rhubarb.

BLOOD PURIFYING

Most diseases can be eliminated through "purifying the blood" and neutralizing excess acidity in the body. The concept of "blood purifying" is an old one in Western folk medicine; it is not a scientific concept. The idea is that the system can become toxic, poisoned, stagnant, and inflamed. When the blood stream is "toxic," it indicates that the lymphatics are stagnant, being glutted with waste materials; the liver is not able to detoxify substances entering the organism from the intestinal blood supply, which is rich with food and toxic wastes; the kidneys are not able to remove uric acid (wastes) from the blood. This stagnation and intoxification results in local tissue irritation, redness, burning, swelling, and skin rashes. Herbs that work on the liver, lymphatics and kidneys are called "blood purifiers" or alteratives.

Some "blood purifiers" include echinacea root, chaparral, red clover, sarsaparilla root, sassafras, cleavers, nettles, burdock root, yellow dock root, and golden seal.

TRANQUILLIZING

Tranquillizing herbs are used when there are conditions of restlessness, nervousness, or spasm accompanying illness. There are three types of tranquillizers: demulcents, nervines, and anti-spasmodics.[2]

Demulcents lubricate the gastrointestinal tract and other mucous linings of our bodies. Herbs such as slippery elm, comfrey root and leaf, and marshmallow root are mucilaginous and serve to lubricate bones and joints as well. *Nervines* or nerve tonics help to balance out the nervous system. These include chamomile, catnip, skullcap, wood betony, hops, spearmint, vervain, and valerian. *Anti-spasmodics* relax tension in muscles; they also help to relieve pain due to tension. Herbal anti-spasmodics include lobelia, hops, vervain, and valerian.

STIMULATING

Herbal stimulants add to the vitality of the various organs by increasing metabolism, circulation, and the breaking up of obstructions in the body.[3] Disease often results through blockages in the blood, lymph system, and digestive tract. When there is decreased vitality, chills, sluggishness, weak digestion, lower back pain, and the beginning of conditions such as colds and flus, stimulation therapy is helpful. Stimulants may be used alone or added to other herbs to increase their activity and help promote circulation and detoxification. For poor digestion, some of the culinary herbs are mild stimulants. These include cardamom, cloves, cumin, coriander, and cayenne. Ginger is another good stimulant and is often used as a tea, in cooking, or as a compress externally.

TONING

Toning or tonification therapy is used to strengthen blood, various organs, and the vitality of the body. It is used after acute diseases, during chronic disease to build the energy for detoxification, and as a recovery facilitator from injuries, childbirth, and surgeries.[4]

After acute diseases, foods such as vegetable juices and broths and other foods high in minerals and vitamins should be used (seaweeds, wheat grass juice, and sprouts). Mild herbal tonics, such as comfrey, nettles, alfalfa, plantain, chickweed, and watercress, may be used in salads or as teas. Later, stronger tonics such as comfrey root, dandelion root, burdock root, or ginseng may be utilized.

Vulnerary herbs promote healing of wounds, cuts and broken bones. These herbs include calendula flowers, marshmallow root, comfrey root and leaf, and aloe vera. They are often added to formulas.

Blood tonics are prescribed for people with anemia and menstrual disorders, and after chronic disease and fatigue. Red clover, sassafras, yellow dock, and parsley are good tonics for the blood.

Everyone has individual organs that need constant attention and toning. This may result from diseased conditions or may simply be congenitally weak areas in our bodies. The following list gives herbs for toning the various organs.

Heart
hawthorn berries
motherwort
borage

Liver
dandelion root
Oregon grape root
mandrake root

Gall Bladder
wild yam
Oregon grape root

Stomach
peppermint
agrimony
wormwood

Spleen
barberry bark
parsley
elecampane

Nerves
catnip
skullcap
hops
lady's slipper
vervain
valerian

Kidney
parsley
prince's pine (pipsissewa)
alfalfa

Colon
comfrey root and leaf
slippery elm

Lungs
mullein
coltsfoot
comfrey
marshmallow root
yerba santa

Pancreas
dandelion root
Jerusalem artichokes
string bean broth

Female Reproductive System
red raspberry leaf
blessed thistle
dong quai
squawvine

Male Reproductive System
ginseng
fo-ti
blessed thistle

THERAPEUTIC CONSTITUENTS OF HERBS

What makes some plants herbs or medicinal plants? Plants contain "active constituents" or chemicals which are recognized by the scientific community to have a known effect on humans and animals. All plants have some or all of these constituents in varying amounts.[5]

1. *CARBOHYDRATES*—includes sugars and starches.
   a. Mucilage—These are slimy, gelatinous materials that are soothing to mucous membranes and skin. They are contained in agar, psyllium seeds, flaxseeds, aloe vera, mullein, coltsfoot, slippery elm, marshmallow root, angelica root and others.
   b. Gums—sticky substances used for many cosmetic preparations because they are soothing and soft.

2. *GLYCOSIDES*—They are made of sugar and a non-sugar compound; they have very pronounced physiological effects on the physical body.
   a. Cardiac glycosides—These have a powerful action on the heart muscle. Foxglove (from which we get the drug digitalis) contains digitoxin, digoxin, digitonin and other glycosides; lily of the valley contains convallatoxin and others. Foxglove has toxic effects, so lily of the valley is preferred.
   b. Anthraquinone glycosides—These have a laxative effect because they stimulate the smooth muscle in the large intestine. Cascara contains barbaloin and chrysaloin; aloe contains barbaloin; rhubarb bark contains emodin; senna contains emodin.
   c. Thiocyanate glycosides—These have an irritating and emetic effect and are found principally in the mustard family. White mustard contains sinalbin; black mustard contains sinigrin.
   d. Phenolic glycosides—These produce a disinfectant, astringent and diuretic action. Uva ursi contains arbutin; iris contains iridin; chimaphila contains arbutin.
   e. Flavonol glycosides—These are circulatory and cardiac stimulants; they are also anti-spasmodic and diuretic. Some, like rutin, hesperidin, and citrin, reduce the fragility of the capillaries and help the body to strengthen the circulatory system and lower blood pressure.[6] These are found in buckwheat. Flavonoids are

also essential to the absorption of vitamin C.

f. Alcohol glycosides—The most important in this group is salicin, found in willow and poplar bark. It oxidizes to salicylic acid in the body, which is what aspirin is.

g. Aldehyde glycosides—They include salinigrin, contained in willow bark, vanillin in vanilla beans, and amygdalin, which is contained in cherry bark, the pits of many fruits, and in bitter almonds.

h. Lactone glycosides—Coumarin and its derivatives are the most important. Coumarin is found in tonka beans, sweet vernal grass, sweet clover and red clover. Coumarin derivatives of scopoletin are found in black haw and cramp bark.

i. Saponin glycosides—These form foaming solutions in water upon shaking. They are irritating to the mucous membranes and can destroy red blood cells. They have an expectorant effect on the body and can be destroyed by heat. Licorice root contains glycyrrhizin; wild yam contains botogenin and diosgenin; ginseng contains many of these glycosides.

j. Cyanophore glycosides—These yield hydrocyanic acid. Amygdalin or laetrile is in bitter almonds, the rose family, and sorghum.

3. *ALKALOIDS*—All alkaloids contain nitrogen. (Alkaloids end in *ine*, but often have prefixes to denote alkaloid from the same source as quinine, quinidine, and hydroquinine.) Lobelia contains 14 alkaloids, lobeline being the strongest. Poison hemlock contains coniine, a powerful poison. Black pepper has alkaloids, as do all of the nightshade vegetables (eggplants, tomatoes, potatoes). Coffee contains caffeine, which is also in cocoa, tea, and kola. Periwinkle is endowed with vincristine, which is being used to treat Hodgkin's disease and other cancers. Coca leaves contain cocaine, used as a local anaesthetic. Golden seal has three alkaloids—hydrastine, berberine, and canadine. Hydrastine acts as an astringent to the mucous membranes. Oregon grape root contains berberine and ocycanthine; berberine also manifests as an astringent on the mucous membranes. Belladonna (nightshade family) contains atropine; it is used prior to surgery to inhibit secretions and relax muscles.

4. *TANNINS*—All plant families are thought to contain tannins,

which can be found in any part of the plant. They precipitate proteins and then combine with them to resist enzyme action. They protect abrased tissue while new tissue forms and are also antiseptic. They are useful for ulcers, diarrhea, bleeding (to constrict capillaries), burns, and wounds. Tannins are powerful astringents. Plants high in tannins include oak bark, rose leaves, uva ursi, peppermint, and sage. Tannins are water soluble but are destroyed by excessive heat and exposure to air.

5. *BITTER PRINCIPLES*—These are not one chemical group but of varied composition. The bitter principles have been shown to have valuable therapeutic effects. Through reflex action via the taste buds, they stimulate the secretion of all the digestive juices, thus stimulating the action of the liver, aiding hepatic elimination. Research is also being conducted on their antibiotic, antifungal, and anti-tumor actions.[7] Bitters can act as nervines as well. Some bitters are hops, gentian, dandelion, chicory, nux vomica, and buckbean.

6. *VOLATILE OILS*—This is the part that gives plants their odors. They are called volatile because they turn from a liquid to a gas quickly. Volatile oils are found in the glandular structure of one or more plant parts; they may attract pollinating insects to the plant. The various actions of volatile oils are:

Antiseptic—thyme, mints, pepper
Antibacterial—garlic, onions
Anthelmintic (expels worms from the digestive tract)—wormwood, wormseed, fennel
Anti-inflammatory—wintergreen, lavender, willow, poplar
Carminative (stimulates peristalsis and relaxes the stomach)—anise, caraway, spearmint, peppermint
Diuretic (increases elimination of urine)—juniper berries
Febrifuge (reduces fevers)—yarrow, chamomile, elder flowers, peppermint
Irritant (to increase circulation)—cayenne, eucalyptus, cinnamon, rosemary, tansy
Insect repellent—citronella, pennyroyal, peppermint

7. *RESINS AND BALSAMS*—Resins are hard, transparent, melt-

able substances, insoluble in water and of a complex chemical nature. They are used in varnishes, inks, and sealing wax. Expectorants include yerba santa, white poplar buds, and asafetida. Cayenne and ginger are carminatives. Balsams are resinous mixtures containing benzoic acid. Benzoin is used as an expectorant, a stimulant, and a diuretic.

8. *STEROIDS*—Steroids are compounds widely distributed in plants: cholesterol in ferns, fungi, algae; hormones in wild yam, black cohosh.

HERBAL PREPARATIONS

TEAS

Herbs for medicinal use may be taken in various forms. The most common form is a tea. Teas include infusions and decoctions. In an *infusion*, 1 ounce of dried herb is steeped in 1 pint (2 cups) boiling water for about 10 minutes (1 teaspoon herb to 1 cup water). It can be steeped in a teapot, or the herb can be put in a tea ball. Leaves, stems, flowers, and berries are infused. Roots and barks are decocted. In a *decoction*, the herbs are simmered in water 15-20 minutes. About 1 teaspoon herb to 1 cup of water is used, but extra water should be added since some of it evaporates.

TINCTURES

A very common method of using herbs is in the form of tinctures. People often find tinctures more convenient to use over teas, though there is some objection to the idea that alcohol is necessary in making a tincture. The alcohol can be removed by placing the tincture in heated water; alcohol boils at a lower temperature than water.

GELATIN CAPSULES AND PILLS

When the herb has a bad taste, one often pulverizes it and puts the powdered form in gelatin capsules. This is done with golden seal powder. The disadvantage of using gelatin capsules is that they are difficult to assimilate. Vegetarians also do not like using them. Pills are more acceptable to many. Herbs do not have to be so finely powdered for pills. A small amount of slippery elm or other mucilaginous herb powder is used and mixed with water until a doughy consistency is reached. Gum arabic dissolved in water is also a good adhesive. The pills can then be dried in the oven at low heat or in the warm air.

SMOKING

For relief of respiratory conditions and bronchial infections, certain herbs are smoked. A small amount of herb is smoked in a pipe or water pipe. The lungs are filled with smoke, and then it's exhaled. For a single treatment, the smoke should be inhaled 6-10 times. Herbs used for this purpose are mullein, lobelia, yerba santa, and coltsfoot.

SYRUPS

Syrups are used for coughs and sore throats. Two ounces of herb are used per quart of water, and this is boiled down to 1 pint. After it is strained, honey or glycerine is used. Syrups may be given in doses of one to two teaspoons daily for several days. Herbs commonly made into syrups include wild cherry bark, licorice root, comfrey root, and small amounts of lobelia for calming.

SALVES

Salves are ointments that are applied to the skin which can be used for burns, cuts, and external injuries and wounds. The best way to make a salve is to extract the herbs in hot oil, starting with roots and barks (about 2 hours), adding leaves and flowers (1 more hour). Afterwards, melted wax is added, and then a small amount of gum benzoin or tincture of benzoin for preservation. Herbs used in salves are comfrey leaves, plantain, chickweed, St. John's wort, golden seal, and myrrh.

LINIMENTS

Liniments are herbal extracts rubbed into the skin for treating strained muscles and ligaments and for inflammatory conditions such as arthritis. Four ounces of dried herbs are placed in a bottle with 1 pint of vinegar, alcohol, or massage oil, and this is allowed to extract for three days. Liniments usually include stimulant herbs, such as cayenne, and oils of aromatic herbs, such as eucalyptus and wintergreen.

POULTICES AND PLASTERS

A poultice is a warm, moist application of powdered or macerated herbs that is applied to the skin to relieve inflammation and to promote cleansing of the affected area. Poultices can draw out infections as well as toxins and foreign bodies. Herbs used include comfrey, plantain, and marshmallow root. To relieve pain and muscle spasm, herbs such as lobelia, catnip, vervain, and valerian can be used.

In a plaster, the herbal materials are placed between two thin pieces of linen or are combined in a thick material and applied to the skin. An example would be a mustard plaster.

FOMENTATIONS OR COMPRESSES

A fomentation or compress is used to treat swellings, pain, cold, and flu. It can stimulate the circulation of the blood or lymph in the area of the body to which it is applied. Sometimes herbs that are too strong to be used internally can be used externally with the body absorbing a small amount.

A compress is prepared by making an herbal tea, dipping a towel or cloth into the tea, and applying it as hot as possible to the affected area. The towel can be covered with a dry flannel cloth or heating pad.

Ginger compresses are helpful in stimulating circulation in certain areas and reducing inflammation. Grate fresh ginger root and put in cheesecloth or a tea ball. Make a strong ginger root tea, and then dip a towel or cloth into this mixture and apply to the affected area. Ginger compresses on the colon are helpful in cases of constipation or blockage.

BOLUS

A bolus is a suppository consisting of powdered herbs added to cocoa butter until the mixture forms a firm consistency. It is then placed in the refrigerator to harden and warmed to room temperature before use. The bolus is rolled into strips about 3/4" thick and cut into segments 1" long. It is inserted into the rectum to treat cysts and into the vagina for infections. Herbs used in boluses include antibiotics, such as garlic, golden seal, or chaparral, and demulcents, such as comfrey root and slippery elm.

HARVESTING HERBS

In order for herbal medicines to be the most effective, herbs should be of high quality. The quality depends on where they are grown, when they are harvested, how they are dried and preserved, how they are stored, and the duration of storage.

Dried herbs bought in stores are generally a couple of years old unless they are harvested locally and brought right to the store. Many of them are imported from other countries and different areas of the United States. To obtain herbs as fresh as possible, one should harvest her/his own herbs (at least those that are available in the area). The time to harvest herbs is when they contain the highest amount of active constituents. This varies from place to place, depending on the growing season, the amount of sunlight and other factors.

Leaves are picked just before the plant is about to flower. At this time, the energy is focused in the upper portion of the plant. The best time of day to pick herbs is after the morning dew has dried, but before the hot Sun has evaporated away the essential oils. Flowers are picked before reaching full bloom. Berries and fruits may be obtained at peak ripeness when they are about to fall from the plant; this is usually late summer.

Barks and twigs of trees are collected in the spring when the sap rises and the leaves first appear. Roots are gathered in the fall when the sap returns to the ground and the berries or seeds are mature.

Several guidelines are important when collecting wild plants:

1. Don't harvest plants which are a protected, endangered, or rare species.

2. Be sure in your identification of the plant. Field guides with col-

ored photographs are helpful. If unsure, check with a local bota-
nist. (For example, the parsley-carrot family has edible and poisonous members which are often difficult to tell apart.)

3. Look for the "grandmother" plant (the largest one). Ask permission of that plant to harvest some of the surrounding plants. Tell
   the plant what you are picking it for. Don't pick tender, young
   plants. Only pick 1 out of 5 plants in an area so that they can
   repopulate.

4. Disturb the area as little as possible when picking. Cover any
   holes, and do not walk on plants.

5. Have clippers or scissors or other cutting tools for leaves and
   stems. Do not pick plants up by the roots unless you are going to
   use the whole root.

6. Collect plants that are far removed from roadsides where there is
   any automobile exhaust. Be aware of areas that may be chemically sprayed.

7. Dry plants immediately upon returning home.

DRYING AND PRESERVING

Plant tops are washed, allowed to dry, and then hung in a well-
ventilated, shaded area. The plant may be tied in bundles and hung
upside down so that the sap runs from the stems into the leaves.
They may also be spread out on a screen and turned each day. Roots
and barks are scrubbed and chopped before drying. The pieces
should not be more than an inch thick. They also may be dried on a
screen and turned daily. Depending on how warm the area is where
the herbs are drying, it takes from three to five days.

It is important to store herbs well since medicinal properties
are destroyed by heat, bright light, exposure to air, bacteria, and
fungi. They should be kept in a cool, dry place with minimum exposure to air and sunlight. After a few days, they should be checked to
be sure there is no mold or moisture in the jar.

Herbs should also be labeled with their name and date collected. After a year, they should be checked and restocked. When

they begin to lose their color and smell, they may be set aside for herbal baths. Herbs with aromatic oils lose potency first; barks, roots, and seeds maintain potency for a longer period.

Oils may last in the refrigerator or another cool place for several years. Salves and lotions may be preserved by adding a small amount of tincture of benzoin.

HERBAL MATERIA MEDICA

ALTERATIVES—also known as "blood cleansers"; cleanse the blood and the lymph and restore the body to its proper functioning.

1. *Echinacea*—It is antiseptic, antibiotic, and anti-toxic. Echinacea is a prime remedy against bacterial and viral attacks; it helps the body rid itself of microbal infections. It is used for infections of the respiratory tract, such as laryngitis and tonsillitis, and catarrhal conditions of the nose and sinuses. It's also beneficial for eczema from blood conditions as well as gastric and duodenal ulcers. As a tincture or decoction, it may be used for pyorrhea and gingivitis.

2. *Yellow dock*—This is used for chronic skin complaints like psoriasis. Yellow dock is also a mild laxative since it increases bile flow; its action on the gall bladder makes it a helpful herb in treating jaundice. It is high in iron and thus used to treat anemia. It combines well with dandelion, burdock, and cleavers. As a salve, it is good for skin diseases and swelling.

3. *Burdock root*—This root is excellent for skin conditions which result from dry and scaly skin, including eczema and psoriasis. Through its bitter principle, it stimulates digestive juices and bile secretion. It is used in the treatment of arthritis, rheumatism, lumbago, and sciatica. It is also used to promote kidney function and works through the kidneys to help clear the blood of harmful acids. Burdock seeds made into a tincture or extraction are good for skin and kidney diseases. Burdock can also be utilized as a fomentation for wounds, swellings, and hemorrhoids.

4. *Sarsaparilla root*—This is used in treating skin problems and is frequently combined with sassafras, yellow dock, and cleavers. Sarsaparilla root is also used to treat rheumatism, arthritis and gout. It contains hormone-like substances and thus is valuable in formulas for glandular balancing to alleviate menopause discomforts and

irregular menstruation.

ANTI-SPASMODICS—ease spasms or cramps in various parts of the body.

1. *Cramp bark*—Cramp bark is helpful in relieving muscle cramps and spasms and also in uterine muscle problems. Thus, it is a good herb for painful cramps associated with menstruation or threatened miscarriage. For uterine cramps, it is often used with black haw and valerian.
2. *Lady's slipper*—A widely used nervine and anti-spasmodic, lady's slipper is used for states of anxiety as well as pains in the nerves. It is a good tonic for exhausted nervous systems, improving circulation and nutrition to the nerves.
3. *Lobelia*—Lobelia is one of the strongest relaxants for the central and autonomic nervous systems. It is often used in combination with other herbs to further their effectiveness. Its particular use is in bronchial asthma where it is often combined with ephedra, cayenne, and grindelia.

ASTRINGENTS—contract tissue and can thus reduce secretions and discharges. Astringents contain tannins.

1. *Eyebright*—Eyebright is excellent for problems of mucous membranes. It is used for eye problems—in inflammatory conditions as well as for stinging and weeping eyes. It is drunk as a tea and also used in compresses. It is an anticatarrhal and may be used for nasal catarrh and sinusitis in combination with golden seal, goldenrod, or elder flowers. Eyebright also aids the liver in cleansing the blood.
2. *Barberry*—Barberry is a bitter tonic with mild laxative effects. It promotes the flow of bile and is indicated where there is inflammation of the gall bladder and where the liver is congested as in jaundice. It is also able to reduce an enlarged spleen.
3. *Golden seal*—One of the most useful of the medicinal plants, golden seal is a powerful toner for the mucous membranes. It is excellent for ulcers, colitis, and gastritis as well as catarrhal conditions of the upper respiratory tract. Externally, as a paste, it may be applied to eczema, poison ivy or oak, acne, ringworm, and other skin

infections. Internally, it may be drunk as a tea or taken powdered in capsules.

CARMINATIVES—stimulate peristalsis in the digestive system and relax the stomach. In doing this, they help to expel gas.

1. *Aniseed*—Aniseed is good for flatulence and intestinal colic. It is usually ground up and mixed with ground fennel seeds, caraway seeds, and dill seeds. Aniseed also works as an expectorant and anti-spasmodic; it is helpful for bronchitis and where there is coughing as in whooping cough. In these conditions, it is often mixed with coltsfoot, white horehound, and lobelia.

2. *Caraway*—Caraway is used for flatulence and intestinal colic; it stimulates the appetite and helps in the treatment of diarrhea. It is often used in combination with aniseed, fennel seed, and dill seed (ground up and made into a tea). Caraway is also used as an anti-spasmodic in bronchitis and bronchial asthma.

3. *Dill*—Dill is another herb also used for flatulence and intestinal colic, especially in children; it is combined with the two herbs listed above and with fennel. In addition, ground dill seeds stimulate the flow of milk in nursing mothers, as does caraway.

4. *Fennel*—This is excellent as a stomach and intestinal remedy to relieve flatulence while also stimulating the appetite and digestion. It has a similarity to aniseed in its calming action on bronchitis and coughs. It is also used to flavor cough remedies and increase the flow of milk in nursing mothers (ground up and made into a tea).

5. *Peppermint*—Peppermint is one of the best carminatives; it stimulates bile and digestive juices, thereby aiding conditions of flatulence, dyspepsia, and intestinal colic; it also helps ulcerative colitis and Crohn's disease. It allays feelings of nausea, especially during pregnancy, and is valuable in the treatment of fevers in colds and flus.

DEMULCENTS—contain mucilage and are soothing to irritated or inflamed internal tissue.

1. *Comfrey*—Comfrey root and leaf is one of the most useful

and versatile herbs. The presence of *allantoin* helps wounds to heal internally and externally. Comfrey is an excellent healing agent in gastric and duodenal ulcers and in ulcerative colitis and hiatus hernia. For these conditions, it is often combined with marshmallow root and meadowsweet. It also used for coughs and bronchitis where it soothes and reduces irritation; in these cases it is often combined with coltsfoot, elecampane, and white horehound. Comfrey is used externally in salves for skin irritations and infections and as a poultice.

2. *Irish moss*—This has a high amount of mucilage and is used for both gastritis and ulcers as a tea (the dried herb is infused). It is also used in the food industry to make jellies and aspic. Its main use, however, is in respiratory problems like bronchitis.

3. *Marshmallow*—Marshmallow root and leaf have a high mucilage content. The root is used for digestive problems and on the skin, while the leaf is used more for the lungs and urinary system. For inflammations of the digestive tract like gastritis, peptic ulcers and colitis, the root is used in combination with comfrey and sometimes slippery elm. For bronchitis and coughs, the leaf is often used with comfrey, licorice root, and white horehound.

4. *Slippery elm*—The bark of slippery elm is soothing and nutritive for inflamed mucous membranes in colitis, ulcers, and gastritis. The powdered bark is used as a nutritive food and may be mixed in juices and cereals. Externally, slippery elm is used as a poultice for boils and abscesses.

5. *Aloe*—The juice from the leaves of the aloe vera plant are helpful in digestive complaints since it soothes the lining of the intestine. It is also helpful for flatulence and constipation; drinking 1/4 or 1/3 cup of this juice will aid elimination. Externally, aloe gel is excellent for burns, sunburn, and insect bites.

DIAPHORETICS—promote sweating and aid the skin in the elimination of toxins.

1. *Cayenne*—Cayenne is one of the most versatile of the stimulating herbs. The powder can be used in soups or salads or in cooking, or it can be infused and drunk with water. For the circulatory system, it regulates blood flow and strengthens the heart and arteries. In the digestive system, it is used for flatulence, dyspepsia, and

colic. It is also a good source of vitamin P, one of the bioflavonoids which helps to assimilate vitamin C.

2. *Elder*—Elder has many uses; the bark, flowers, berries and leaves are utilized. The leaves, flowers, and berries are used for treatment of colds and flu as well as for inflammation of the upper respiratory tract like sinusitis. Elder is also a good diuretic. It may be combined with peppermint, yarrow, or hyssop for colds and flus, and with goldenrod for nasal catarrh.

3. *Garlic*—Garlic is the most universally used of the medicinal herbs. It is effective against bacteria, parasites, and viruses. It aids the immune system and is often used in combination with echinacea. In the digestive tract, it supports natural flora while killing pathogenic bacteria. It helps circulation and is used for colds and flus. Garlic can be eaten as cloves, cooked with food, or taken in capsules of garlic oil.

4. *Ginger*—Ginger is used in feverish conditions to promote perspiration. It is also used to stimulate circulation in cases of chilblains or cramps. As a carminative, it promotes gastric secretions and is used for dyspepsia, flatulence and colic. It is also helpful for motion sickness. Ginger root is simmered, often with other herbs, and used as a tea.

DIURETICS—increase the secretion and elimination of urine.

1. *Corn silk*—Corn silk is the fine soft threads from the flowering corn; it is best used fresh but may be dried. It is helpful in irritations of the urinary system. Combined with other herbs like couchgrass, bearberry, or yarrow, it treats cystitis, urethritis, and prostatitis.

2. *Cleavers*—Cleavers is one of the finest diuretics. It is used for all kidney and bladder problems, particularly for stones and gravel. It is also an excellent alterative as well as a toner for the lymphatic system (used for swollen glands, tonsillitis and adenoid problems). Cleavers is beneficial for skin conditions where it is often combined with yellow dock and burdock.

3. *Dandelion*—Dandelion root and leaves are used. It is an excellent diuretic because it is a natural source of potassium; therefore, it stimulates the kidney function without the loss of potassium. Dandelion root is also used as a *cholagogue* in inflammation and con-

gestion of the liver and gall bladder. It is the best tonic for the liver and may be used with barberry or balmony.

4. *Gravel root*—Gravel root is used primarily for kidney stones or gravel. It may be used in urinary infections like cystitis and urethritis as well as in the treatment of rheumatism or gout. It is often used with parsley piert or hydrangea for kidney stones or gravel.

5. *Juniper berries*—Juniper berries are an excellent antiseptic in conditions such as cystitis. They should be avoided in kidney disease as they are stimulating to the kidney nephrons. They may also be used in conditions of rheumatism or arthritis.

6. *Nettles*—Nettle leaves are one of the most useful herbs available. They are high in iron, potassium, silicon, and vitamin C. Nettles are used for anemia, as a "blood purifier," and for nosebleeds and other hemorrhage in the body. The tea is also an expectorant for the lungs in combination with comfrey, mullein and white horehound.

7. *Parsley*—Parsley has many usages; primarily, it is a diuretic, an *emmenagogue*, stimulating the menstrual cycle, and a *carminative* to ease flatulence. Parsley is a good source of vitamin C, potassium, and other nutrients.

NERVINES—tone and strengthen the nervous system. Some act as relaxants; some act as stimulants.

1. *Chamomile*—One of the most widely used herbs, chamomile is calming for restlessness, anxiety, nervous stomach, and insomnia. It is especially good for children who suffer from digestive upsets. It eases flatulence and dyspeptic pain and is also helpful in cases like gastritis. As an inhalant over a steam bath, it helps nasal catarrh.

2. *Hops*—Hops have a strong effect on the central nervous system and are, therefore, used in the treatment of insomnia, often combined with valerian and passion flower. Hops also have an effect on the liver and gall bladder and increase the flow of bile.

3. *Passion flower*—Passion flower treats insomnia and also is used as an anti-spasmodic in Parkinson's disease and seizures. It is effective in neuralgia and in shingles (infection of nerves).

4. *Scullcap*—Scullcap is one of the most widely used nervines. It is used in the treatment of nervous tension, seizures, epilepsy, and

hysteria. It has the quality of renewing the entire nervous system.

5. *St. John's wort*—St. John's wort is a very versatile plant. It has a sedative effect internally and thus is used for anxiety, restlessness, and irritability (particularly the irritability that often accompanies menopause). Externally, it is an anti-inflammatory for use in healing wounds and bruises, mild burns, and varicose veins.

6. *Valerian*—Valerian is one of the most effective relaxing nervines and is often used in orthodox medicine. It relieves tension and anxiety, is used for insomnia (often with hops and passion flower), and has an anti-spasmodic effect which is helpful in relieving cramps (including menstrual cramps) and intestinal colic.

7. *Vervain*—This herb is helpful in cases of depression and melancholy and is often mixed with scullcap, oats and lady's slipper for this. It is also used for seizures and hysteria in addition to acting as a *diaphoretic* in the early stages of fever.

STIMULANTS—quicken the physiological functions of the body.

1. *Cayenne*—see *DIAPHORETICS*
2. *Ginger*—see *DIAPHORETICS*
3. *Mustard*—Internally, mustard is used as a stimulant for colds, fevers, and flus. The mustard flour is infused as a tea and drunk. Externally, mustard stimulates the circulation to a particular area of the body, which relieves muscular and skeletal pain. A poultice of mustard will also help bronchitis.

TONERS—tone various organs or the whole body. There are specific tonic herbs for various body systems.

Circulatory System

1. *Hawthorn berries*—Hawthorn berries tone the heart and circulatory system, either stimulating or depressing the heart, depending on its need. They may be used for heart palpitations and also for treatment of high blood pressure, arteriosclerosis and recurrent chest pains.

2. *Motherwort*—Motherwort is a good tonic to strengthen the heart; it is used for rapid heartbeat as well as conditions associated with anxiety and tension. This herb is also useful in certain men-

strual conditions, such as delayed menstruation, and is a good tonic for menopausal changes.

Digestive System
1. *Comfrey root*—see DEMULCENTS
2. *Marshmallow root*—see DEMULCENTS
3. *Slippery elm*—see DEMULCENTS
4. *Agrimony*—Agrimony's combination of bitter and astringent properties make it a good toner for the digestive system since it can stimulate liver and digestive secretions. In cases of mucous colitis, diarrhea, and appendicitis, agrimony works well.
5. *Dandelion root*—see DIURETICS

Nervous System
1. *Chamomile*—see NERVINES
2. *Vervain*—see NERVINES
3. *Lady's slipper*—see ANTI-SPASMODICS
4 *Scullcap*—see NERVINES

Respiratory System
1. *Coltsfoot*—Coltsfoot is soothing to the mucous linings and has an expectorant and anti-spasmodic action as well. This makes it helpful in respiratory conditions, bronchitis, asthma and whooping cough. For coughs, it is often used with white horehound and mullein.
2. *Comfrey root and leaves*—see DEMULCENTS
3. *Elecampane*—Elecampane has an expectorant action, is soothing to the mucous linings, relaxing them, and is antibacterial. It may be used where there is catarrh formed as in bronchitis and emphysema. Its bitter quality also helps to stimulate digestion. It is often used in combination with coltsfoot, yarrow, and white horehound.

Reproductive System
1. *Black cohosh*—Black cohosh is an excellent herb for toning the female reproductive system. It balances the sex hormones and is used in cases of delayed menstruation, painful menstruation, and menopausal conditions. It is also a relaxing nervine utilized in the treatment of rheumatic as well as muscular and neurological pains.
2. *Ginseng*—Ginseng root comes from the Orient; it is a toner

for the male hormonal system and generally raises the vitality. It helps normalize blood pressure and reduces blood cholesterol. It also reduces blood sugar levels and is thus helpful in diabetes.

3. *Dong quai*—Dong quai is an herb from China that tones the female reproductive system. It is helpful for menstrual cramps, irregular menstruation, and menopause. It is also a good "blood purifier" and is used in treating anemia as well as circulatory problems.

4. *Raspberry*—These leaves create a wonderful tea for the female organs. Used throughout pregnancy, it eases cramps and pain in childbirth. It is also used for menstrual cramps and normalizing the menstrual cycle. Raspberry leaf is combined with other herbs like uva ursi and squawvine to treat vaginal discharge.

5. *Squawvine*—Squawvine was used by Native American women during pregnancy to assure proper development of the child and to help promote proper lactation. It is excellent for painful and irregular menstruation, relieving congestion in the ovaries and uterus. It is often combined with raspberry leaf. If the berries are crushed and added to a tincture of myrrh for a few days, it will provide a good fomentation for sore nipples.

Urinary System
1. *Gravel*—see DIURETICS
2. *Nettles*—see DIURETICS
3. *Parsley*—see DIURETICS

NOTES

1. Michael Tierra, *The Way of Herbs* (Berkeley, CA: Unity Press, 1980), p. 10.
2. Ibid., p. 14.
3. Ibid., p. 13.
4. Ibid., p. 17.
5. Cascade Anderson, "Therapeutic Constituents of Medicinal Plants."
6. David Hoffman, *The Holistic Herbal* (Dorset, England: Element Books, 1989), p. 132.
7. Ibid., p. 134.

HOMEOPATHY

In order to understand the basis of homeopathic medicine, we need to understand the workings of *vibrational medicine* (see chapter 19). The electromagnetic field of the body has been defined by the new Physics (see Fritjof Capra's *The Tao of Physics* [Bantam, 1977]) and photographed through the use of Kirlian photography. This electromagnetic field has been referred to as the "etheric body." There are channels of energy which flow from the physical to the etheric body. These are the meridians of the acupuncture system. Along these meridians are points where the vital force enters (called *chi* by the Chinese, *prana* by the Hindus).

According to George Vithoulkas, a contemporary practitioner of homeopathy and author of many books on the subject, the aspect of the vital force which establishes balance in states of disease is known as the "defense mechanism."[1] Samuel Hahnemann, the 19th-century German physician who developed the science of homeopathy, theorized that when disease occurs, the first disturbance occurs on the dynamic electromagnetic field of the body which then brings into play the "defense mechanism."[2] Hahnemann believed that a therapeutic agent could act directly upon the electrodynamic field and thereby strengthen the defense mechanism.

Hahnemann's search consisted of finding a substance whose frequency had a similar resonance to the individual's own and thus could affect the electromagnetic field. He sought substances that would produce similar symptoms.[3] He believed that any substance which could produce a totality of symptoms in a healthy human being could cure those symptoms in a sick human being. This cure had to affect all levels of being—the mental/spiritual, the emotional/psychic, and the physical.

The "law of similars" is basic to homeopathic practice; it is utilized in immunizations and vaccines against diseases like smallpox, diphtheria, and typhoid, as well as in allergy treatment where small doses of allergens are used to create an anti-body response. In the 4th century B.C., Hippocrates worked with the law of similars. He stated, "Through the like, disease is produced, and through the application of the like it is cured."[4]

The usage of micro-doses is also basic to homeopathy. Hahnemann believed that a person's inherent healing powers were strong enough so that only a small stimulus was needed to catalyze the healing process. After many years of experimentation, Hahnemann found a method of diluting substances that kept the toxic properties at a minimum. This method called *potentization* is a process of successive dilution. If the medicine is soluble, one part is diluted in 10 parts water or alcohol, and the mixture is mixed vigorously. If it is insoluble, it is finely ground or triturated in the same proportions with powdered lactose (milk sugar). One part of the diluted medicine is diluted again in the same manner, and the process is repeated until the desired strength is obtained. A remedy that has been diluted fewer times has a lower potency. It has been found that the more a substance is potentized, the deeper and longer it acts and the fewer number of doses are needed in treatment.

Potentization has stirred controversy among certain scientists who believe that if a substance is potentized to a very high dose, there will be little of the physical remedy left. Dana Ullman, however, reports in his book *Homeopathy: Medicine for the 21st Century* (North Atlantic Books, 1988) that evidence for the efficacy of small doses was given in *Science News*. A study engaged in by chemists noted that when they shook coupled molecules of nitric oxide the units did not weaken and break into parts, but developed stronger molecular buds. The homeopathic process of dilution and succussion (shaking) therefore created superstrong molecules.[5]

In prescribing a certain homeopathic medicine, a patient's symptoms are noted. Symptoms of most importance concern the patient's relationship to her/his environment, food, sleep, sex, and habit patterns rather than the clinical details of her/his physical symptoms. Hahnemann derived his system of remedies for specific symptoms through "provings." Provings is the systematic procedure of testing substances on healthy human beings in order to elucidate that the symptoms reflect the action of the substance. The remedy is tried on a healthy person in toxic as well as diluted doses. Symptoms on all three levels are noted, as well as those symptoms that have disappeared from the patient after a cure has been produced.[6]

Homeopathic remedies are catalogued in books known as *Materia Medicas*, which are compilations of these drug provings that associate certain symptom pictures as well as physical and emotional characteristics with various substances. There are also *Repertories* available—books which list certain symptoms and the remedies known to heal them. Most well-known of the *Repertories* is that of Dr. J. T. Kent (B. Jain Publishers, 1986), which has a word index including all parts of the body and all types of conditions that affect these parts.

After the administration of a homeopathic remedy, symptoms on the deeper levels improve while those on more external, superficial levels may temporarily get worse. The principles of the homeopathic healing process were first observed by Constantine Hering, a German homeopath who emigrated to the U.S. in the 1830s. These principles are known as *Hering's Law*, or the "Law of Direction of Cure." Hering observed that *the body seeks to externalize disease*, to dislodge it from more serious internal levels to more external levels. As an example, a person with asthma may find her/his lungs getting better, but s/he may develop a skin rash.

The first aspect of Hering's Law states that *healing progresses from the mental and emotional levels and the vital organs to the external parts* like the skin and the extremities. Eventually, even the superficial symptoms are alleviated. A cure is in progress if psychological symptoms lessen and physiological symptoms increase. As a guide to this law, George Vithoulkas has provided the following list of symptoms. Symptoms from each level, in order of depth, are as follows:

Physical: brain, heart, endocrine, liver, lung, kidney, bone, muscle, skin

Emotional: suicide, apathy, sadness, anguish, phobias, anxiety, irritability

Mental: confusion, delirium, paranoia, delusions,
               lethargy, dullness, lack of concentration,
               forgetfulness, absent-mindedness

The second aspect of Hering's Law states that *healing progresses from the upper to the lower parts of the body.* Pains in the neck and chest area might appear in the legs, but the person would be considered to be on the mend.

The third aspect says that *symptoms appear and disappear in the reverse of their original order of appearance.* It has been observed by homeopathic doctors that patients experience symptoms from past conditions, especially in dealing with chronic illnesses. The symptoms may be from illnesses ranging from six months to many years. In homeopathy, when symptoms become worse, it is referred to as a "healing crisis." This is often necessary to achieve a complete healing on a deep level. While s/he is undergoing the healing crisis, the individual's vital force is becoming stronger.

These laws are not always observed in each person's healing process. Symptoms may also proceed upward in the body. The important thing is that the individual begins to feel stronger, that old symptoms disappear, and that a change in the psychological make-up of the individual is apparent.

Depending on the symptoms present, the homeopath may choose to administer a second dose of the same remedy or another remedy. Sometimes one remedy clears out certain symptoms and paves the way for another remedy.

ADMINISTERING REMEDIES

Depending on the form of the remedy, one dose would consist of one drop of the liquid, about 10 of the tiny little granules, or three to four of the larger tablets. It is best not to touch the remedy but to pour it onto or under the tongue. It is also important not to take water or food with the remedy for 15-20 minutes before or after administering.

Certain substances have been found to antidote homeopathic remedies, particularly coffee and products containing camphor (cosmetics, lip balm, nail polish, Vick's, Noxema, etc.). These substances do not always antidote the remedy, but if the original symptoms return after drinking coffee or using products with camphor, it is best to repeat the remedy.

CHOOSING THE CORRECT REMEDY

In order to choose the correct homeopathic remedy, it is important to make careful observations of the person and to note all his physical and psychological symptoms. Physical symptoms include general strength and energy level, muscular coordination, restlessness, sleep patterns, response to temperature changes, thirst and appetite, food cravings, color of skin and tongue, pulse, and type of body odor. Psychological symptoms include mood changes, state of mind, desire to be with others or left alone, neatness and orderliness, self-image, and efficiency in completing projects.

After studying a person's symptoms, a homeopath attempts to find a remedy that matches a person's totality of symptoms. Certain symptom patterns are identified with medicines that have healed them; for example, the "Nux Vomica" type, the "Phosphorus" type.[7] Treatment may consist of a repetition of the same remedy in a different potency or another remedy.

In Europe, certain homeopathic practitioners utilize several remedies for different sets of symptoms. This practice is known as *Pluralism*; there is no formal research comparing it with classical homeopathy.[8]

In addition to the "constitutional remedy," there are also remedies for many acute conditions like burns, bee stings, colds, coughs, sprains, etc. It is possible for the layperson to prescribe these remedies for her/himself with the help of a book, such as Stephen Cummings' and Dana Ullmann's *Everybody's Guide to Homeopathic Medicines* (J. P. Tarcher, 1984) or Maesimund Panos' *Homeopathic Medicine At Home* (J. P. Tarcher, 1980).

COMMON REMEDIES

There are certain common homeopathic remedies that are included in homeopathic first-aid kits and should be available in each household. A short description of each of these follows.

Aconitum napellus (monkshood) Aconite is useful in the early stages of inflammation or fever or the first stage of a cold. Typical is hot, red skin, strong thirst, sometimes a throbbing headache. There is anxiety and restlessness with the physical symptoms and ailments stemming from fright with sudden onset and intense symptoms.

Allium cepa (red onion) This remedy is good for colds, respiratory allergies, sneezing, runny nose and eyes, stuffed nose, hoarseness and beginning laryngitis, neuralgic pains, and sinus headaches.

Apis mellifica (honeybee) Apis relieves insect bites, bee stings, hives, and other injuries with stinging, burning pain.

Arnica montana (leopard's bane) Arnica is used for bruises, falls, injuries, pain after dental extractions, soreness of muscles, joint sprains, and shock from injuries.

Arsenicum album (arsenic) Arsenicum is used for burning pains, especially of the throat, stomach, or eyes. Discharge of the nose or diarrhea often burns and irritates the skin. Heat and warm drinks are helpful. There is often restlessness and fear as well as severe weakness and exhaustion.

Belladonna (deadly nightshade) Belladonna is called for in the acute early stages of inflammatory illnesses characterized by high fever and severe pain which begin suddenly and end abruptly. Intense heat, redness, throbbing, and swelling are key symptoms. Fevers, sore throats, earaches and skin eruptions are treated with belladonna.

Bryonia alba (wild hops) The person requiring bryonia is irritable, easily angered, and often wants to be left alone. There may be a dry, hard cough, headaches, a strong thirst for large amounts of liquid, and often constipation with dry, hard stools. Motion aggravates any of these conditions.

Calcarea phosphorica (phosphate of lime) Calc phos aids the healing of bones and is good for fractures, teething, pains in bones and joints, colic in babies, and promoting milk in breast-feeding mothers.

Cantharis (Spanish fly) Cantharis alleviates pain from burns and scalds; it is also helpful for painful, burning urination and cystitis.

Carbo vegetabilis (vegetable charcoal) Carbo veg is an important remedy for stomach gas. There is often heartburn, regurgitation of food, and burning in the stomach. It is also good for one whose energy is low after a serious illness.

Chamomilla (German chamomile) Chamomile is soothing to the nervous system; it is good for sleeplessness, nervous conditions, and pain. It is often given to irritable, fussy children, especially during teething.

Ferrum phosphoricum (phosphate of iron) Ferrum phos is a great remedy in the beginning stages of inflammatory conditions such as colds, flu, rheumatism, or bronchitis. It is good for those suffering from allergies and anemia.

Gelsemium (yellow jasmine) Gelsemium is often recommended in damp weather. The person requiring this remedy often feels heavy and tired and mentally sluggish. They often experience chills running up and down the body. Anxiety and anticipation may bring on these symptoms.

Hypericum perfoliatum (St. John's wort) This is a good remedy for injuries to the nerves. It is also helpful for injuries to the fingertips, nails, toes, and tailbone, as well as in treating severe concussions and eye injuries.

Ignatia amara (St. Ignatius bean) Conditions calling for ignatia are those that are precipitated by emotional stress, such as grief, anger, or disappointment. It is used for unstrung conditions of the nervous system due to strong emotions and overstimulation.

Ipecacuanha (ipecac root) Ipecac relieves nausea with or without vomiting; it also helps to stop nosebleed or bleeding from any part of the body.

Ledum palustre (marsh tea) Ledum is the chief remedy for puncture wounds, stings, and bites.

Magnesia phosphorica (phosphate of magnesium) Mag phos eases any pains or cramps, such as menstrual cramps, leg cramps, or colic. It is good for severe nervous conditions and sleeplessness.

Mercurius vivus (quicksilver) Mercury is required during acute conditions where there is inflammation of the skin and mucous membranes along with pus formation and open sores; urinary infections; and skin infections such as boils and herpes.

Nux vomica (poison nut) Nux vomica is used after overindulgence in food, alcohol and drugs. It is also used for irritable bowel syndrome and intermittent peristaltic action. People requiring this remedy are usually irritable and quick-tempered.

Pulsatilla (wind flower) Pulsatilla is a remedy that is often used for menstrual problems—delayed menstruation, PMS, and menopausal symptoms. Those needing pulsatilla tend to be sensitive, vulnerable, moody, and desire attention. It also a good remedy for certain cases of allergies, digestive upsets, ear infections, and colds.

Rhus toxicodendron (poison ivy) Rhus tox is helpful for inflamed skin blisters from poison ivy and oak, chickenpox, and herpes. It also works well for achy and sore muscle and joint pains that are relieved by motion.

Ruta graveolus (rue) Ruta is helpful for injured, bruised bones and for sprains after arnica is used. It is also beneficial for sciatica and headaches due to eyestrain.

Sulphur Sulphur is used most often for chronic conditions. Sometimes these conditions involve dry, scaly skin, sometimes constipation with dry, hard stools. There is usually a great deal of thirst, flushes of heat, and improvement from the open air.

CELL SALTS OR TISSUE SALTS

The biochemic system of medicine was developed by Dr. W. H. Scheussler of Germany in the late 1800s. Dr. Scheussler explained disease and body imbalance as a result of the molecular disturbance in certain cell salts or trace minerals in the body. He found 12 of these to be the most abundant constituents of cremated human remains. He therefore theorized that an adequate supply of all 12 was necessary to prevent disease.[9]

Although Dr. Scheussler's explanations are overly simplistic, the 12 cell salts, which are homeopathically prepared, have been extremely useful in balancing conditions in the body. Dr. Hahnemann and his colleagues have included provings of these in the *Materia Medica*. The cell salts are obtainable in low potencies such as 3x, 6x, 12x, and 30x, but they are also available in higher potencies.

Since each person's chemistry and metabolism are different, so the proportion of tissue salts varies in each of our bodies. We may have an inherent tendency to lack one or more of the salts, and at various times in our life we may develop deficiencies of any of the salts. We also may have more of the tissue salts.

Some of the salts seem to be more useful than others, as proved by the testing of individuals. For example, two of the three sodium salts are rarely needed because most people have too much sodium in their bodies. On the other hand, the potassium salts are called for a great deal.

Descriptions of the 12 salts follow.

Kali Phos (potassium phosphate) Kali Phos is found in all the tissues and fluids of the body, particularly the brain and nerve cells. It is a great nutrient for the nerves. A deficiency of Kali Phos may produce irritability, timidity, fearfulness, and sleeplessness. It is a good remedy for headaches, depressions, insomnia, and conditions of nervous origin.

Nat Sulph (sodium sulphate) The principal function of this salt is to regulate intracellular fluids in the body by eliminating excess water. It is important in the proper functioning of the kidneys and bladder.

Kali Mur (potassium chloride) This salt unites with albumin, forming fibrin, which is found in every tissue of the body with the exception of the bones. Fibrin helps cells retain their shape. Kali Mur is helpful in treating any respiratory problem, such as colds, hay fever, allergies, bronchitis, sore throats, and tonsillitis. It is often taken in a high dose at the first sign of a cold or flu.

Calc Fl (calcium fluoride) Calc Fl appears in the surface of the bones, the enamel of the teeth, and the elastic fibers of the muscle tissues. Its deficiency causes these tissues to lose their elasticity. It is useful in treating diseases of the teeth, bones, hardening of the arteries, and conditions such as arthritis and rheumatism.

Mag Phos (magnesium phosphate) Mag Phos is anti-spasmodic as its work relates to the nerves. A deficiency of this salt causes the body to contract, producing spasms and cramps. The contraction puts pressure on the sensory nerves, which give rise to sharp, shooting pains. Mag Phos is good for cramps associated with menstruation, muscle spasms, epileptic conditions, and heart conditions. A larger dose of magnesium is required for all these, but as a first-aid measure Mag Phos can be very helpful.

Kali Sulph (potassium sulphate) Kali Sulph carries oxygen to the cells of the skin and distributes oil in the body which aids in perspiration and the elimination of body poisons. Kali Sulph is excellent in the treatment of acne and other skin conditions, including dandruff.

Nat Phos (sodium phosphate) Nat Phos maintains the acid/alkaline balance in the blood. Lack of this salt may produce a yellow coating on the tongue. Nat Phos is helpful in relieving acid stomach and in treating ulcers.

Calc Sulph (calcium sulphate) Calc Sulph is a blood purifier which builds the epithelial tissue in the body. It is effective in the healing processes of the bones, joints, and teeth and is used in elimination problems such as constipation.

Silica (silicon dioxide) Silica is present in the blood, bile, skin, hair, and nails. It is also found in connective tissue, bones, nerve sheaths and mucous membranes. In proper amounts it gives fingernails, hair, and teeth a glossy appearance. It helps to minimize scar tissue formation after surgery or injury. It needs to be used with the appropriate amount of calcium to be effective.

Calc Phos (calcium phosphate) Calc Phos is a constituent of the bone tissue. The body requires large amounts when it is growing or recovering from fractures. It also plays an important role in the clotting mechanism of the blood. Lack of Calc Phos causes skeletal problems such as rickets, curvature of the spine, and swollen or painful joints. Calc Phos is helpful for teething and all problems of teeth and bone where calcium is required.

Nat Mur (sodium chloride or table salt) The most useful of the sodium salts, Nat Mur is found in every cell and fluid; one of its most important roles is to maintain the proper degree of moisture within the body. A deficiency of this salt may cause an imbalance of water in the body in which the individual may appear very bloated and sometimes may suffer the opposite condition of excessive dryness. It is useful in watery blisters, insect bites and stings where it is applied externally in a solution. It is also indicated for dryness of tear ducts, sneezing and post-nasal drip.

Ferrum Phos (iron phosphate) Found in the blood, Ferrum Phos is an essential component of the hemoglobin which carries oxygen to all parts of the body. It is the most frequently needed of all the tissue salts because most diseases start with inflammation of one kind or another. Ferrum Phos is essential for red blood cells and its lack can cause anemia. Due to the difficulty of assimilation of iron, Ferrum Phos in all potencies is a most helpful remedy.

NOTES

1. George Vithoulkas, *The Science of Homeopathy* (Athens: George Vithoulkas, Athenian School of Homeopathic Medicine, 1978), p. 76.
2. Ibid., p. 109.

3. Ibid., p. 112.
4. Ibid., p. 113.
5. Dana Ullmann, *Homeopathy: Medicine for the 21st Century* (Berkeley, CA: North Atlantic Books, 1988), p. 15.
6. Vithoulkas, p. 118.
7. Ullmann, p. 19.
8. Ibid., p. 23.
9. J. B. Chapman, M.D., *Dr. Schuessler's Biochemistry* (London: New Era Laboratories, 1961), p. 6.

TRADITIONAL CHINESE MEDICINE

Traditional Chinese medicine is based on the belief that all humanity is a part of the natural environment and that health or balance can only be achieved when one follows natural law, adapting to the changes of the seasons and the surrounding environment. Chinese medicine has its philosophical basis in *Taoism* (the Way of the Tao, or the Way of Life). Taoism teaches that all phenomena exist within interrelated space. It also expounds that everything has an energy field or vibration and is in a constant state of flux.

What activates all phenomena is the movement of energy between two poles, *yin* and *yang*. Yin is the tendency toward contraction and centripetality; yang, the tendency towards expansion and centrifugality. Yin is receptive and feminine; yang, active and masculine. Yin is the Earth force; yang is the force of Heaven. The Chinese character for yin refers to the shady side of a slope. It is associated with qualities like cold, rest, passivity, darkness, interiority, downwardness, inwardness, and decrease. The character for yang is the sunny side of a slope. It is associated with heat, stimulation, movement, activity, excitement, vigor, light, upwardness, outwardness, and increase.[1]

The front part of the body is considered yin and the back, yang. The upper part is more yang than the lower part. Illnesses that are characterized by weakness, slowness, coldness, and underactivity are yin. Illnesses that manifest strength, forceful movements, heat and overactivity are yang.

CHI

The dynamic vital energy present in all things is called *chi* by the Chinese. When a person is in good health or balance (physically, emotionally, and spiritually), her/his chi is maximized, and s/he resonates with the environment. When out of balance, her/his chi is low or deficient.

The Chinese have three sources of chi. Original or pre-natal chi is transmitted by parents to children; this is the inherited constitution. The second source is grain chi, derived from the digestion of food. The third is the natural air chi, which is extracted by the lungs from the air we breathe.

Chi has five major functions in the body. The first is movement (including involuntary movements and activities like thinking and dreaming). Chi is in constant motion in the body. Secondly, chi protects the body from pathological and environmental agents. Thirdly, chi transforms food into blood and urine. It also governs retention of the body's substance by holding organs in their proper place and preventing excessive loss of bodily fluids. Finally, chi warms the body.[2]

BLOOD

Blood in Chinese medicine is a broader concept than in Western medicine. Its main activity is to circulate throughout the body, nourishing and maintaining its various parts. Blood moves through the blood vessels and also the meridians.[3] It originates through the transformation of food. After the stomach receives food, the spleen distills a purified essence from it. The spleen transports this essence up to the lungs. Here it is combined with air to form blood, which is then propelled through the body by the heart chi in combination with the chest chi.

The heart, liver, and spleen all have special relationships to the blood. Blood depends on the heart for its continuous circulation throughout the body. The liver stores the inactive blood, and the spleen keeps it within the blood vessels.[4]

JING

Jing or "essence" is the substance that underlies all organic life.

Jing is like a fluid and is the basis of reproduction and development. Pre-natal jing is the essence we inherit from our parents, and post-natal jing is derived from the purified parts of ingested food.[5]

Jing is the material that imbues an organism with development from conception to birth. Disharmonies of jing might involve improper motivation, sexual dysfunction, and premature aging. Jing is different from chi in that chi is involved with movement, but jing is associated with the slow movement of organic change.[6]

SHEN

Shen means "spirit"; it is the substance of human life. Shen is associated with the ability to think, to discriminate and to choose. Shen also has a material aspect. It is the mind's ability to form ideas and the desire of the personality to live. When shen is out of harmony, one's thinking may be muddled or one may suffer from insomnia, unconsciousness, or incoherent speech.[7]

ORGANS

The Chinese organs are different from the Western organs in that they are defined by their *function*, not their structure.[8] The Chinese recognize the *triple burner* as an organ, but it is not a physical entity. The triple burner is a relationship between various organs that regulate water. It is the pathway that makes these organs a complete system; since fire controls water, the triple burner implies fire.[9]

Organs are divided into yin and yang. The function of the yin organs is to produce, transform, regulate, and store the fundamental substances—chi, blood, jing, shen, and fluids. The function of the yang organs is to receive, break down, and absorb that part of the food that will be transformed into fundamental substance and excrete the unused part.[10]

Yin Organs	Yang Organs
heart	small intestine
lungs	large intestine
spleen	stomach
liver	gall bladder
kidneys	bladder
pericardium	triple burner

MERIDIANS AND ACUPUNCTURE

Meridians are the channels that carry chi and blood through the body; they connect the interior of the body with the exterior. The philosophy of acupuncture is that working with points on the outside of the body affects the substances that are traveling through the meridians.[11]

The meridian system is comprised of the 12 regular meridians that correspond to the 6 yin and 6 yang organs. There are also eight extra meridians, only two of which, the Governing vessel and the Conception vessel, are considered major meridians. They have points that are not on any of the 12 regular meridians. The paths of the other six meridians intersect with the 12 meridians and have no independent points.[12]

Disorder within a meridian creates disharmony on its pathway and could result in problems in the meridian's connecting organ. For example, disorder in the stomach meridian may cause a toothache in the upper gums because the meridian passes through this area.[13] Disharmony in an organ may also manifest in the corresponding meridian. Understanding the connections between the substances, organs and meridians is the essence of Chinese medicine. Chinese medicine uses acupuncture and herbs to rebalance yin and yang in the meridians and organs. An example of imbalance is excess anger, which would indicate too much liver chi.

The idea behind acupuncture is that the insertion of fine needles into points along the meridians can rebalance bodily disharmonies. The action of the needle affects the chi and the blood in the meridians, thus affecting the substances and organs.[14] The needles help to reduce excesses, increase deficiencies, warm cold areas, cool down fire, circulate stagnant energy and move congealed energy. There are about 365 points on the surface meridians of the body, but in practice, a doctor may use only about 150 points.[15] Each acupuncture point has a defined therapeutic action—a combination of points is, therefore, always chosen. Needles are made of stainless steel and produce relatively little pain when inserted. The depth to which a needle penetrates depends on the particular point.

In addition to acupuncture, a related technique called *moxibustion* is employed. Moxibustion applies the heat from burning substances at certain acupuncture points. The heating substance, or *moxa*, is mugwort (artemisia vulgaris).[16] This helps to increase the effect of the acupuncture treatment.

HERBOLOGY

Chinese herbology is an extensive body of knowledge that has been developed over several millenia into an organized system of medicine. Substances used in the Chinese *materia medica* span a great range of materials from herbs and minerals to strange animal products. Each entry is usually defined in terms of how the various herbs and their combinations affect imbalances in the body.[17]

There are many classical prescriptions that can rebalance disharmonies in the body. These prescriptions are found in the pharmacopoeias and manuals. Most of the herbs are used as teas, but herbal tablets, powders and tinctures are also utilized.

PATTERNS OF DISEASE

The Chinese do not speak of causes of disease in the same way as does Western medicine. Cause implies a linear progression; Chinese medicine works in a *circular* way, believing that there are many factors that create a pattern of imbalance, disharmony or dis-ease. These factors are categorized under environment, emotional outlook, and way of life.[18]

Environmental factors are spoken of as the "six pernicious influences." These six are Wind, Cold, Fire or Heat, Dryness, Dampness, and Summer Heat. When weakened by an imbalance of yin and yang, a climatic phenomenon can invade the body. If the protective chi is strong, the influence is expelled and the individual recovers. But if the chi is weak, the influence may go deep and become involved with the internal organs. Illnesses generated by any of the "pernicious factors" come on suddenly. When the pernicious influences arise internally, symptoms come on gradually. This is the case with chronic disease as opposed to acute disease.[19]

All the climatic influences are images for body processes.[20] The body does not have to experience damp climate to have damp in the lungs; our emotional and mental states can create the same condition.

SEVEN EMOTIONS

The seven emotions that particularly affect the body are joy, anger, sadness, grief, pensiveness (worry), fear, and fright .[21] Sadness and grief as well as fear and fright are often combined as one emotion. The seven emotions correspond to the five yin organs:

> heart—joy
> liver—anger
> lungs—sadness and grief
> spleen—pensiveness or worry
> kidneys—fear and fright

The two organs most susceptible to emotions are the heart and the liver. The heart stores the shen; imbalances may lead to insomnia, crying or laughing, and extreme hysteria.[22] Imbalances in the liver can result in excess anger or emotional frustration.

Organ	Out of Balance	In Balance
liver, gall bladder	anger	patience
heart, small intestine	excitement	joy
spleen, stomach	worry	sympathy
kidney, bladder	fear	confidence
lung, large intestine	grief	happiness

WAY OF LIFE

Several factors that the Chinese refer to as Way of Life are important in determining a person's state of health. These include diet, sexual activity, and physical activity. Diet is important because the stomach receives food and the spleen transforms it into chi and blood. Preferences for certain types of food can cause disharmonies. For example, too much raw food can strain the yang aspect of the spleen and generate intense cold. [23] Fatty and greasy foods can produce dampness and heat.

Many of the principles of Chinese medicine have been utilized by the Japanese philosopher George Ohsawa in creating the Macrobiotic Diet. Macrobiotics, however, is not a part of Chinese medicine though it is often practiced and used along with acupuncture and herbs (see chapter 4).

Excessive sexual activity is often considered a precipitating factor of disease. Overindulgence affects the kidneys and reduces vitality; giving birth too many times weakens the jing and the blood.[24]

Physical activity is important, but excess can strain the spleen's ability to produce chi and blood. Inactivity can weaken the vitality of chi and blood; excess use of a part of the body can also weaken it.[25]

THE FOUR EXAMINATIONS

Before making a diagnosis, the Chinese physician performs four examinations—Looking, Listening and Smelling, Asking, and Touching.[26]

In the Looking examination, the first factor is the patient's general appearance: how s/he looks, her/his manner and the state of her/his shen. Lack of interest, apathy, and depression can indicate an imbalanced shen. The second factor is facial color. The third concerns the tongue, including the material of the tongue itself, its coating, and its shape and movement. The fourth is the bodily secretions and excretions.[27]

A person whose appearance is strong is more likely to have disharmonies of excess. One who is frail and weak-looking will tend to have disharmonies of deficiency. One who is agitated, talkative, aggressive, and unstable usually manifests a yang tendency. A more inward, quiet manner is usually yin. The color of the face and its moistness are related to the chi and blood. If the face is healthy, the indications are that the chi and the blood are not weakened and the illness is not serious.[28]

Tongue observation is a central point of the Four Examinations. The tongue can be various shades of red and can have varying degrees of moisture. A normal tongue is pale red and somewhat moist which indicates that the chi and blood are normal. A pale tongue indicates deficient blood or chi or excess cold. A red tongue points to a heat condition in the body.[29]

The coating on the surface of the tongue is the result of spleen activity. During its vaporization of essences, the spleen causes small amounts of impure substances to ascend which come out on the tongue. This is related to digestion. The coating varies in thickness, color, and appearance.

The most important of the examinations is *touching*, and it consists of *pulse taking*. Chinese medicine takes the pulses at the radial artery near the wrist. Many years of experience are required to get the feel of the differences between pulses. The three middle fingers are used, one at each position near the radial artery. The pulse is palpitated at three levels of pressure—first, a light superficial touch, then a moderate amount of pressure is applied, and third, a very deep pressure. A balanced pulse is felt mostly at the middle level. Normal speed is between four and five beats per complete respiration (one inhale and one exhale), which amounts to 70-75 beats per minute.[30] A normal pulse may vary according to the type of work a person does, her/his age, and body type such as thin or heavy. Chinese texts describe about 28 different types of pulses, though most people are a combination of types.

THE FIVE PHASES

The five phases in Chinese philosophy and medicine have been misunderstood in the Western world. They are commonly referred to as the Five Elements, which is an incorrect translation of the Chinese; they are five *movements* or phases.[31] The phases are a system of correspondences that explain the dynamics of events or relationships. Each phase describes certain functions and qualities. The phase called *Wood* is associated with active functions that are in a growing phase. *Fire* designates functions that have reached a maximal state of activity and are about to begin a decline or resting period. *Earth* designates balance or neutrality. *Metal* represents functions in a declining state. *Water* represents functions that have reached a maximal state of rest and are about to change the direction of their activity.[32]

The five phases were originally related to the seasons with Wood-Spring, Fire-Summer, Earth-Indian summer, Metal-Autumn; and Water-Winter. In time, they were related to color, odor, emotions, and many other correspondences were added. They were also associated with the organs, and thus they became connected with the system of Chinese medicine.

The organs are placed in the five phases in what is known as the Mutual Control or Mutual Checking sequence. In this sequence, each organ controls the next one so that there will not be any excesses or deficiencies. Thus, Wood-liver controls Earth-spleen, which controls Water-kidneys, which controls Fire-heart, which controls Metal-lungs. Disharmonies may be produced if Wood does not produce enough Fire, which means the liver is not sending blood to the heart, or if Wood overcontrols the spleen, which indicates excess blood from the liver invading the spleen.

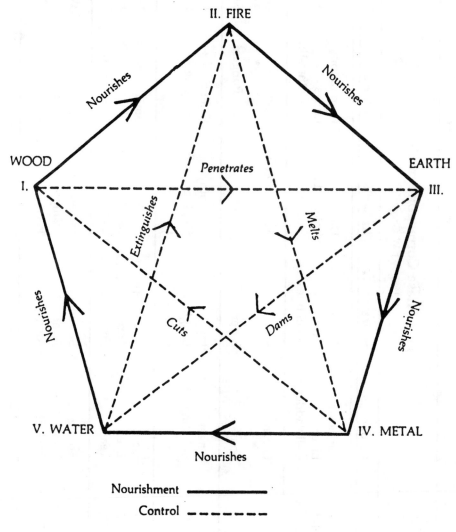

Cycles of Nourishment & Control

Five Phase Correspondences

© 1983 by J. W. Garvy, Jr.

	I Wood	II Fire	III Earth	IV Metal	V Water
Function	Purification	Circulation	Digestion	Respiration	Elimination
Organ/Solid	Liver	Heart	Spleen/Pancreas	Lungs	Kidneys
Organ/Hollow	Gallbladder	Small Intestine	Stomach	Large Intestine	Bladder
Color	Green	Red	Yellow (Orange)	White	Gray, Deep Blue, Brown, Black
Flavor	Sour	Bitter	Sweet	Hot, Pungent	Salty
Emotion	Anger	Joy	Sympathy	Grief	Fear
Sound	Shouting	Laughter	Singing	Weeping	Groaning
Direction	Up	Outward	Horizontal	Down	Inward
Sense	Sight	Touch/Speech	Taste	Smell	Hearing
Head Part	Eyes	Tongue	Mouth	Nose	Ears
Secretion	Tears	Sweat	Saliva	Nasal Fluid	Urine
Season	Spring	Summer	Indian Summer	Autumn	Winter
Climate	Wind	Heat	Dampness	Dryness	Cold
Injurious Entrance	Back of Neck	Mouth	Feet	Nose	Shins

NOTES

1. Manfred Porkert, *The Essentials of Chinese Diagnostics* (Zurich: Chinese Medicine Publications, Ltd., 1983), pp. 22-24.
2. Ted Kaptchuk, *The Web That Has No Weaver: Understanding Chinese Medicine* (New York: Congdon & Weed, 1983), p. 38.
3. Ibid., p. 41.
4. Ibid., p. 42.
5. Ibid., p. 43.
6. Ibid., p. 44.
7. Ibid., p. 46.
8. Ibid., p. 51.
9. Ibid., p. 68.
10. Ibid., p. 53.
11. Ibid., p. 77.
12. Ibid., p. 78.
13. Ibid., p. 71.
14. Ibid., p. 79.
15. Ibid., p. 80.
16. Ibid., p. 79.
17. Dan Bensky, *Chinese Herbal Medicine: Materia Medica* (Seattle, WA: Eastland Press, 1986), pp. 6-8.
18. Porkert, p. 121.
19. Kaptchuk, p. 119.
20. Ibid.
21. Ibid., p. 129.
22. Ibid., p. 130.
23. Ibid., p. 132.
24. Ibid.
25. Ibid., p. 133.
26. Ibid., p. 143.
27. Ibid., p. 144.
28. Ibid., p. 146.
29. Ibid., p. 148.
30. Ibid., p. 160.
31. Porkert, p. 43.
32. Kaptchuk, p. 344.

AYURVEDIC MEDICINE

Ayurvedic medicine is the ancient Hindu system of healing; like Chinese medicine, it views health as a continuous relationship between the individual and the cosmos. In Sanskrit, *aya* means "life" or "daily living"; *veda* means "knowledge." The science of Ayurveda encompasses many diagnostic techniques (pulse diagnosis, nail diagnosis, facial diagnosis), various types of cleansing, herbs and homeopathic remedies, an extensive dietary regimen based on the different tastes and their attributes, yoga postures, and various *mudras* (hand gestures) and *mantras* (chants) that help balance out specific energies. It is a comprehensive and holistic system.

The *theory of the five elements* forms the basis for the Ayurvedic system. *Ether* is the first element; it is the medium through which sound is transmitted and is related to the ear and the actions of speech and hearing. *Air* is created from Ether and refers to the sense of touch and the skin. The organ for the sense of touch is the hand and its action is holding. *Fire* or heat came about through the friction of Ether. Fire manifests as light, heat, and color and is related to vision. (The eye, the organ of sight, governs the action of walking.) Through the heat of Fire, certain elements dissolved and liquified (Water) and solidified to form *Earth*. *Water* is related to taste and the tongue. The tongue in Ayurvedic medicine is associated with the genitals—the clitoris and penis and the action of procreation. Earth refers to the sense of smell, and the nose, the sensory organ of smell, is associated with the anus and the action of excretion.[1]

TRIDOSHA

Ayurvedic medicine is organized around three humors or *doshas* which form the core of the system.

Vata is the first dosha; it is the principle of movement and is formed from Ether and Air. Vata governs breathing, movements of the muscles and tissues, pulsations in the heart, expansion and contraction, as well as the motion of cytoplasm and impulses to nerve cells. Feelings and emotions governed by Vata include nervousness, fear, anxiety, pain, tremors, and spasm. The large intestine, pelvic cavity, bones, skin, ears, and thighs are the seats of Vata; excesses of Vata will accumulate in these areas.

Pitta, the second humor, is formed from Fire and Water; it is akin to bile. Pitta refers to metabolism, nutrition, digestion, absorption, assimilation, body temperature, and skin coloration. Psychologically, Pitta arouses anger, hate, and jealousy. The small intestine, stomach, sweat glands, blood, fat, eyes, and skin are the seats of Pitta.

Kapha originates from Water and Earth. Kapha cements the elements in the body; it lubricates the joints, provides moisture to the skin, helps to heal wounds, and maintains immunity. Kapha is the mucus secretion present in the chest, throat, head, sinuses, nose, mouth, and joints. Psychologically, Kapha is related to the emotions of attachment, greed and envy; it is also expressed in tendencies toward calmness, forgiveness, and love.

The tridosha governs all metabolic processes—anabolism or building up (Kapha), catabolism or breaking down (Vata), and metabolism (Pitta). When one dosha is out of balance, the metabolism will be disturbed.[2]

CONSTITUTIONAL TYPES

Vata types may be too tall or too short; their complexion is dark and their skin is usually cold, dry, rough, and cracked. Hair is often curly with thin eyelashes; nails are rough and brittle and noses may be turned up. Physiological tendencies of Vata people vary. They often crave sweet, sour, and salty tastes and like hot drinks. Their urine is more scanty, and feces tend to be dry, hard, and small. They perspire less than other types. Their hands and feet are often cold, and they tend toward constipation. Vata types are alert, active, restless, sleep less and talk fast. Their appetites are irregular; they have bursts of energy and often have difficulty sleeping. Psychologically, they have short memories but quick mental understanding. They can be nervous, fearful, and anxious at times.

Pitta types tend toward medium height. Their complexion may be yellowish or reddish with skin soft, warm, and less wrinkled than Vata skin. They blush easily and are sensitive to the Sun. Physiologically, they have a strong metabolism and good digestion. They often crave sweet, bitter, and astringent tastes and enjoy cold drinks. Their sleep is generally uninterrupted. They produce a large volume of urine and their feces are liquid and soft. There may be a tendency toward excessive perspiring. Body temperature runs high and hands and feet tend to be warm. Psychologically, they have good powers of comprehension and are intelligent and sharp. Their emotional traits tend toward hate, anger, and jealousy. Pitta people are ambitious, like to be leaders, and display impatience.

Those of *Kapha constitution* have well-developed bodies though they tend to carry excess weight. When exercising properly, they are good athletes. Kapha types have fair and bright complexions; their skin is soft and oily and tends to be pale; their hair is thick, soft, and wavy. Physiologically, Kapha people have regular appetites—their digestion functions slowly and there is less intake of food. They tend to move slowly and crave pungent, bitter, and astringent foods. Stools are soft and may be pale in color with slow evacuation. Their sleep is sound, and they possess a strong vitality with good stamina. Psychologically, Kapha types are tolerant, calm, forgiving, and loving when balanced. They may also be greedy, envious and possessive, stubborn, reactionary, and complacent. Their comprehension is slow, but they retain knowledge well. They need motivation and stimulation, just as Vatas require balance and relaxation, and Pittas need a challenge.

Vata-Pitta people have poor circulation, characteristic of Vata types, but cannot handle heat as well due to their Pitta qualities. They often have wavy hair, resulting from Vata's curliness and Pitta's straightness. When their energy is out of balance, fear alternates with anger as a response to stress; they can be bullying and domineering. Both Vata and Pitta have lightness and intensity. When unbalanced, Vata's tendency to addiction for pain control and Pitta's intensity combine to stronger addictive states. If directed, they can work with intensive self-development. They need to be weighted down with the heaviness of Kapha.

Pitta-Kapha types have the stability of Kapha with the adaptability of Pitta. They usually enjoy good physical health due to Kapha's strong body and Pitta's good metabolism. Pitta's danger can be balanced by Kapha's cautiousness. The negative side is seen in Pitta's arrogance and Kapha's self-satisfaction. Both of these types have a share of oiliness or wetness and need the dryness of introspection or spiritual disciplines.

Vata-Kapha types suffer from cold; their lack of heat may manifest in digestive disorders like constipation or respiratory disease with a lot of mucus. They can be overzealous about what they do and often overdo things. Emotional hurts go deep with the strong emotional nature of Kapha and the overactive and sporadic nature of Vata.[3]

DISEASE CLASSIFICATION

In Ayurvedic medicine, disease is classified according to its origin—psychological, spiritual, or physical. Disease is also classified according to the site of manifestation and the imbalance of the doshas—Vata, Pitta, or Kapha. Vata disease originates in the large intestine; Vata types often have gas, low back pain, arthritis, sciatica, and neuralgia. Pitta disease originates in the small intestine; these types often have gall bladder and liver disorders, ulcers, acidic conditions, and gastritis. Kapha diseases start in the stomach; they may experience tonsillitis, sinusitis, bronchitis, and congestion of the lungs.

In terms of emotions, repressed fear creates an imbalance of Vata, anger causes excess Pitta, while envy and greed aggravate Kapha. If physical conditions, improper diet and environmental toxins create an imbalance in the body, then the corresponding emotions will also be present—distorted Vata creates fear, depression, and nervousness; excess Pitta causes anger, hate, and jealousy, and too much Kapha may create possessiveness, greed, and attachment. Fear and anxiety alter the flora of the large intestine, and problems with gas or bloating may result. Repressed anger changes the flora of the gall bladder and bile duct and may cause inflammation on the walls of the small intestine. Excess envy and greed may affect the mucous membranes of the stomach. Repressed emotions affect *agni*, the biological fire that governs metabolism. When agni is low, the body's auto-immune response is affected, and this may lead to allergies—pollens, dust, and other substances.

TREATMENT

The most important treatment in Ayurvedic medicine is the elimination of toxins through various cleansing procedures. Ayurveda uses the term *panchakarma* to include the five basic cleansing processes; these are vomiting, laxatives, medicated enemas, nasal administration of medicine, and purification of the blood. When there is excess mucus in the chest, bile in the small intestine, or gas accumulation in the colon, elimination therapies are helpful.

When there is congestion in the lungs causing repeated attacks of bronchitis, coughs, or asthma, *therapeutic vomiting* is used. Three or four glasses of an herb tea or two glasses of salt water is administered first. Then the tongue is rubbed to induce vomiting. Therapeutic vomiting is also indicated for skin diseases, chronic sinus problems, and chronic indigestion.

When allergies, rashes, or skin inflammations develop, it is due to bile accumulation in the gall bladder, liver or intestines. For these conditions, Ayurveda uses *purgatives* or *laxatives*. Herbs like senna, flaxseed, and psyllium seed husks as well as castor oil are used.

Enema treatments are taken for various Vata disorders such as chronic gas, constipation, hyperacidity, arthritis, rheumatism, and gout. There are several types of enemas—oil enemas where 1/2 cup of sesame or olive oil is heated and put into the enema bag; decoction enemas where various herbs are decocted; and nutritive enemas where a cup of warm milk or bone marrow soup are added to the enema.

Another cleansing process involves nasal administration of medication, or *nasya*. Nasal administration helps to correct the disorders of *prana* affecting the cerebral, sensory, and motor functions. It is indicated for dryness of the nose, sinus congestion, hoarseness, migraine, as well as eye and ear problems. Breathing can also be improved through nasal massage. In this technique, the inner walls of the nostril are massaged with oils, ghee, or the juice of various herbs like gota-kola or aloe vera.

Bloodletting is used in various Pitta disorders like rashes and acne where toxins are circulated in the blood stream. The Ayurvedic physician extracts a small amount of blood from the vein which relieves the tension created by the toxins in the blood. Bloodletting stimulates antitoxic substances in the blood stream which help develop the auto-immune mechanism. Blood purifying herbs include burdock root tea, saffron, turmeric, and calamus root powder.[4]

BALANCING THE BODY

In order to heal and balance the body, three things must be in equilibrium. These are *prana*, life force, called *chi* in Chinese medicine, which brings body, mind and spirit together on a single strand of breath and causes them to work as a single organism; *tejas*, the force of transmutation which permits body, mind, and spirit to influence one another; and *ojas*, the subtle manifestation or the glue that cements body, mind, and spirit together. Vata, Pitta, and Kapha are the gross manifestation of prana, tejas, and ojas. When physical, mental and spiritual digestion are at their peak, Vata, Pitta, and Kapha are produced from bodily functions.[5]

Prana is obtained from our food and the atmosphere; breathing recharges prana; nourishment and water also carry prana. While most nutrients are absorbed from the small intestine, prana is absorbed from the colon. The health of our lungs and colon determine how much prana we can absorb. When the lungs or colon are not healthy, too much Vata is generated, which can then cause disease; Vata especially affects the bone. Cigarette smokers often lose more calcium from their bones due to the effect of carbon monoxide on blood chemistry.[6]

Tejas is fire; prana inflames tejas. When the mind is clear and stable, tejas burns cleanly; when the mind is agitated by emotion, tejas is imbalanced and produces too much Pitta. Chemical toxins are transported by the blood; the ability of tejas to nurture the digestive system depends upon the blood, the liver and spleen, which control the blood, and the brain.[7]

Ojas is the medium through which the force of tejas is transmitted. Ojas is a substance, unlike prana and tejas; it can be produced, collected and stored. When there is good digestion of food and other sensory impressions, ojas is efficiently produced. Ojas is a living force which protects the integrity of the individual. Ojas has a negative counterpart called *Ama*, which is a living substance in the sense that it is a collection of nutrients for alien invaders like bacteria, viruses, and cancer cells. Ojas is the foundation of physical immunity and produces the aura. The aura is the first line of defense from intrusions and a buffer against negative vibrations.[8]

Indigestion is the main cause of disease; physical indigestion causes mental indigestion, and vice versa; the two usually exist together. If the body is purified as much as possible, then one can begin working with the mind. Vata-caused indigestion mainly affects the large intestine. Usually, constipation alternates with loose stools and there is intestinal gas. Pitta-caused indigestion affects mainly the small intestine and usually causes loose stools. Burning sensations such as heartburn are common. Kapha-caused indigestion affects mainly the stomach; there is usually heaviness in the upper abdomen and in the limbs with constipation.[9]

Ayurvedic medicine works to remove the cause of the indigestion, eliminate the excess energy from the doshas, balance the doshas, rekindle the digestive fires, and then rebuild the organism.

The first treatments concern the *elimination of Ama*. Fasting is the most basic way to cleanse the body. Vata types should not fast on just water for more than a day or two; they may fast on vegetable juices, or for a prolonged fast they should choose a single food like cooked vegetables. Pitta types do well to fast on vegetable or fruit juices or raw vegetables or fruit. Kapha people may fast on water for several days or raw vegetable and fruit juices.

Medicated enemas are an important treatment in cleansing the body. Sweats in a sauna or in a wet steam bath are beneficial, depending on which doshas are out of balance.

If the patient is strong and the disease weak, the "panchakarmas" or cleansings should be used. If the patient is weak and the disease strong, the doshas should be balanced first and the patient strengthened before doing the cleansings.[10]

After cleansing the body, there are ways to balance the doshas. If the imbalance is due to excess Vata, tea made from ginger with ground-up fennel and dill seeds is helpful. Ginger and garlic are good to rekindle digestive fire. Light, well-cooked foods and warm liquids are soothing. Yoga stretches are good as well as regular sunbathing. To balance excess Pitta, fennel may be used. Psyllium seed husks or bitter herbs like gentian or Oregon grape root help to light the digestive fire. Light and raw foods and juices with coriander and sandalwood tea are good. Also, walks in the open air and sunbathing early or late in the day are helpful. If Kapha is in excess, dry ginger, black pepper, or cumin is helpful to digest Ama. Bitter or pungent herbs like garlic or black pepper will activate the digestive fire. Small quantities of roasted food may be taken with as little liquid as possible. Vigorous exercise and extensive sunbathing to encourage sweating is good as well as wind-bathing, well-wrapped to encourage body heat.[11]

DIET

Ayurvedic diet is based on the individual constitution. The taste of food is taken into account—whether it is sweet, sour, salty, pungent, bitter, or astringent—and also whether it is heavy or light, hot or cold, oily or dry, liquid or solid. The seasons of the year are also considered in choosing diet. During summer when the temperature is hot, people perspire readily. Since Pitta predominates in the summer, it is not good to eat spicy, pungent foods because they aggravate this dosha. In autumn when the wind is high and dry, Vata predominates. At this time one should avoid dry fruits, high protein foods, and other foods that increase Vata. Winter is the season to avoid cold drinks, cheese, yogurt, and dairy products as they increase Kapha.

There are six basic tastes in Ayurveda: sweet, sour, salty, pungent, bitter, and astringent. These tastes are derived from the five elements. Sweet contains Earth and Water elements; sour, Earth and Fire; and salty, Water and Fire. The pungent taste contains Fire and Air; bitter, Air and Ether; and astringent, Air and Earth.

See chapter 4 for specific foods for Vata, Pitta, and Kapha types.

MENTAL BALANCE

Once the body is cleansed and balanced, attention should be given to mental states. Vata types tend to worry and be fearful, so they need to keep their minds occupied. Meditation as well as being engaged in projects where they utilize mental energy is helpful. Pitta types tend to anger, especially when they are impatient. Pittas need complex projects to engage their energy so they do not become too restless. Kapha types tend to be complacent and often want to consume and possess things. They also become lazy in caring for their health. It is important for them to be strongly motivated and to concentrate on one activity at a time.[12]

YOGA

The practice of yoga works with Ayurveda in maintaining health and preventing disease. Yoga postures and exercise balance the nervous system, improve the metabolism, and help the body to handle stress. Certain postures move accumulated energies that have stagnated in various organs of the body. Ayurveda indicates which type of yoga is suitable for each individual according to her/his constitution. See chapter 17 for more details on yoga.

NOTES

1. Vasant Lad, M.D., *Ayurveda: The Science of Self-Healing* (Santa Fe, NM: Lotus Press, 1984), pp. 23-25.
2. Ibid., pp. 29-30.
3. Robert Svoboda, *Prakruti: Your Ayurvedic Constitution* (Albuquerque, NM: Geocom Ltd., 1988), pp. 50-52.
4. Lad, pp. 69-70.
5. Svoboda, p. 124.
6. Ibid.
7. Ibid., p. 125.
8. Ibid.
9. Ibid., p. 121.
10. Ibid., p. 132.
11. Ibid., pp. 136-37.
12. Ibid., pp. 138-39.

BODYWORK THERAPIES

Bodywork therapies are designed to make one sensitive to her/his elemental being. We all contain within our bodies each of the elements. Earth may be seen in the structure of the body—our bones and joints, the way our body is held together. Body techniques as chiropractic and osteopathy help us with our Earth. Water, our emotional body that contains our deepest feelings, may be penetrated and balanced through energetic massage like rolfing and bio-energetics which break up old patterns. Air, the breath of life, can be deepened through Reichian work as well as through techniques like rolfing and bioenergetics. Fire, magnetism, may be transmitted through all of these therapies, particularly through the therapies that work with the meridians and subtle energies such as acupressure, shiatsu, jin shinn, reiki and polarity therapy.

The most important thing in choosing a particular bodywork therapy is the alchemy between the healer (toucher) and the one being healed (receiver). Through this alchemy, the vital force (*prana, chi*) is transmitted. It is helpful to work with a healer who knows several different therapies so s/he can use them in combination; often one technique opens up the body for another stronger or deeper one.

Bodywork therapies may be divided into five general categories:

1. Those that work with the body structure, such as osteopathy and chiropractic

2. Massage techniques for releasing stress based on deep tissue work which breaks down body armor and releases pent-up emotions

3. Techniques which work with the electromagnetic currents in the body and balance the chi or vital energy

4. Sensual and relaxing types of massage like Swedish massage and lomi-lomi

5. Vibrational healing techniques that work with the subtle body

BODY STRUCTURE TECHNIQUES

OSTEOPATHY

Osteopathy was the first structural or manipulative therapy. Osteopathy contends that when spinal problems exist, biochemical changes occur which interfere with normal nerve transmission and circulation. This affects not only the muscles and skeleton but also the circulation and all the organs of the body. Osteopathy was developed by Dr. Andrew Taylor Still, a physician from Missouri, and the first college of osteopathy was established in Missouri in 1897.

The *interdependence between structure and function* is the basis of osteopathic work; if the structure of the body is abnormal in any way, then the function also becomes altered. Osteopaths believe that abnormalities in spinal structure cause the arteries to become pressed as they leave the spine; chiropractors hold that it is the nerves that are being pressed. Osteopathy does not concern itself with just the spine; all parts of the body are studied. Osteopaths emphasize the rib cage as well as the thoracic and pelvic diaphragms in respiratory and digestive problems.

Dr. Still's system is not just a system of manipulation; it also takes into consideration diet and other natural measures to help balance the body. However, osteopaths believe that health cannot be restored without correcting anatomical abnormalities.

CHIROPRACTIC

Chiropractic work is based on the theory that when the vertebrae of the spine are not in alignment an unlimited amount of symptoms can occur. Chiropractic was developed by Dr. David Palmer and was practiced in the U.S. as early as 1895. Palmer believed that misaligned spinal segments interfere with the passage of vital forces or nerve impulses. Manual adjustments of parts of the spine promote the health of the tissues supplied by the appropriate nerves. Chiropractors use the term *adjustment* rather than manipulation because it suggests a discriminatory approach. Some chiropractors use a rapid manual thrust aimed at inducing a sudden force across an individual joint, causing the release of a fixed and immobile joint.

The spine needs to be kept *moving and aligned* for the vital energy to flow. If the energy in the spine is stagnant, the life force is lost. Chiropractic works with the 31 pairs of spinal nerves which travel with an artery and a vein. The nervous system is the communicator which uses electrical energy to send impulses to the blood. Blockages in the spine thus affect our entire being since blood carries nutrients to the body.

Chiropractic has become more scientifically oriented with colleges throughout the world. Although it is licensed in the United States and included in health insurance, there is still much controversy between chiropractors and traditional medical practitioners who consider chiropractic unorthodox.

CRANIO-SACRAL THERAPY

Cranio-sacral therapy manipulates the skull bones so that they move in sync with one another, allowing the cerebrospinal fluid to circulate freely. During the manipulation process, practitioners of cranio-sacral therapy remove the stresses that accumulate in the membranes supporting the brain and spinal column.

All of the bruises and blows to our head we have ever received, including the birth process, have probably pushed some of the skull bones out of alignment so that they move improperly. This interferes with the quality of our energy and often gives us headaches and other problems related to the *temporo mandibular joint* (TMJ).

A cranio-sacral therapist holds the skull gently in her/his hands and attunes her/himself to the rhythm of the individual patient. With gentle movements, s/he begins her/his balancing work. It may consist of rebalancing the fluid or balancing the bones. The treatment is very relaxing to the patient, who may doze off or go into a deep state of consciousness.

Two pioneers in this work have been Dr. James Sutherland and Dr. John Upledger. Dr. Sutherland experimented by wrapping his head with bandages so that his skull bones could not move. In so doing, he found an immediate change in the function of respiration. He felt that the cranial respiratory system was the primary one with the skull designed to expand and contract. He concluded that restrictions in the cranio-sacral rhythm may be implicated in conditions such as migraines and depression.

Dr. John Upledger has a school where he teaches cranio-sacral therapy. Most of his students are physical therapists, chiropractors, M.D.'s and D.O.'s (doctors of osteopathy).

A cranio-sacral therapy session takes 45 minutes to an hour. It has proven effective in relieving migraine headaches, ringing in the ears, and TMJ-related joint pain. Many problems in other parts of the body have also been helped by this therapeutic method.

TECHNIQUES INVOLVING DEEP TISSUE WORK

ROLFING

Rolfing, also known as structural integration, was developed by Dr. Ida Rolf in the 1930s. It is not just massage but a technique of freeing the body, mind, and emotions from their conditioning. Dr. Rolf believes that muscular imbalance in the body can be a shield or armoring protecting a person from certain deep hurts that have occurred throughout her/his life. These armorings or tense areas pull on the body, causing a limitation of movement and rigidity. The body's rigid patterns reflect mental and emotional attitudes.

Another important concept in rolfing is that of gravity. Distortion of the body is accentuated by gravity. The practice of rolfing involves the loosening and lengthening of specific muscles and the fascia(the envelope of connective tissue which houses muscles, tendons, ligaments, nerves, etc.). Misalignments, which may have been distorted by previous accidents or illness, by fear and other conditioning, thus resume their normal functions.

A rolfing treatment usually involves 10 sessions. The first seven sessions work on removing old patterns of stress and relating to the world through the freeing of specific muscles and connective tissue. The focus of the last three sessions is to integrate the loosened body into new patterns of movement. As old muscle patterns are broken up, tensions and resistance surface and the individual experiences fixed attitudes from childhood and other emotions which have kept her/him bound up. Then s/he is free to change these habitual ways of thinking and to adopt new perspectives.

ASTON PATTERNING

Aston patterning is a combination of bodywork with movement. Judith Aston began working with Ida Rolf in doing deep tissue work. Then she added her own ideas which relate to what she terms the "asymmetrical movements of our bodies." She felt that bodies moved like spirals in space, not straight. Each person has her/his own unique pattern of movement.

In Aston patterning, the practitioner looks for areas of tension in the body and maps these on a body chart. Then, each person stands and moves; a videotape is made to show her/him how s/he is walking and moving. The bodywork involves connective tissue massage with gentle strokes that move the tissue in an asymmetrical spiral.

REICHIAN THERAPY

Wilhelm Reich was an Austrian-born disciple of Sigmund Freud who believed that the body's energy, which he called *orgone*, could be trapped in muscular contractions, which he referred to as the *armor* of the body. Reich's aim in breaking chronic muscular armoring was to permit the release of repressed emotions and to re-establish the free flow of orgone. With the flow re-established, he believed the individual could experience an *orgasm reflex*, a spontaneous pulsation of the entire body at the time of orgasm, allowing full energetic discharge.

Today there are many Reichian-based therapies; the two most practiced are orgonomy and bioenergetics.

An *orgonomy session* consists of a patient lying on a couch (usually in underwear or a thin gown), discussing the present issues in her/his life. The patient is encouraged to do some deep breathing. Afterwards, there could be some work on the body armor from the head to the pelvis, combined with emotional release and discussion.

The long-range goal of orgonomy is to reach *genitality*, which is defined as "the ability to be what you would have been if the world hadn't interfered with your mental development."[1]

Bioenergetics was developed by Alexander Lowen, a pupil of Wilhelm Reich. Lowen used breathing techniques, body postures, and exercise to help people become aware of their patterns of tension. Bioenergetics deals with the relationship between somatic functions and psychological trauma. It seeks to bring about a healthy integration of body and mind so that energy is freed for pleasure rather than used in a defensive manner. The techniques utilized work on releasing physical tensions while dealing with psychological problems.

Three areas included in bioenergetics work are grounding, breathing, and character structure. *Grounding* is related to emotional security and personal authority. To be in a particular stance with feet firmly on the ground allows the energy to flow. Where one has problems of insecurity or problems with authority, there will be difficulty grounding.

Breathing patterns are unconsciously established over the years and caused by chronic muscle tension, often due to emotional suffering. Developing a loose and flowing breathing pattern charges the body with energy and releases many old physical patterns.

Character structure is the third aspect of bioenergetics. The system divides the personality into five different types and relates certain emotional patterns to muscular patterns as well as the way the body is held. Through getting in touch with these emotions and breaking them up, a new way of body posturing evolves.

TECHNIQUES THAT WORK WITH ELECTROMAGNETIC ENERGY

Perhaps the most exciting kinds of body therapies are those techniques that deal with electromagnetic energy, seeking to polarize the various electrical currents in the body. The system of meridians or lines of force running through the body derives from ancient Oriental systems of healing. Each meridian is connected to one of the vital organs. Each organ is also connected to another organ in another part of the body by reflex action, setting up a polarity. These body therapies deal with the *chi* energy (also called *prana*, universal life force). Illness is created through stagnation of the flow of chi energy. When the chi is made to flow again, the body heals itself. The body receives chi energy through the air we breathe, the food we eat, and everything visible and invisible in our environment, including our thoughts. Acupressure, acupuncture, shiatsu, polarity therapy, jin shinn, and reflexology are all techniques that work with balancing the chi energy. Various pressure points along the meridians of the body are used to release bottled-up energy and muscular tension.

ACUPUNCTURE AND ACUPRESSURE

Acupressure applies finger pressure to the *tsubos* (points along the meridians where the energy flows may become blocked), whereas acupuncture uses needles under the skin. Acupuncture is utilized for chronic conditions and for treating diseases of the internal organs. It is also used as an anesthetic by some surgeons in China. Acupressure is used for aches and pains, menstrual cramps, preventing colds and flu, treating headaches and backaches, and generally boosting the energy level. (Acupuncture is used for these conditions as well; some people may prefer one or the other.) If a point is sore, it indicates a blockage of chi. By stimulating that point, chi is released and the soreness usually disappears. With acupressure, pressure is generally applied for five seconds, and then released for five seconds. While the points are being pressed, the patient should do some deep breathing to release the energy.

SHIATSU

Shiatsu is the Japanese method of stimulating the flow of chi. Shiatsu practitioners use a combination of fingers (mostly thumbs), elbows and knees to press the points. There is also stroking and twisting of the body, much like regular massage. Shiatsu and acupressure release muscular tension, enabling the blood to flow freely; an increase of circulation brings more oxygen to affected areas.

POLARITY THERAPY

Polarity therapy was developed by Dr. Randolph Stone, who wrote many books as a result of extensive travel and research in India. Polarity therapy is based on the balancing of energy circuits and fields within the body. Dr. Stone classifies anatomical relationships as positive and negative polarities. He also deals with the elements—Earth, Air, Fire, and Water—and has designed charts for the energy flow of each element in the body.

A polarity treatment involves subtle finger pressure on various areas of the body. The polarity therapist usually starts out by standing behind the head of the person and later moves to the feet. Gentle manipulations are also included. Dr. Stone wrote much about structural balance, especially regarding the sacrum, the bone at the base of the spine housing the *kundalini* energy (the basic root of the vital force or power for each individual).

In addition, polarity therapy involves instruction on diet; Dr. Stone's diet involves a fairly balanced vegetarian menu incorporating dairy products and eliminating eggs.

JIN SHINN

Jin shinn has two forms—jin shin jitsu, which was developed by Jiro Murai in Japan, and jin shin do. Its basis is the synchronization of pulses utilizing the eight extra meridians of the acupuncture meridian system. (Acupuncture, acupressure, shiatsu and other techniques use the organ meridian system of healing energies and include two of the extra meridians. Jin shinn uses eight.)

The 12 organ meridians are like rivers or streams, with the eight extra meridians like reservoirs or lakes. When the river becomes full, it spills into the reservoir; when deficient, it draws from it, offering a system of checks and balances. The chi or vital energy flows through these channels; when the flow becomes stagnant, an imbalance results, creating stress or tension, and eventually illness. Jin shinn releases this stagnation by using these eight meridians within a system of 26 to 30 pressure points. Instead of the heavier pressures used in acupressure and shiatsu, jin shinn uses a pulse-taking pressure and works through clothing. When necessary, jin shinn can avoid physical contact, using the hands over a particular area to remove pain. As the energies are unblocked and made to flow, the body can then heal itself.

REFLEXOLOGY

The principles behind reflexology or zone therapy were known in ancient China and used by some American Indian tribes.

Eunice D. Ingram systematized the techniques and brought them to the American public. Reflexology states that whenever an organ is out of balance, the corresponding reflex in the feet will be very tender. As one releases tension by working on the reflex points in the feet, the blood supply returns to that organ.

There are 10 zones which divide the body longitudinally. The hands have the same reflexes as the feet and can be used instead of the feet. There are also cross reflexes linking shoulder and hip, elbow and knee, hands and feet. The pressure applied to the reflex points varies according to the age of the person being treated and her/his sensitivity. By working on these points, the energy begins to flow in each organ, increasing the chi or vital force.

SENSUAL AND RELAXING MASSAGE TECHNIQUES

SWEDISH MASSAGE

When most people talk about massage, they generally mean Swedish massage. Peter Long of Sweden developed a system of massage strokes that integrates ancient Oriental techniques with more modern principles of anatomy and physiology. The system was introduced into the United States by Dr. S. W. Mitchell.[2]

Swedish massage emphasizes several basic strokes applied to the soft tissue of the body, often quite vigorously. There are many benefits of this type of massage. It helps improve circulation by encouraging the movement of blood through the veins toward the heart. It aids in balancing the musculature, relieving tensions in the body and soreness in the shoulders, neck, and back. Massage also has a tranquillizing effect on the central nervous system. It enables people to become aware of where tensions exist in the body and how to prevent them. Massage can loosen up emotional blocks and help one to deal with these emotions once they are brought to the surface.

LOMI-LOMI

Lomi-lomi is a type of massage practiced by the Hawaiian Kahunas. (*Kahuna* means "keepers of the secret.") It incorporates techniques like Swedish massage combined with some manipulation, as in chiropractic and osteopathy, and also the laying on of hands. Lomi-lomi practitioners use their elbows and forearms as well as hands. Today, most of the practitioners of lomi-lomi focus more on massage techniques and not so much on the more subtle aspects.

TECHNIQUES THAT WORK WITH THE SUBTLE BODIES

LAYING ON OF HANDS

Throughout the ages, people have been healed simply through touch, through the energy of love that is channeled through the hands. Anyone is capable of doing this, especially to their loved ones or ones they feel close to. Some people have a natural gift for channeling heat through their hands and tuning in to the blocks in the being. There are many techniques that have been developed to utilize the energy of touching.

REIKI

Reiki ("universal life energy" in Japanese) is an ancient form of natural healing involving the laying on of hands. Reiki treatments follow the energy flows in the body; the practitioner acts as a channel for the energy using his hands as electrodes.

To learn reiki, you need to study with a master. There are seven levels or degrees in reiki training in the West; as one becomes more proficient, s/he may study further and attain another degree. In the United States, reiki training is known as The Radiance Technique and is being promoted by Barbara Weber Ray, Ph.D., in Santa Monica.[3] Reiki works on the level of the subtle body to remove physical, emotional, and spiritual blocks.

THERAPEUTIC TOUCH

Therapeutic touch, developed by Dr. Dolores Kreiger of New York University, is another way of transmitting energy through the laying on of hands. The technique has four phases; the first is to center oneself physically and psychologically; the second is to exercise the sensitivity of the hand to assess the energy field of the patient; third, to mobilize the areas in the patient's energy field that the healer perceives as congested or blocked; and the fourth is directing the healer's energy to help the patient repattern her/his own energy. Therapeutic touch uses sweeping motions to cleanse the aura of the body before working on specific areas.

Immediate effects of therapeutic touch are relaxation and pain relief. It has been helpful in working with those who are continuously depressed and those who are terminally ill.

NOTES

1. John Feltman, ed., *Hands-on Healing* (Emmaus, PA: Rodale Press, Inc., 1989), p. 258.
2. Ibid., p. 282.
3. Ibid., p. 132.

___

EXERCISE

Physical exercise is one of the most important ingredients in maintaining health and balance. The amount of exercise affects metabolism, digestion, circulation, and all other bodily processes. Remaining sedentary for extensive time periods leads to a sluggish metabolism, poor digestion, and impaired circulation. Exercise helps the body to burn off toxins as well as assimilate important minerals like calcium, magnesium, and iron.

Exercise has many functions; one of its primary functions is to *stretch* and *reshape the body*. There are several types of exercise that stretch the body—Hatha yoga, gymnastics, dance, as well as Feldenkrais and Alexander work which also help to reshape the body. Another function of exercise is to *increase vital force*. Aerobic exercise (which includes running, jogging, aerobic dance and aerobic walking) increases the heart rate and circulation, thereby warming the body. The martial arts strengthen the vital force through focusing and working with the breath.

There are many forms of exercise available. Individual and team sports like tennis, basketball, racquetball, golf, and swimming have been popular throughout the years. Many of our ancient cultures, such as the Greeks, Romans, and Mayans, held games which were not just vehicles for exercise but also a means to re-enact certain deep truths and higher wisdom. The Sioux Indians also had a game (called Tapa Wanka Yap, the "throwing of the ball") in which the presence of the Great Spirit was revealed to the players. China, Japan, and Korea developed the martial arts which focus on mastering higher states of consciousness as well as developing physical prowess. In Tibet there were walks which lasted for many days and nights that were used to attain elevated mental states.

Exercise is also a way of *appreciating nature*; hiking, swimming, canoeing, and sailing enable one to connect with the forces of nature and become invigorated through this interchange of energy.

Recently, many forms of exercise have been introduced into the Western world from the East to develop higher states of awareness through the use of physical disciplines. The most popular of these are the various yoga systems from India and tai chi from China, as well as the martial arts—aikido, karate, and judo—from the Orient.

YOGA

Yoga itself is a philosophy that encompasses physical, mental, emotional, and spiritual disciplines. It is a system of conscious evolution or self-improvement. There are five forms of yoga—Gnana (spiritual), Raja (mental), Bhakti (emotional), Karma (social responsibility), and Hatha (physical). Hatha yoga has become increasingly popular in the West. It includes various physical postures along with breathing exercises (*pranayama*), and some stress on diet, cleansing (*kriyas*) and meditation. The aim of Hatha yoga is relaxation and balance of spirit, mind, and body.

The *asanas*, or yoga postures, are not exercises; they stretch the muscles and work on balancing the spine, endocrine system, and autonomic nervous system. Pranayama, or breathing which is done along with yoga, is controlled breathing in which there is a constant ratio between the number of breaths inhaled, retained, and exhaled. The kriyas include cleansing of the nasal passages, stomach, and bowel areas with water, cotton, or rubber tubes.

TAI CHI CHU'AN

Tai chi chu'an or tai chi (tai = "great" or "original," chi = "force" or "energy," and chu'an = "fist" or "boxing") is a series of flowing movements which imitate movements of nature such as birds, animals, clouds, and wind. The movements are used to restore vitality while maintaining a deep state of inner consciousness. They are designed to help the *chi* or energy flow through the organs, thus preventing any energy blocks and disease states.

MARTIAL ARTS

There are many forms of martial arts—aikido, judo, karate, kung fu—but their essence is similar. Weaponless forms of combat existed in China back in the days of Huang Ti, the "Yellow Emperor," whose army used them in battle as long ago as 2674 B.C.[1] Most scholars believe that the ancient precursor of the martial arts was developed by Bodidharma, who also originated Zen Buddhism. He was an Indian monk who arrived in China about 520 A.D.[2]

Some of the sources that led to the martial arts are ancient Indian and Chinese weaponless fighting, Buddhism and its non-violent philosophy, yoga exercises and movements, I-Ching and its principles of harmonizing with change, and Taoism and its respiratory techniques. The Taoists began exercises with deep in-and-out breathing exercises designed to stimulate circulation.

The martial arts were originally called *kung fu* in China. (*Kung* means "master" and *fu* means "man," so kung fu is a master of man.) *Karate* developed in Okinawa in the 17th century as an outgrowth of the Japanese subjugation of the island and the prohibition of weapons.[3] (*Kara te* means "empty hand.") *Aikido* developed in Japan along with Zen Buddhism about 800 years ago; it includes tactics with swords and spears. *Judo* is an outgrowth of the ancient art of *jujitsu*, which was created by Professor Jigoro Kan in 1882 in Japan.

The object of the martial arts is to defend oneself and overcome another without any use of weapons but through mastery of many movements or forms along with one's own skill and resourcefulness. A student of any of the martial arts is gradually taught these stances and then works with a partner in developing her/his strength. Breath is an important part of the training since deep breathing empties the mind of thought and allows the *chi* to flow through the body. The body is kept very soft and relaxed through deep breathing until the moment of impact, and then specific sets of muscles are contracted. One aim of the martial arts is to acquire the ability to focus all one's energy on an isolated area of the body and then relax it again.

AEROBIC EXERCISE

Aerobic exercise makes the heart work more efficiently and increases the blood's oxygen-carrying capacity. When the heart is able to pump blood with less effort, it has more time to rest between beats. One is, therefore, able to exercise for longer periods without getting tired. The effect of aerobic exercise is to create new blood vessels, which helps to prevent heart disease when some of the existing arteries are clogged with plaque. Aerobic exercise also lengthens blood clotting time, lowers blood pressure and prevents gout by lowering uric acid levels.[4]

There are many types of aerobic exercise. The most common, generally referred to as "aerobics" or "aerobic dance," consists of exercises which are done to music that involve different movements of the legs and feet, arms and torso. Each set of exercises is repeated several times, and then the pace is increased. Usually there is a warm-up and various stretches before beginning the aerobics. Every few sets of exercises, one stops and checks her/his pulse rate. (To find one's "normal" pulse rate, assuming s/he is in good health, one subtracts her/his age from 220. This figure is multiplied by .075 to get the average pulse. The pulse is taken at the wrist or at the neck artery for 6 seconds and then multiplied by 10.) There is also a cooldown or simple stretches at the end of the series. A class in aerobics usually runs from 45 minutes to an hour.

"Aerobic dance" or "dance aerobics" may involve more complex steps and movements, but the principles are the same.

The most common forms of aerobic exercise are walking, jogging, and running. Aerobic walking is walking at a faster pace until one has her/his heart rate increased to where s/he wants it. Then more miles may be added at the same rate. From walking, one often begins jogging. Joggers need to do warm-up stretches, especially for the knees, which are a sensitive area. They also need to wear the right kind of shoes. Jogging and running can provide a tremendous release of tension, as well as a kind of euphoria or high. They increase the flow of *epinephrine* (often mistaken for adrenaline), a hormone that causes a surge of energy to the brain. Another exercise that may be done aerobically is swimming. One swims so many laps in a certain amount of time in order to increase the heart rate.

ALEXANDER TECHNIQUE

The Alexander technique (which takes its name from F. Matthias Alexander) is not a series of exercises as such but rather the creation of a new awareness in breaking old habit patterns and becoming more conscious of the way we stand, walk, and carry our bodies. The posture of many individuals places a strain on the heart, lungs, digestive organs, and certain muscles. To learn to adapt to a different posture takes much time but ultimately frees the body as well as the mind and emotions. Working with this technique, individuals have achieved lower blood pressure, deeper states of relaxation, and increased mental alertness.

FELDENKRAIS WORK

Moshe Feldenkrais had similar ideas to Alexander. He saw that muscle tension was related to neurological functioning and that in order to break old physical habit patterns a reprogramming of the brain was necessary. Feldenkrais worked individually with people and also designed specific exercises to create an awareness of the way we stand, walk, and move. This system of body therapy, exercise, and movement is also known as Functional Integration.

Feldenkrais believed that stress causes muscular reaction in the body, which often leads to serious structural problems and disease. By reprogramming the mind along with the body, these patterns can be changed and a more relaxed and balanced state may emerge.

DANCE THERAPY

Through the ages, dance has provided a release of physical and emotional energies and has opened the door to more transcendent states of consciousness. In Asia there are the trance dances of Bali; in the Arabic countries, the Whirling Dervishes; in Africa and Native American culture, all-night dance dramas performed with drums and other instruments.

Western therapeutic dance was started by Rudolph Laban (1879-1959). He started with theater dance in Germany, but then fled to England during the war where he worked with freer movements to create better emotional and mental states. Dance therapy is used with many psychiatric patients to help them express their emotions and achieve a better balance between mind and body.

NOTES

1. W. Scott Russell, *Karate: The Energy Connection* (New York: Delacorte Press, 1976), p. 21.
2. Ibid., p. 20.
3. Ibid., p. 26.
4. Nathan Pritikin, *Pritikin Program for Diet & Exercise* (New York: Bantam Books, 1979), p. 69.

MENTAL AND
SPIRITUAL THERAPIES

In order for total healing to occur, it is important that the mind be trained in various techniques so that it can control and direct the body in a conscious way. The spirit in reality is the higher mind, and as one learns to reach the deeper levels of the mind (alpha and theta brain waves), a connection with the higher mind or spiritual self begins to develop.

Meditation techniques show us how to open up to these deeper states of consciousness. *Autogenics* serves to relax the body so that we may enter these higher mental states. *Biofeedback* teaches us how to monitor brain waves in order to ascertain when we have accessed alpha and theta waves. *Visualization* enables us to work with images to influence our thought processes and bodily functions. *Hypnosis,* now referred to as hypnotherapy, is a process where a therapist guides us into a deep state of consciousness and then works with guided imagery to change old habit patterns and break up mental and emotional programming.

RELAXATION

Relaxation involves withdrawing the mind and body from external stimulation in order to reach deeper levels of consciousness. The aim in relaxation is to induce a light trance; in this state the brain operates at the frequency of 8-12 cycles per second (alpha waves), which is much slower than our normal beta waves.

In his book *The Relaxation Response* (Avon Books, 1976), Dr.

Herbert Benson was the first to discuss the purposes of relaxation in medicine and healing. Relaxation is necessary in order for meditation and visualization to occur.

AUTOGENICS

Autogenics was developed by the German psychiatrist Johannes Schultz in the 1920s; his work is in seven volumes edited by Wolfgang Luthe. Specific exercises are used which induce states of deep physiological and mental relaxation.

Having worked with hypnosis, Schultz noticed that people in a hypnotic trance experienced certain physical sensations—a feeling of heaviness in the limbs and torso as well as a feeling of warmth in the limbs. He, therefore, designed specific exercises to induce these conditions where the individual would be in a passive state, not exercising conscious will. After these preliminary exercises have been mastered, specific exercises can be taught to deal with certain organic diseases such as asthma, injuries, and other conditions.

The six specific exercises are done in a sequence. The first is to imagine that the right arm is heavy; the second is to feel warmth in the arms and legs; the third is to feel the heart beat calm and regular; the fourth focuses on breathing; the fifth warms the solar plexus; and the sixth cools the forehead. Schultz and Luthe were careful that inappropriate visualization not occur; for example, imaging the stomach area warm with a patient suffering from gastric disturbances.

Autogenics has been successful in causing physical changes in blood pressure, blood sugar, heart rate, hormone secretion, brain waves, and white blood cell count.

After achieving physical relaxation, the individual can advance to the more subtle psychological aspects of autogenic training through which higher states of consciousness may be developed as well as a marked degree of autonomic control. Feats similar to that of Eastern yogis have been reported, such as self-anesthetization against a third-degree burn produced by a lighted cigarette on the back of a hand. The appeal of autogenic training to many Westerners is that it begins on an easily understandable level and slowly progresses to a more esoteric state.

MEDITATION

Meditation is not just relaxation, though it produces certain marked physiological effects, such as slowing down the breath and reduced oxygen consumption. Meditation is a way of clearing the mind so all the ripples on the surface dissipate and one can begin to see into the depths. This clearing results in calmness and stillness, making one's perceptions more acute.

When the mind is able to loosen its hold on moral and social judgments and can begin to perceive natural law and harmony, one is able to tap into her/his own creative flow. By expressing this creativity, we can maintain a constant state of physical and emotional well-being.

There are many techniques that are helpful in entering a meditative state. Focusing on a single image such as a candle or a mandala is a simple one; repeating a sound is another easy method; this is done in many Hindu practices where there may be several different sounds or patterns of sounds referred to as a *mantra*. Most commonly, concentration is centered on the ebb and flow of breath as one sits in a certain position without moving. Meditation improves concentration, and in time, can lead to experiences that are deeply spiritual.

Physical benefits of meditation have been well documented. In his book *The Relaxation Response* (Avon Books, 1976), Dr. Benson showed that meditation tends to lower or normalize blood pressure, pulse rate, and the levels of stress hormone in the blood. It also produces changes in brain-wave patterns. In 1976, a research study was conducted by Gurucharan Singh Khalso, founder of Boston's Kundalini Research Institute. The study was conducted at the Veterans Administration Hospital in La Jolla, California and showed that regular yoga and meditation increased blood levels of three important immune-system hormones by 100 per cent.[1] In 1980, psychologist Alberto Villoldo of San Francisco State College showed that meditation and self-healing visualization improved white blood cell response and the efficiency of hormone response to a standard test of physical stress—immersing one arm in ice water. Those trained in meditation withstood the pain of the test better than those who did not meditate.[2]

VISUALIZATION

Visualization is an important technique for healing that evolved out of meditative states. The ability of the mind to bring forth positive images and to visualize the body as healed is very powerful. Visualization therapy was developed by Dr. Carl Simonton through his work and treatment of cancer patients. Dr. Simonton, working together with his wife Stephanie, had patients mentally picture their disease to see how their bodies were interacting with the treatment so they could hasten the recovery process. For example, he would have them visualize an army of healthy cells overcoming the cancer cells. Jeanne Achterberg, with her husband Frank Lawlis, continued and expanded the work of the Simontons, incorporating more spiritual imagery and not just aggressive visualizations of attacking cells. Jeanne has written a monumental book in the history and use of images in healing called *Imagery in Healing: Shamanism and Modern Medicine* (Shambhala Pubns., 1985).

Visualization is based on the body's lack of ability to distinguish between a physical and a mental experience. Dr. Bernie Siegel reports in his book *Love, Medicine and Miracles* (Harper & Row, 1990) that cancer survivors who worked with visualization had the ability to enter states of mind that enabled their bodies to perform like those of athletes. He mentions the work of psychologist Charles Garfield at the University of California Medical Center who noted similar techniques used by cancer survivors as by Soviet and Eastern European athletes enjoying success in the Olympics.[3]

Other tools like calming music or working with drawings or paintings may enhance the process of visualization. Dr. Bernie Siegel and Louise Hay have both been using guided visualization with many who are successfully healing themselves. (See Louise Hay's *You Can Heal Your Life* [Hay House, Inc., 1988]).

HYPNOSIS

Hypnosis is a state of consciousness whereby the critical factor of the mind, the left hemisphere of the brain, is put to sleep, allowing suggestions to be accepted and repressed memories recalled into consciousness.

Dr. James Braid (1795-1860), a Scottish physician who practiced in Manchester, England, published a book called *Neurypnology or The Rationale of Nervous Sleep.* In it he suggested that the combined state of physical relaxation and altered conscious awareness entered into by patients should be called *hypnosis* (from the Greek word *hypnos,* meaning "sleep").

Hypnosis has been especially important in the treatment of psycho-neuroses and in relieving pain. In 1958, the British Medical Association recommended that all doctors and medical students receive training in its application. A similar recommendation was made by the American Medical Association.

More modern forms of hypnosis, or hypnotherapy as it is now called, take the patient through some guided imagery, allowing her/him to choose her/his own images. This differs from the more authoritarian hypnotist who used his own suggestions and assumed total control. Jeanne Achterberg states that the more authoritarian hypnotist is akin to the shaman who would choose images for his patient. Whereas some people respond to that type of treatment more strongly, others need the freedom to choose their own images.

Achterberg also reports on evidence compiled by Dr. Howard Hall, a psychologist working at Pennsylvania State University. In experiments conducted with hypnosis and visualization on two age groups, the younger group showed significant increase in their lymphocyte count. This showed the effects of hypnosis in stimulating immune functioning.[4]

The reason that medical hypnosis has not become more widespread is that there are still fears concerning it. There is the fear of being unconscious and not remembering what has transpired in a session, divulging information that one does not want to share, and being unable to return to a "normal" state of consciousness after a session. The facts are that no one can be hypnotized against her/his will and that under hypnosis a patient is aware of what is happening at all times. Hypnosis is simply a deep state of consciousness, and one is able to return quickly to her/his normal state.

BIOFEEDBACK

Biofeedback is based on the principle that if we can learn to become aware of some body function of which we normally overlook, then we can learn to control that function. Technical biofeedback implies the use of sophisticated instruments that can measure brain-wave activity, blood pressure level, skin temperature, heart rate, etc.

Jeanne Achterberg reports that every clinical function that can be measured can be brought under control.[5]

The brain generates electrical rhythms which occur in four groups, each of which can be correlated with a state of awareness or particular brain activity.

1. *beta waves*—Beta waves are the normal working rhythm of the brain; they are faster and indicate more frenetic activity. A relaxed person shows very little beta.

2. *alpha waves*—Alpha waves are building blocks for higher levels of awareness. In conjunction with theta, they indicate a calming down or emptying of the mind, usually with physical relaxation.

3. *theta waves*—These occur during creative inspiration and meditation.

4. *delta waves*—This is the rhythm of sleep, but they are found in many people in response to new ideas.

Among those who pioneered biofeedback techniques were Elmer and Alyce Green, who wrote the definitive book, *Beyond Biofeedback* (Delta), in 1975. Biofeedback techniques were also pioneered by Dr. Joe Kamiya in San Francisco. He monitored a subject's alpha rhythms with an EEG (electroencephalogram) device. When alpha rhythms were being generated, a pleasant sound would be produced. Alpha was related to a feeling of well-being, and most subjects could learn to turn it on or off.

In addition to the EEG to measure brain waves, biofeedback also uses the ESR (electrical skin resistance meter), which indicates physical arousal and relaxation. This is connected to the palm of the hand, and the meter readings relate to the behavior of the autonomic system. The rate of blood flow varies with body tone and causes change of polarization of the sweat gland membranes. The polarization varies according to how tense or relaxed we are. The reactions which make us tense or relaxed are reflected in the "fight or flight" response or in the "relaxation response."

Stress increases the blood pressure and heart rate, the amount of muscle tension, and oxygen usage. Relaxation increases circulation to skin and organs and lowers heart rate and muscle tension.

Using the data from both the EEG machine and ESR device, beta rhythms and low skin resistance accompany panic states while alpha rhythms and high skin resistance indicate relaxed states. Separating physical and mental states is the purpose of many meditation techniques. Thus, we can have a relaxed body and an alert mind when we need to or an active body and a relaxed mind.

Biofeedback has been used effectively to teach subjects to control abnormal heart rhythms, to indicate stomach acidity in the case of ulcers, to control migraines and headaches, to help in retraining the muscles, and to benefit a wide range of diseases. Jeanne Achterberg states that those who are most successful in using biofeedback techniques are those who have a strong ability to visualize and those who are highly motivated.[6]

PAST LIFE THERAPY AND REGRESSION

Past life therapy is a general term that includes various techniques for accessing information from past lives and understanding how the emotional "root patterns" that we bring in with us correlate with patterns in other lifetimes. When we understand these roots, we can work further on our patterns this lifetime. The specific circumstances of the past life—time, place, and other details—are not important in themselves. It is the emotional patterns that we are trying to ascertain.

Regression to the past is one of the tools used by a therapist working with accessing past life information. The client is put into a deep meditative state through the use of relaxation and guided imagery techniques. The therapist or facilitator then takes the client through a process where the client describes places and people from a particular lifetime. Some individuals are able to do this easier than others. Many do not trust the information they are getting and feel it might be coming from their imagination.

In other types of past life therapy, the therapist tunes in to the information her/himself. S/he may be trained in various techniques that enable her/him to tune in to this. One technique uses a dowsing rod to determine the time, place, and circumstances of the lifetime; other techniques read the chakras or energy centers of the body. The therapist then shares the information s/he has accessed with the client. They then work together on how this information is relevant to the client's life now and what s/he can do to change old emotional patterns and habits. Even if the details of the lifetimes were not literally correct, they would still be a symbolic way for the individual to attune to her/his emotional patterns. This type of therapy is helpful in working out many blocks and in enabling an individual to transform old patterns of behavior.

NOTES

1. Bernie Siegel, M.D., *Love, Medicine, & Miracles* (New York: Harper & Row, 1990), p. 150.
2. Ibid.
3. Ibid., p. 153.
4. Jeanne Achterberg, *Imagery in Healing: Shamanism in Modern Medicine* (Boulder, CO: Shambhala Pubns., 1985), p. 196.
5. Ibid., p. 99.
6. Ibid., p. 101.

SUBTLE AND
VIBRATIONAL HEALING

Vibrational healing is the oldest form of healing on the planet. Primitive people used sounds and tones, colors and crystals, and both the essence and aroma of flowers and plants in their healing ceremonies. The present Holistic Health movement has reacquainted us with the principles of electromagnetic energy which surrounds our subtle bodies. *Acupuncture*, the ancient Chinese form of healing, utilizes the meridian system which conducts electrical energy to the organs. Many of the *body therapies* now being practiced—jin shin do, shiatsu, polarity therapy, and reiki—use this same energy.

Homeopathic medicine is based on the principle of vibration; remedies have little physical substance but carry the vibrational quality of the substance in a pellet or globule which has a milk sugar base.

Colors emit vibrations, ranging from infrared to ultraviolet. *Sounds* also have vibrations; each note of the scale vibrates at a different frequency. *Crystals and gems* are part of the mineral kingdom; different crystals have their own unique vibration according to which crystal family they belong, how they are cut and what size they are. *Flower essences and aromas* project vibrations, depending on the plants or flowers from which they are derived.

Vibrational medicines tend to manipulate subtle energy fields by directing energy into the body rather than manipulating cells and organs through physical substances like foods and vitamin supplements or through body adjustments or therapies.

One of the tools that has opened up the whole field of vibrational medicine is Kirlian photography. Through the use of electromagnetic apparatus, the film surface is charged, enabling the electrical energy or magnetic field surrounding the body (often called the "etheric body") to be photographed.

THE HIGHER BODIES AND THE CHAKRA SYSTEM

In addition to our physical body, we have six other bodies that are not visible but whose energy currents can be detected. (New technologies that enable us to make these bodies visible have not yet been refined.) The etheric body looks quite similar to the physical body on which it is superimposed. Within the etheric body is information which *guides the growth of the physical structure* of the body. It carries specifics on how the developing fetus is to unfold in utero and the data for growth and repair of the organism if disease occurs. The physical body is dependent on the etheric body for cellular guidance; if the etheric field becomes disturbed, physical disease follows.[1]

There are channels of energy which flow from the physical to the etheric body. These channels are synonymous with the meridian system in Chinese medicine; the points along these meridians are where the *chi* enters (called *prana* by the Hindus).

There are also centers of energy called *chakras* (wheels), which are whirling vortices of subtle energy. Chakras are involved with the flow of higher energy via energetic channels into the cellular structure of the physical body.[2] There are seven major chakras; each is associated with a major nerve plexus and a major endocrine gland. They are in a vertical line, ascending from the base of the spine to the head.

The chakras are connected to each other and to portions of the physical cellular structure via fine subtle energy channels known as *nadis*. The nadis parallel the nerves; there are about 72,000 nadis interwoven with the physical nervous system. The dysfunction of the chakras and nadis is associated with pathological changes in the nervous system.[3]

Above the etheric body is the *astral* or *emotional body*, which has its own set of chakras. Medical science has begun to see relationships between emotional stress and physical illness. The astral body is the seat of our desires, longings, fears, and appetites. The astral

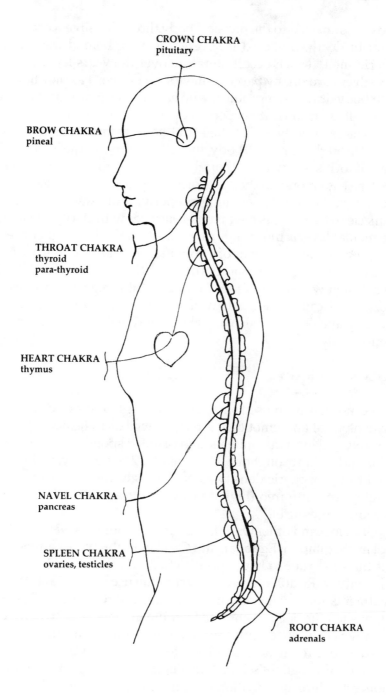

Chakras and Endocrine Glands

body is connected to the physical body through a silver cord. At the point of death, this cord is severed, leaving behind the physical etheric shell. (Much occult literature over the years has written of this silver cord; many psychics have seen this cord as they have left their body during sleep; others who have undergone what has come to be called "near death experiences" have also seen this cord.)

The next body above the astral body is known as the *mental body*. Through the mental body, the self experiences the intellect. Energetic forms known as "thought forms" originate in the mental body just as emotional thoughts originate on the astral level.[4] When the mental body is functioning properly, it allows individuals to think clearly and focus their mental energies with clarity. Healing at the mental level is more enduring than at the astral or etheric level.

Beyond the frequency of the mental body is the *causal body*. The causal body deals with concepts or ideas, the essence behind the details. When we want to program important things in our lives, we work on the causal plane. Many of the roots of disease stem from the causal plane. There is also a higher emotional body and a higher mental body.

COLOR THERAPY

Color has been used since ancient times for producing certain psychological and emotional effects as well as to heal and balance the body. All humans, animals, and plants respond to differences of color and light throughout the cycle of a 24-hour day. Color is related to atmospheric density as well as light though its spectrum, ranging from infrared (high density) to ultraviolet (subtle density and lower pressure).

In Tibet and other Oriental countries, color rays were used as a tool in meditation. Egyptian and Greek temples were painted various hues in order to have specific effects on their worshippers. In this century, Rudolf Steiner suggested the use of color and form as treatments for certain conditions. Dinshah P. Ghadali (1873-1966) established the Spectro-chrome Institute in Malaga, NJ where color therapy is combined with sound and rhythm and a color machine called a Spectro-chrome is utilized to beam the various colors onto portions of a patient's body. In England, the Hygeia studios in Gloucestershire use a color rhythm beamer developed by Theo Gimbel.

Color healing can be done in many ways—through beaming the colors onto the body in a special machine or through using a slide projector with various colored gels, by drinking colored water, by wearing certain colors or decorating our rooms with them, and through simply visualizing certain colors to surround the body or a certain part of it.

The meanings of the individual colors when used in healing are as follows:

Red is a warm color and, therefore, a stimulant. It improves circulation and stimulates the nervous system, which energizes the senses of sight, smell, taste, hearing, and touch. It also is used in cases of anemia since it increases the hemoglobin in the blood. It causes expulsion of toxins through the skin and may bring in skin redness, itching, and pimples until the cleansing is complete.

Scarlet is considered a brain as well as a kidney stimulant. It raises blood pressure by contracting the blood vessels. It also increases the heart rate and stimulates the menstrual function.

Orange is related to calcium and is used to treat calcium deficiencies as well as to build bones. It is also a lung builder and respiratory stimulant. As an anti-spasmodic, it is helpful for cramps and spasm. As a digestive stimulant, it relieves flatulence in the digestive tract. It stimulates the thyroid and depresses the parathyroids. It also stimulates the mammary glands to increase milk production and increases eliminative discharges, bringing boils and abscesses to a head.

Yellow stimulates the motor nervous system, which energizes the muscles. It stimulates the production of bile, thus acting as a laxative. It also helps to increase hydrochloric acid and pancreatic juices. Yellow depresses the spleen and is helpful in expelling worms and parasites.

Lemon is a blood purifier; it helps to eliminate mucus throughout the body and has been effective in treating colds. It builds bones through phosphorus and stimulates the brain and thymus area.

Green has been considered the master healer. It stimulates the pituitary (which in turn stimulates the other glands); dissolves blood clots; builds muscles, tissues and skin; destroys micro-organisms like germs and bacteria; and breaks up congestion and hardened cell masses.

Turquoise is an excellent tranquillizer; it is cooling and relaxing and helps headaches and swelling. It is also a skin tonic and rebuilds burned skin.

Blue is an antidote of red because of its cooling qualities. It relieves itching and irritation. It is used for fevers, fast pulse, and pain, and combats inflammatory conditions. Blue is also a stimulant to the pineal gland; it is a good antiseptic for bleeding of the lungs, dysentery, jaundice, cysts, burns, and bruises.

Indigo, a combination of blue and violet, is used to stimulate the parathyroids, depress the thyroid, purify the blood stream, and treat convulsions and nervous ailments, as well as bronchial, lung, and nasal disturbances. It is also a mammary depressant.

Violet stimulates the spleen and promotes production of white blood cells. It depresses the lymphatic glands and decreases muscular activity, including the heart. It also decreases the activity of the motor nervous system. Violet helps to maintain the sodium/potassium balance in the body. It is used for bladder trouble, overactive kidneys, neuralgia, nervous and mental disorders, and sciatica and skin problems. Violet is a good remedy for diarrhea and induces deep, relaxing sleep.

Purple increases the activity of the veins and lowers blood pressure by dilating the blood vessels and reducing the heart rate. It also drops body temperature and controls fever and high blood pressure. Purple is a kidney depressant and decreases sensitivity to pain, inducing relaxation and sleep.

Magenta, a combination of red and violet, is an important color for all heart disorders. It energizes the heart and stimulates the circulatory system and adrenal glands. It also helps to dissolve kidney stones as well as regulate blood pressure and arteries.

Various colors are found in the auras of individuals. The colors in the aura impart information concerning spiritual development as well as health and emotions. The major color indicating spiritual development seems to be stable, whereas the colors indicating physical health and emotional states appear to fluctuate. When the physical vitality is strong, the colors are clear. When the vitality is low, the colors may appear diluted; when fear, depression, or anxiety are present, they may be muddy.

The meanings of colors found in the aura are as follows:

white—purifying and uplifting, a symbol of wisdom and divine power, kindness, gentleness, and forgiveness
red—energy, strength, courage, vitality
pink—universal love, warmth, companionship, artistry
orange—thoughtfulness, consideration, leadership, wisdom, energy, balance
yellow—health of body and mind, optimism
blue—inspiration, artistry, a harmonious nature. Deep blue shows a high degree of spirituality, serenity, and wisdom. Blue mixed with black or brown indicates depression.
green—abundance, healing, cooperation, serenity, faith
aqua or turquoise—peace, healing; a high vibration
purple—ability to deal with practical or worldly matters
violet and indigo—spirituality
gray—illness, grief, sorrow, loss
brown—earthiness, industriousness, organizational ability
black—depression; a low vibration

MUSIC THERAPY

The healing qualities of music have been known from earliest times. Paracelsus used music to cure a variety of mental, emotional, and physical ailments. He prescribed special compositions for certain illnesses in accordance with the law of vibrations.

Music therapy is now being used to heal many psychiatric patients, handicapped children, and in less severe cases, to transform various emotions such as pain, fear, depression, and anxiety.

After World War I, some experiments were conducted by Margaret Anderton, a musician and nurse, among wounded Canadian soldiers. She found that it was most beneficial to administer music for any form of war neurosis, which was predominantly mental, but have the person himself produce the music in orthopedic cases or paralysis.[5] She reported that memories were brought back to men suffering from amnesia, insanity departed, and paralyzed muscles were restored.

Experiments have also been performed with the human voice at the New York State Hospital for the Insane on Ward's Island. They have shown that a tired brain and nerves were soothed by song and that vocal music was more effective than instrumental music in treating the insane.[6]

Harriet Ayes Seymour, chairman of the music division of the Hospital Visiting Committee of New York, is also a pioneer in music therapy. She has compiled a list of various medical prescriptions for different ailments.[7]

Dr. Paul Nordoff, an American composer, and Clive Robbins, a special educator working with handicapped children, used music therapy with autistic, mongoloid, and brain-damaged children. The therapy which they developed has been used at a hospital in London for "sub-normal" children. When working with an individual child, the therapist improvises vocally and at the piano to try to present the child with an experience of her/his mood—frustration, rage, or anxiety. The child is encouraged to respond on percussion instruments, on the piano, or with her/his own voice.[8]

Music in certain keys proves beneficial in various types of emotional and mental states. Music therapy aims to quiet the mind and re-establish the natural balance of the individual. For example, compositions in the scale of F and F-sharp are grounding; in certain esoteric systems, F is considered the key relating to Earth. There are many systems of musical correspondence to color and to astrological signs.

TONING

Another modern form of music therapy is toning, originated by Laurel Keyes. The tone of a person's voice is indicative of her/his state of health; if a person is whiny or has a gasping sound, s/he is often ill and feeling discouraged and hopeless. S/he draws to her/himself negative conditions by the voice's sound. Another type of tone might carry hostility and resentment, so the individual constantly attracts fighting into her/his life.

Toning involves a cleansing of the whole being and a tuning in of the higher self as to what one is really feeling and experiencing. To tone, one stands with eyes closed, relaxing the jaws and letting the sounds come out. One may groan or sigh or express her/his feelings verbally. Toning stimulates the energy flowing in the body. (The phrase we use is "body tone.") One may do toning along with certain exercises like yoga or stretching.

Toning can also be done in groups for healing. One of the objectives of toning groups has been to send healing to those in need of it. The effects have been quite dramatic, and there are many case histories of those who have been healed through toning.[9] A nurse who had been a diabetic with uremic poisoning and multiple sclerosis for years came to see Laurel Keyes with her sister. Laurel and her sister toned for her for 20 minutes. She experienced a real breakthrough of sobbing and understanding what was going on in her body. As she began to tone for herself, the uremic condition cleared up, her vision improved, and the multiple sclerosis was halted.[10]

HEALING WITH CRYSTALS AND GEMS

Crystals and gems have been used in many ancient cultures for various types of healing. In Egypt, the Ebers Papyrus recommends the use of certain astringent substances such as lapis lazuli as ingredients for eye salves. Hematite, an iron oxide, was used for checking hemorrhages and reducing inflammation. Later, the potency of these gems was enhanced by engraving the images of certain gods on them. In Roman times, Pliny compiled material on gems, categorizing them by color and constitution as to which diseases they could cure. A distinction was made between the talismanic quality of stones for the cure and prevention of disease and the medicinal use of them as mineral substances. In the former case, they were simply worn on the person, while in the latter, they were ground in water or some other liquid.

Some stones were prized for their variety; others, because certain planetary and spiritual influences were latent in them. The symbolism of color also was important in recommending particular stones for diseases. *Red stones*, like the ruby, garnet, carnelian and bloodstone, were considered remedies for hemorrhages and inflammatory diseases. This was based upon the principle of like curing like. *Yellow stones* were prescribed for bilious disorders, jaundice and other diseases of the liver. Stones of *green hue* relieved diseases of the eye due to the beneficial influence exerted by this color upon sight. The lapis lazuli, sapphire, and other *blue stones* were believed to counteract the spirits of darkness and invoke the aid of the spirits of light and wisdom. *Amethyst* was said to counteract the effects of indulgence in intoxicating beverages.

Gemstones have been used for healing both externally and internally. Externally, they are either worn directly on the body or in a setting of a precious metal like gold or silver. They may be placed on the affected area of the body or on one of the chakras. They may also be held in the hand and used on the affected area.

Gemstones were also worn in the form of talismans for healing. The stones were engraved with a symbol or figure at a certain time of the day and month when various planetary forces were operative to give maximum benefit to the wearer. The Star of David, the pyramid, the ankh, and the cross were common symbols since they carried a certain vibratory character in addition to the stone's.

Internally, they can be used in a number of ways. In Europe, they were pulverized and small amounts were mixed in wine or some other liquid and drunk. Ayurvedic physicians in India used the ashes of the gemstones which had been pulverized in preparing special medicines. A less expensive way to use them is to place the stone in liquid, alcohol or water for several days and then drink it. This liquid contains the vibrations of the particular stone. One way to do this is to place the stone and some liquid in the sunlight for several days and then use this as a mother tincture for making future remedies.

Crystals can amplify energy and have been used for their amplification qualities in various types of healing. Different shapes were important for healing purposes. Circular, square, and triangular shapes were faceted in specific forms and numbers. The odd number of facets were used for particular diseases, while the even numbers were used for those already on the road to recovery.

Physicians prescribed energy crystals to treat various ailments and to raise the vibrations of the bodies themselves. Color played an important role. *Lavender* crystals were used for treating cancer. *Aqua* crystals were used to treat bone disease. *White* ones were used for the eyes. *Green* crystals were used for the internal organs, such as the liver, kidney, and pancreas. The shape of the crystal was also important in determining the direction of energy flow.

Presently, the use of crystals in healing is being revived. Many healers find that since crystals carry electromagnetic energy they amplify the energy field and can be placed on the body during massage and other work. A child receiving third-degree burns on her legs was healed by the use of a crystal and therapeutic touch. The red areas started to shrink, all of the blisters disappeared, and then a filmy substance covered the burn area.[11]

A description of the most important gems and their uses follows.

AMETHYST: The amethyst has long been associated with royalty because of its purple regal color. It has the ability to purify and amplify all healing rays. It draws to it the forces being directed to a particular body and is able to repel those vibrations which the body does not need. It is extremely helpful in treating thrombosis or a clot in the vein which needs to be dissolved.

BLOODSTONE: Bloodstone is a member of the chalcedony family; it is a deep green stone with bright splotches of red jasper in it and has been associated with mysticism in India, where much of it is mined. It has been used to staunch hemorrhages and to prevent nosebleed. It affects the kundalini center strongly and has long been used to move energy up and down the spine and to align the centers.

CARNELIAN: Carnelian is a translucent chalcedony that is red to orange in color. It is thought to be the stone referred to as "sardius" in the Bible (Revelations 21:20) and the stone in the breastplate of the high priest called "sard" or "odem." Carnelian is used to remove lethargy for those who are lazy, languid, and inactive. It causes a release in the individual so that energy can be focused outward. It is also helpful in stimulating the liver to throw off impurities.

CORAL: Coral is an important gem since it is a gift from the sea. Dark red coral is a stimulant and tonic to the blood stream. It is also used as a remedy against melancholy, an astringent and a heart stimulant. Coral in general raises a person's vibrations and enables her/him to attune to nature and creative forces.

DIAMOND: Diamond is the hardest of the gemstones and it has been symbolically associated with the marriage ceremony. The stone amplifies the searching or seeking within the soul. It also emphasizes a total openness of being and an attaining of spiritual clarity where one is not swayed by material values. Diamonds are used for general healing and taken internally when pulverized and mixed with wine or water. They are said to strengthen the body, nourish the tissues and improve the complexion. They also help in attunement with God.

Diamonds are used in conjunction with other stones to amplify them. They are particularly helpful when used with the emerald and amethyst and aid in opening up the two higher chakras.

EMERALD: The emerald is a superior stone for healing. Its green color is effective in grounding one on the Earth plane, in quieting the emotions, and in balancing the aura. Physically, it strengthens the heart and spine, helps alleviate problems associated with diabetes, and strengthens the adrenals. It has a strong love vibration and causes one to give love to others. It also enhances wisdom from the mental plane.

The main use of emeralds in ancient times was in bathing the eyes. The stones would be steeped in water for several hours and infusion used to bathe the eyes. They were also used to enhance memory and mental powers and to develop clairvoyance. In some ancient societies, emeralds were the guardians of spring and symbolized the processes of generation and ripening.

GARNET: The garnet has the highest crystallographic symmetry of all the gemstones and is a strong crystal former. Since it grows well-developed crystals, it may keep some of its powers within itself. Red garnets were generally thought to counteract melancholy and act as a heart stimulant. Physically, garnets are useful in cleansing and purifying the body and should be held over the spleen for the best effect. They are also thought to be useful to the pituitary gland as well as to enable a person to recall past life memories when worn on the third eye. The green garnet is a strong healing stone and is used to purify thoughts in healing others.

JADE: Jade is considered to be the most precious of stones in China and Japan. The Chinese believe that it provides a link between the spiritual and the worldly. In ancient Egypt, jade was used in amulets and endowed with mystical powers. Jade is a good stone for meditation; it strongly influences the heart center and draws impurities from the glands, thus cleansing them. Red jade can bring forth emotional problems such as anger so that they can be better defined. Yellow jade stimulates the solar plexus and works on the bile flow, aiding digestion. Blue jade has an effect upon the mental body and is very calming. Green jade works particularly with the emotions.

LAPIS LAZULI: Found in Afghanistan and Russia, it is a stone of deep blue color often mixed with white calcite, containing flecks of gold or pyrite. Lapis has a strong spiritual vibration and has been significant in religions throughout the ages. It was one of the stones in the high priest's breastplate, and it is reported that Moses inscribed the Ten Commandments on blocks of this material. In ancient Egypt, it was the stone used for the image of truth, and the high priest wore an amulet of the goddess of truth around his neck. Lapis is also one of the seven precious stones in Buddhism.

It is important for attunement and spiritual purification; this blue stone can help to develop mental images for telepathic communication, especially when taped over the third eye. It also affects the kundalini and heart centers and helps to bring forth that which is contained within the person.

MALACHITE: Malachite is one of the basic ores of copper and is often found along with azurite. It was used in ancient Egypt to treat cholera and rheumatism and to protect children from evil spirits. It was also used for cosmetic purposes when ground and mixed with water and painted on the eyelids. As a healing stone, malachite was used for degenerative diseases like cancer since it acts as a deterrent to abnormal cellular growth.

MOONSTONE: Moonstone is a variety of feldspar associated with the Moon and its powers. It absorbs the healing properties of the Moon and acts a reflection of the wearer. Moonstone helps a person to see her/himself clearly, protects her/him while traveling, and keeps the mind clear and uncluttered.

OPAL: The qualities given to the opal are predominantly mystical, and in ancient times it was rarely used for physical healing except for the eyes. Opals are classified as common, precious, black, or fire.

They are said to be seductive, stimulating the erotic nature. Opals work on the third eye center and enhance memory.

PEARL: Pearls are found in the shells of oysters as well as in conch shells and abalone. Cultured pearls are created by the insertion of a bead of mother of pearl along with pieces of tissue from the mantle into the body of the oyster. The oysters are left from three to six years at depths of seven to ten feet in the ocean.

Vibrations from pearls are healing as well as creative because of the way they are produced—from irritation of the organism which defends itself by secreting self-protecting material. Thus, the formation of beauty occurs by overcoming hardship. Wearing pearls helps to develop an even temper and gives strength and purity. Pearls affect the abdominal area and the absorption of toxins in the body. They can become discolored from absorbing vibrations. Pearls have been used throughout history to increase fertility. At one time, pulverized pearls were stirred in milk and drunk by an individual to cure irritability. Pearls have been used for acid indigestion in pulverized form.

RUBY: Rubies aid in circulation of the blood and in cleansing the blood of infection. They are also beneficial in dissolving blood clots if used in conjunction with a prism. Rubies signify courage; they strengthen the adrenal glands and have been used to staunch the flow of blood when ground up with water as a paste. Rubies have often been taped to the forehead to influence the thoughts or placed under the pillow to induce pleasant dreams.

SAPPHIRE: Like the ruby, the sapphire is a variety of conundrum. The sapphire was a respected stone by the Buddhists who ascribed magical powers to it. It was believed to be a powerful influence for purity and was used in the ecclesiastical rings in the Catholic Church. Ayurvedic physicians use the ashes of sapphire to treat rheumatism, colic, and mental illness.

The blue stone is best for healing; the black is worn for protection or as a centering stone. White sapphire acts a focal point to center the mind and is of high spiritual quality. The star sapphire is a special sapphire and is used to balance the chakras.

TOPAZ: Topaz had religious significance in ancient Egypt where it was the symbol of the Sun god Ra, the giver of life and fertility. It has sacred associations for the Burmese and is one of the gems set in the Nan-Ratan, a piece of jewelry which is an important part of the regalia of Burma. Topaz is considered a source of strength because of its color and clarity. In healing, it is used in treating tension headaches since it helps bring about the relaxation of cells within the head. It also acts as a protection against depression and insomnia.

TURQUOISE: Turquoise has been an important gem for American Indians in the Southwest. It is considered a holy mineral. In the East it was used for protection and symbolic of prosperity. It was thought to have magical powers and is still used today for amulets. The blue-green color is important in healing a number of conditions. It has been used to treat eye problems as well as ailments of an inflammatory or feverish origin. Turquoise draws to itself poisons and other dangerous elements and thus protects the person wearing it. It also helps to impart wisdom and sensitivity to the wearer and should be set in silver to enhance its qualities.

FLOWER REMEDIES

Flower remedies or flower essences are subtle remedies derived from wildflowers. They use the healing power of the flowers to create within us a condition in which we are more emotionally balanced and less prone to disease.

Essences are prepared from a mother tincture which is made by infusing flowers with water out in the sunshine. The Sun acts as a catalyst to draw out the aura or etheric body of the flower. This liquid is then preserved with alcohol (usually brandy) and used as the mother tincture from which stock bottles are made. Remedies may be taken internally through the mouth in a dropper or placed in a bath where they penetrate the whole body. Several remedies may be taken at once in combination.

Flower remedies penetrate the circulatory system first, entering the blood stream, and then the nervous system, where they are transmitted through electromagnetic energy to the meridians and in turn to the subtle bodies and the chakras.

There are several different ways of determining which flower remedies should be utilized at a certain time period. An interview and consultation should take into account the patient's emotional history, noting any fears, anxieties, or personality dysfunctions that exist. Some practitioners use radiesthesia, the pendulum, or a dowsing rod to determine which remedies are best for the person (see chapter 20 on Diagnostic Techniques).

The first flower essences were developed by Dr. Edward Bach, an English physician who worked in bacteriology in a London hospital. After experimenting with vaccines of toxic substances to boost the immune system, he turned to homeopathy. Bach developed homeopathic *nosodes* (potentized extractions of diseased matter, tissue or discharges) for the seven types of bacteria associated with chronic illness. He discovered that patients carrying each of the seven types of intestinal bacterial pathogens displayed particular personality characteristics. This led him to further research on emotional factors and personality types contributing to illness. Since he did not like giving nosodes prepared from disease-producing agents, he went out to nature to look for flowers whose essence would work with emotional patterns. Bach stated, "Providential means have placed in nature the prevention and cure of disease by means of divinely enriched herbs and plants and trees. They have been given the power to heal all types of illness and suffering."[12]

Dr. Bach felt that illness was a reflection of disharmony between the personality and the higher self; this disharmony causes dysfunctional energetic patterns in the subtle bodies. The flower essences realign emotional patterns so that patients increased their physical vitality and thus could fight their disease. Patients suffering from an unknown fear would be given aspen; those from a known fear or phobia, mimulus; those who were in shock, a combination of remedies known as "Rescue Remedy" containing star-of-Bethlehem for shock, rockrose for terror and panic, impatiens for mental stress and tension, cherry plum for desperation, and clematis for faraway, out-of-the-body feelings.

Following Dr. Bach's footsteps, an American healer named Richard Katz began experimenting with flower remedies made in the Sierras and at Mount Shasta in California. Many of the essences he developed work on removing blockages involving sexuality, issues of intimacy in relationships, spiritual transformations, and achieving higher states of conscious awareness. Mr. Katz developed the Flower Essence Society with his wife, Patricia Kaminski. Purposes of the Flower Essence Society include utilizing the healing power of plants, establishing a network of communication with practitioners around the world who are utilizing flower remedies, researching new remedies, and conducting classes and retreats on the essences. To date, the Flower Essence Society has four kits which include 72 essences. They also have a number of publications available including *Flower Essence Repertory* (Flower Essence Society, 1986), which lists different emotions and categorizes all the remedies (including the Bach Remedies) under their appropriate emotions.

Another researcher and healer named Gurudas published a text in 1983 on *Flower Essences and Vibrational Healing* (Brotherhood of Life, Inc.). The book contains detailed descriptions of 108 new flower essences, some of which had been made and described by the Flower Essence Society. Much of the information in the book comes from channeled material by a man named Kevin Ryerson who met with Gurudas and Richard Katz and others. The book goes into the history of flower remedies, their preparation, and detailed descriptions on all the essences. It also explains how flower essences penetrate the subtle bodies.

AROMATHERAPY

The term *aromatherapy* was coined about 50 years ago by René Maurice Gottefosse, a French chemist. Aromatic oils are used in foods, toiletries, and medicines. In foods, they are used as natural flavorings, such as oil of lemon and orange. In cosmetics, they are incorporated in perfumes and in toothpaste flavorings. In medicines, they are used as therapeutic agents; for example, clove oil for toothache, peppermint for indigestion, and eucalyptus oil for respiratory problems.

Essential oils are odorous and readily evaporate in the open air. They are soluble in alcohol and ether and partially soluble in water. They are present in tiny droplets in a large number of plants and are responsible for the scent from flowers and herbs. They move from one part of the plant to another according to the time of day and season.

Essences are extracted by distillation. This involves placing the plant material in a vat and passing steam through it. The essence escapes along with water and other substances. The distillate is cooled, and the essence is then separated from the water.

Heat, light, air and moisture have a damaging effect on essential oils. They should be kept in dark airtight bottles and in cool, dry conditions.

Essential oils are taken from herbs and plants. Certain flowers emit a strong fragrance or scent as part of their reproductive process. Once they become impregnated, the fragrance ceases.

Essences have a long history. They were used by the Egyptians who put them in cosmetics, massage oils, and medicines. Priests were the first to use the aromatics, and later they were also used by physicians. The aromatics used in Egypt included myrrh, frankincense, cedarwood, origanum, bitter almond, spikenard, henna, juniper, coriander, calamus, and other indigenous plants. Cedarwood oil was also used in the process of mummification.

The ancient Hebrews used essential oils in many of their religious rituals. Women were given a 12-month purification with myrrh oil.

Learning from the Egyptians, the Greeks attributed the origin of aromatics to the gods and used various oils in their perfumes as well as to anoint specific parts of the body. The Greek physicians recognized the difference between stimulating and sedative properties in the essences. The Romans were even more lavish in their use of perfumes than the Greeks. The knowledge of distillation, however, remained forgotten since Egyptian times. An Arabian physician known as Avicenna is credited with this invention in the 10th century. Avicenna first used the rose and later distilled other essences.

The Chinese used aromatics with their acupuncture, and many essences are written about in the Hindu Ayurvedas. Sandalwood was one that was used as an incense and an unguent. In the Middle Ages, the herbalists and alchemists worked with essential oils and were familiar with the process of distillation.

In modern times, research has been carried out in regard to the antiseptic properties of essences. This research has been conducted primarily by chemists and pharmacists. René Maurice Gottefosse was a chemist interested in the cosmetic use of essences. He soon gathered enough information to convince him that many essential oils had even greater antiseptic properties than some of the antiseptic chemicals in use. Then, one of Gottefosse's hands was badly burned as a result of a small explosion in his laboratory. He immersed it in lavender oil and found that the burn healed at a phenomenal rate with no infection or scarring.[13]

A colleague of Gottefosse named Godissart set up an aromatherapy clinic in Los Angeles. He was successful in achieving cures for skin cancer, gangrene, osteomalacia (softening of the bones as a result of imbalance in calcium and phosphorous metabolism), facial ulcers, and bites from black widow spiders using lavender oil.[14]

Gottefosse published his first book *Aromatherapie* in 1928. Meanwhile, another Frenchman, a medical doctor named Jean Valnet, began to use essences in his treatments. He used them during the war in treating battle wounds and in many pathological conditions. Dr. Valnet administered the oils orally—a few drops in a little sugar.

Marguerite Maury, author of *The Secret of Life and Youth* and a French biochemist, treated the whole person—mind, body, and psyche—with essential oils. She dissolved the oils in vegetable oil and used them in massage so that they absorbed through the tissues of the body; in this way, they worked on internal problems as well. She found that bergamot, chamomile, and lavender stimulated the production of white blood cells when rubbed on the skin or inhaled.[15]

Italy has also produced some researchers in the field. Doctors Gatti and Cajoa, working in the 1920s and 1930s, realized the scope of therapy with essential oil. Paolo Roveti of Milan worked with citrus oils indigenous to Italy—bergamot, lemon, and orange—and also demonstrated clinically the benefit of certain essences in states of anxiety and depression.[16]

PSYCHIC SURGERY

The vibrational therapies thus far discussed—color therapy, music therapy, crystals and gems, flower essences and aromatherapy—create vibrations which move into the energy field of the body. Psychic surgery, which has been so successful in the Philippines as well as in Brazil and other countries, is also based upon the principle of an energy body. The energy body was discovered back in 1935 by Harold Burr, professor of anatomy at Yale. The energy body is a blueprint of the physical body; it determines the function of cells and organs as well as the shape, size, and color of the physical body. The energy body is affected by the mind and emotions of the individual.[17]

In psychic surgery, the energy body is disconnected from the physical body so that the tissues become an amorphous jellylike mass. The diseased tissues are removed and afterwards the two bodies are reconnected. The surgery itself takes only a few minutes; the patient does not feel anything at all. The healer actually penetrates the body with his hands; no instruments are used to make the incisions. There is blood surrounding the spot where the healer is working. This is washed off quickly and the diseased part of the organ is removed. Afterwards, the patient feels perfectly normal; s/he gets off the table and walks away without having undergone any shock at all.

I experienced psychic surgery by one of the Filipino healers. After penetrating the skin with his hands, there was quite a bit of blood. When this was washed away, a small piece of tissue was removed from the colon. The whole process, including a prayer and balancing of the energy centers, took about seven minutes.

The psychic surgeons themselves are very simple, devout, and sensitive individuals. They all practice some type of spiritual religion and are guided by higher level beings. They are trained as healers from early childhood and are motivated by love and a sense of service.

NOTES

1. Dr. Richard Gerber, *Vibrational Medicine* (Santa Fe, NM: Bear & Co., 1988), p. 121.
2. Ibid., p. 128.
3. Ibid., p. 131.
4. Ibid., p. 153.
5. Corinne Heline, *Healing and Regeneration through Music* (Santa Barbara, CA: J. F. Rowny Press, 1968), p. 20.
6. Ibid., p. 21.
7. Ibid.
8. Ann Hill, ed., *A Visual Encyclopedia of Unconventional Medicine* (New York: Crown Publishers, Inc., 1978), p. 220.
9. Laurel Elizabeth Keyes, *Toning: The Creative Power of the Voice* (Marina del Rey, CA: De Vorss and Co., 1964), p. 45.

10. Ibid.
11. Caroline Myss, "Oh-Shinnah: A Healer Using Crystals," in *Expansion* 2 (July-Aug. 1981), 1.
12. Gerber, p. 245.
13. Robert B. Tisserand, *The Art of Aromatherapy* (New York: Destiny Books, 1977), p. 41.
14. Ibid., p. 42.
15. Ibid., p. 43.
16. Ibid.
17. Hill., p. 180.

DIAGNOSTIC TECHNIQUES

There are many diagnostic techniques available in alternative medicine to audit the body in figuring out which organs and what systems are out of balance. These techniques help to see the biological changes taking place in the body so that the practitioner can spot a change before there is any pain or discomfort.

IRIDOLOGY

Iridology is the science that analyzes the iris of the eye in order to determine physical constitution, tissue weaknesses, and psychological traits. The iris is the portion of the eye that carries the color. (Iris was the goddess of the rainbow in Greek mythology.) The fibers of the iris comprise a huge communication network. The iris is connected to every organ and tissue of the body by way of the brain and nervous system. The nerve fibers receive their impulses through connections to the optic nerve, the optic thalami, and spinal cord.[1] Thus, the eye not only enables us to bring images of the outside world within, it also shows images of what is within our bodies and psyches to the outside world.

Iridology dates back to the early 1800s when a young Hungarian, Ignatz von Peczely, caught an owl in his garden. While struggling with the owl, he accidentally broke its leg. When he looked into the owl's eyes, he saw a black stripe appear. As he nursed it back to health, the black stripe was replaced by white lines. Years later, von Peczely became a doctor and observed changes in his patient's eyes after accidents, surgeries, and illnesses. He created the first chart of the iris based on these findings.

Modern iridology was pioneered by Dr. Bernard Jensen, who developed a map of the iris that represents the placement of organs and tissues. The iris is divided into seven zones; the right iris is comparable to the right side of the body; the left, to the left side. There are 90 known specific areas on each iris (see p. 242) and each iris is different.[2]

When observing the iris, the first impression is its overall appearance—how light or dark it is, its color, whether there are any black holes or lesions on it. This gives an idea of constitutional strength.

Colored spots on the eye include psora and drug deposits. *Psora* are heavy dark patches which are usually inherited. Drug spots are smaller and different in color. Chemical deposits, including drugs, show up as bright yellow, red, orange, and other colors. They are usually scattered about and found mostly in the digestive zone and the glandular zone.[3]

By observing the shape of the pupil and its size, it is possible to learn where major stresses are occurring in the body. The pupil is not located in the center of the iris. It is slightly down from the geometric center. If it is small and pinched down, a condition of extreme nervous tension is indicated. When it is wide and open beyond its usual perimeter, a condition of nerve depletion and exhaustion is present. The response to light is also an indication of tension or stress.

On the map of the iris, the digestive system is the hub, the stomach being in the first area and the intestines in the second (see p. 241). This is because all nutrients that sustain body tissue are obtained from the digestive process. The second zone is usually darker than other parts of the iris as this is where the greatest amount of toxicity is found. Dark areas on the colon usually indicate pockets or diverticula that do not remove waste materials very well. It is easy for infections to get started there. Often a change of diet and cleansing will help to remove these pockets.

Healing can be observed through the iris when white lines come forth.[4] Healing lines often appear in the intestinal area and lead to healing in other areas.

METHOD OF ANALYSIS

To make an accurate analysis, an iridologist photographs each iris. Then s/he can compare them with photographs taken later for signs of healing and change. A transparent overlay of the iris chart is placed over the photograph of each iris and correspondences made. An iridologist will also make a personal observation of the irides with a magnifying glass and a light.

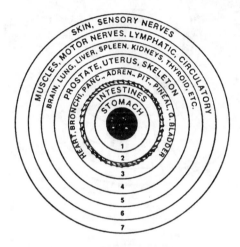

The iris is divided into 7 zones.

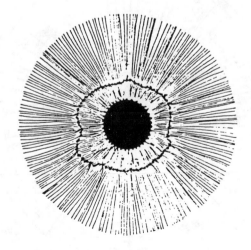

The autonomic nerve wreath is a major landmark.

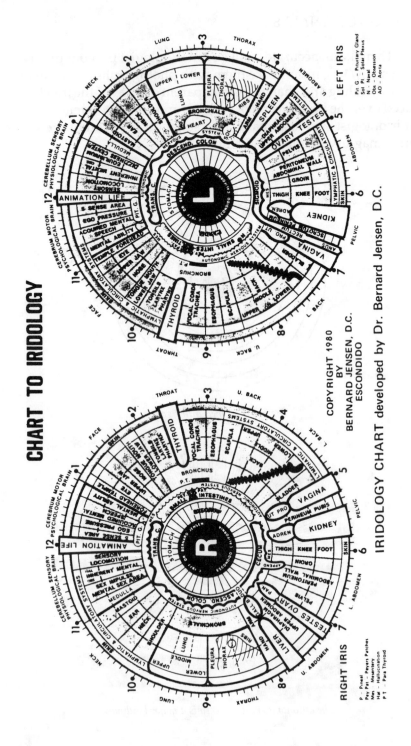

CHART TO IRIDOLOGY

IRIDOLOGY CHART developed by Dr. Bernard Jensen, D.C.

COPYRIGHT 1980
BY
BERNARD JENSEN, D.C.
ESCONDIDO

TRADITIONAL CHINESE DIAGNOSIS

See material in chapter 14 under The Four Examinations.

MACROBIOTIC ORIENTAL DIAGNOSIS

In Macrobiotics, traditional Oriental diagnostic techniques are used which are similar to the Chinese system. The emphasis, however, is slightly different. It includes the taking of the pulses, facial diagnosis, and the study of the hands and feet, the nails, the tongue, the eyes, and the ears. Macrobiotic diagnosis takes into consideration these seven things:

1. Destiny—whether a person is or will become happy or not.
2. Personality—what kind of ideals, view of life, nature and character s/he has.
3. Constitution—what kind of constitution s/he has, both physically and mentally.
4. Disorders—what kind of disorders s/he has developed and suffers at present.
5. Recommendations—what changes are required to turn her/his disorders into health and well-being.
6. Orientation—what kind of future s/he should be oriented to for the realization of happiness.
7. Inspiration—what encouragement should be given to develop her/his possibility to achieve happiness.

In determining constitution, family, social and cultural influences are noted—as well as the date of conception and birth since Orientals look at the astrological horoscope to see the planetary influences and what effects they have upon the individual in terms of potential health problems, mental abilities, emotional make-up, and spiritual aspirations.

To evaluate the organs, s/he works with several different pulses on the wrist. Studying the pulses and the nuances in their rhythm takes many years to develop.

right hand   1. deep: lungs
surface: large intestine
2. deep: spleen and pancreas

surface: stomach
3. deep: sex/circulation (pericardium)
surface: triple burner

left hand
1. deep: heart
surface: small intestine
2. deep: liver
surface: gall bladder
3. deep: kidneys
surface: bladder

After the pulses are determined, a general study of the face is made. The face and the head represent the conditions of the internal organs.

The *cheeks* show the condition of the lungs and their functions.

The *tip of the nose* represents the heart, while the *nostrils* represent the bronchi connecting the lungs. The *middle part* of the nose signifies the stomach, while the *upper part* reveals the condition of the pancreas.

The *eyes* portray the kidneys as well as the condition of the ovaries in the case of a woman and the testicles in the case of a man. Also, the *left eye* represents the spleen and pancreas, while the *right eye* represents the liver and gall bladder.

The *area between the eyebrows* shows the condition of the liver, and the *temples* on both sides show the condition of the spleen.

The *forehead* as a whole represents the small intestines, and the *peripheral region* of the forehead, the large intestine. The *upper part* of the forehead shows the condition of the bladder.

The *ears* represent the kidneys: the *left ear*, the left kidney; the *right ear*, the right kidney.

The *mouth* as a whole shows the condition of the entire digestive vessel. The *upper lip* shows the stomach; the lower lip, the small intestines at the inner part of the lip and the large intestines at the more peripheral part of the lip. The *corners* of the lip show the condition of the duodenum.

The *area around the mouth* represents the sexual organs and their functions.

The *palms* and *hands* are also studied in assessing organ balance (see illustration on p. 245).

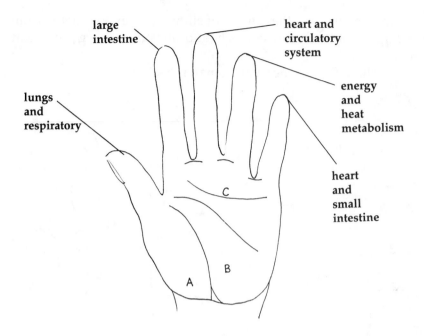

large
intestine

heart and
circulatory
system

energy
and
heat
metabolism

lungs
and
respiratory

heart
and
small
intestine

C

B

A

Palm and Fingers

Line A and its related area on the palm at the base of the thumb signifies the digestive and respiratory functions, including the state of the esophagus, stomach, small intestine, large intestine, and lungs.

Line B and its area represent the nervous system, including the brain and central nervous system as well as the peripheral nerves.

Line C and the upper palm represent the circulatory and excretory systems, which include the heart, kidneys, and bladder.

THE FINGERS

The fingers represent the organs and functions located in the upper part of the body, namely the lungs and heart. They also are connected to the small intestine and large intestine as well as their related functions such as circulation and heat metabolism. Each finger corresponds to a certain function:

the thumb—functions of the lungs and respiratory activities

the index finger—large intestines and their functions

the middle finger—heart and circulatory functions, including reproductive vitality the ring finger—the activity of eliminating excess energy from the regions of the heart, stomach, and intestines; energy and heat metabolism

the little finger—heart and small intestine

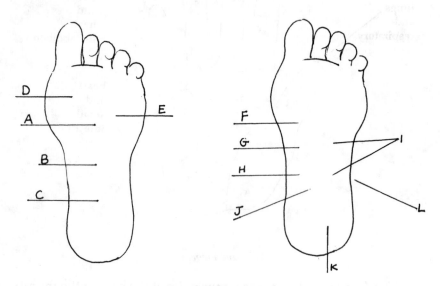

Foot—Body correlations

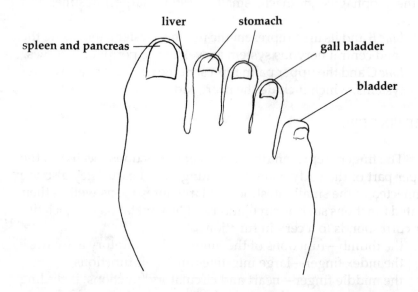

Toes—Organ correlations

THE FEET AND TOES

Studying the feet and toes is another way to determine the condition of the organs and their functions (see illustrations on p. 246).

Points A, B, and C correlate to the kidneys, heart, and stomach, and the abdominal center. The inside ball of the foot (D) under the big toe corresponds to the shoulders and shoulder blades, while the outside ball (E) corresponds to the lungs and respiratory functions.

The inside middle region of the foot (F) represents the nose and mouth cavity, (G) the throat and vocal cords, and (H) the bronchi and diaphragm region.

The outer middle region of the foot (I) signifies the stomach, duodenum, and upper intestinal region.

The inner lower region (J) corresponds to the intestinal region, especially the middle part of the intestines.

The heel (K) as a whole correlates to the lower intestinal region, the rectum, and the uterus.

The line running along the bottom outside of the foot (L) represents the spine and the muscles along the spine, as well as the meridian related to the bladder functions.

The *toes* and *toenails* represent the functions and the organs which are located in the middle region of the body, namely the spleen and pancreas, liver, stomach, gall bladder, and bladder.

The *first toe* and its nail, especially the outer area, correspond to the spleen and pancreas. At the inner area, they also correspond to the liver and its functions.

The *second* and *third toes* and their nails represent the stomach and its functions. The second toe represents the stomach organ with the third toe signifying the functions of the stomach sphincter and duodenum.

The *fourth toe* and its nail correspond to the gall bladder and its functions.

The *fifth toe* and its nail relate to the bladder and its processes.

These are just some of the ways the Oriental practitioner assesses the conditions of the body organs. S/he also studies the eyes, the ears, and the tongue. Then s/he is able to evaluate the temperament of the individual as well as the status of the organs and their functions. Thus, s/he is able to help the patient balance her/his body and psyche to prepare for the goals s/he wishes to achieve.

MEDICAL RADIESTHESIA

Medical radiesthesia is a good diagnostic tool for assessing imbalances within various organs of the body. It is also extremely helpful in testing for food allergies, preparing herbal formulas and flower remedies, and in checking vitamin and mineral supplements.

Waves of force (commonly called *vibrations*) emanate from all objects in the physical universe and from levels of consciousness that lie beyond the range of physical sense perception. Various instruments like the dowsing rod and the pendulum have been used to detect and measure these forces. These instruments can be used by any individual who takes the time to develop this ability.

A *pendulum* or *dowsing rod* is a way of bringing higher information into conscious awareness. These tools act to amplify the neuromuscular response in providing a clear set of signals. *Witnesses* or substances symbolizing the person are often used—a photograph, a lock of hair, a blood spot, saliva, the name of the person written on a piece of paper, or an astrological chart.

When testing foods or remedies, the physical substance itself can be utilized or its name can be written on a piece of paper. The pendulum alone can be used for a yes/no or neutral valuation of the food or remedy. Further information as to how positive or negative the substance in question is can be determined by the size of the swing of the pendulum.

Remedies can also be placed on a circular scale of 360 degrees to measure their potency. Most often, however, the practitioner uses a specific geometric pattern or chart for diagnostic purposes. Certain points in the chart indicate health or disease of different types. Placing a witness on one end of the chart, one can determine the vitality level of the patient. Witnesses of various organs and diseases are also used, and when the causative factors have been found, certain remedies may also be placed on one part of the pattern. When the right remedy or group of remedies is thus placed, they cancel out the disease and the pendulum returns to the normal swing.

RADIONICS

Radionics is based on the same principle as radiesthesia but uses a machine to determine the cause of disease and to project various remedies to the patient in order to restore health.

As a healing discipline, radionics developed from the research of the American physician, Dr. Albert Abrams. Abrams, who was a specialist in nervous disease, discovered that certain areas of the abdomen gave a dull note on percussion when particular diseases were present. In order to identify these disease reflexes from each other, he devised an instrument with calibrated dials to measure intensities. In 1924, his instruments were tested in England and their diagnostic value was upheld.[5]

Ruth Drown, an American chiropractor, developed a more sophisticated form of radionic instrumentation in the 1930s. She found that it was possible to diagnose as well as treat the disease of a patient from a distance using a sample of blood as a link. In the 1940s and 1950s, extensive research into radionics was done in Oxford, England by George and Marjorie De La Ware. In the 1970s, Malcolm Rae, an American, added a new dimension through using magnetically energized geometric patterns and electronically pulsed distance treatment.[6]

In radionics, all diseases, organs, and remedies have their own special frequency or vibration. These are expressed in numerical values known as *rates*. The radionics machine has calibrated dials upon which the frequencies or rates can be placed.

Usually, a patient sends a blood spot or hair sample to the practitioner. S/he places that on the radionics instrument and adjusts the dials (like tuning a radio to receive a transmission). The practitioner then goes through a series of questions to get a picture of the patient's health. S/he selects those rates which will counteract the imbalance and broadcasts to the patient a homeopathic medicine, color, flower remedy, vitamin or mineral supplement. S/he may also refer her/him to other treatments, such as structural work or acupuncture, and suggest dietary changes as well.

One of the advantages of radionics is that it assesses the underlying causes which give rise to pathological states and prevents these from developing further.

APPLIED KINESIOLOGY

Applied kinesiology uses a system of simple muscle-testing procedures to assess the energy levels in the different organs and body systems. Dr. George Goodheart, a chiropractor in the U.S., discovered that the tests used in kinesiology to determine muscle strength and tone over the range of movement of the joints could also determine the balance of energy in each of the body's systems. With further research, he established the relationship between each muscle group, the particular organs, and the acupuncture meridians.

Many chiropractors and other healers are now using applied kinesiology to discern structural imbalances, to determine dietary deficiencies and allergies, and to detect various organ dysfunctions. Once imbalances have been found by muscle testing, any treatment may be carried out and the effects monitored by repeating the muscle test and comparing the results. Muscle testing can reveal how effective the treatment has been, how often it is required, and the dosage of any remedies or supplements the body needs.

MEDICAL ASTROLOGY

The astrological horoscope is one of the oldest diagnostic tools in both the Eastern and Western worlds. Hippocrates, the father of modern medicine, stated, "A physician without a knowledge of astrology cannot rightly call himself a physician." Following the Hermetic axiom, "As above, so below," Hippocrates contended that one could not know the disposition and temperament of a man without an understanding of the greater environment in which he was born.

Certain planetary configurations dispose us to have weaknesses in particular organs of our body which correspond to emotional states. By being aware of these areas, we can work not only with our psychological patterns but also with physical exercise, diet, herbs, and supplements to maintain our bodies in a state of vitality and health.

Understanding the cycles of the planets can also show us why we may lack certain minerals or vitamins at particular time periods and when these time periods occur. Thus, we can work preventively to maintain ourselves in a state of physiological and psychological balance.

What to Look for in the Horoscope:

1. First look at the *Sun* and its aspects (distances from other planets). The Sun shows the constitutional vitality and

vigor. Its aspects to other planets indicate metabolic tendencies—whether one burns energy quickly or slowly.

2. The *Moon* is the "amperage"—how the vital forces flow through the body. Certain types of aspects from the Moon may make the individual ill from time to time though her/his vital force may be strong. This indicates a need for more rest and slowing down.

3. The *Ascendant* or rising sign is the conductor of energy. Fire and Air signs are the strongest conductors, less so Earth and Water. This can be changed if a strong Fire planet like Mars is near one of the angles of the chart. One may be more physically sensitive if a Water planet like the Moon or Neptune is near one of the angles.

4. The *element balance* in the horoscope should be perused. In determining the element balance, the planets and houses are considered as well as the signs. The first, fifth, and ninth houses are Fire houses; second, sixth, and tenth, Earth; third, seventh, and eleventh, Air; and fourth, eighth and twelfth, Water. The Sun, Mars, and Jupiter are Fire planets; Saturn, Earth; Mercury and Uranus, Air; Moon, Venus and Neptune, Water. Pluto may be considered a combination of Fire and Water. When these planets are angular or in close hard aspect to the Sun and Moon, they may balance other factors in the horoscope.

    With a lack of planets in *Fire* signs (Aries, Leo, Sagittarius), there is less physical vitality and a tendency to lethargy and depression. These individuals need much physical exercise. A preponderance of planets in Fire indicates a person who often burns her/himself out, not conserving physical energy. These people are constantly on the go and rarely take time to reflect on life.

    A lack of the *Earth* element (Taurus, Virgo, Capricorn) frequently leads one to ignore the physical body. Often these individuals have pale, sensitive skin, unless they spend enough time outdoors. An abundance of the Earth element usually indicates those who enjoy taking care of their physical needs by exercising, cooking, and other activities. Sometimes they tend to be too focused on their physical bodies, especially with a strong Virgo or sixth house emphasis.

Lack of the *Air* element (Gemini, Libra, Aquarius) may point to a weak nervous system and difficulty in communicating. Many planets in Air tend to make one mentally active. These people habitually overdo mental projects and often develop symptoms that relate to the nervous system and respiratory ailments. Working with yoga, exercise, and breathing techniques can be very helpful for them.

An individual having few planets in *Water* (Cancer, Scorpio, Pisces) may find difficulty expressing her/his emotions; s/he also tends to lack fluids in the body. If this is not balanced out, toxins may accumulate. Drinking more liquids and frequent juice fasts are helpful. With an excess of the Water element, emotionally caused conditions are prominent. These individuals are supersensitive and tend to absorb negative feelings from others as well. They need to learn detachment from personal feelings.

5. The next thing to consider is planetary placement in Cardinal, Fixed, and Mutable signs and in Angular, Succedent, and Cadent houses (which correspond to Cardinal, Fixed, and Mutable signs). *Cardinal* signs (Aries, Cancer, Libra, and Capricorn) relate to body structure, the gastrointestinal system, the eyes, and the kidneys. With an emphasis of Cardinal signs or Angular houses, these areas of the body may be affected. *Fixed* signs (Taurus, Leo, Scorpio, Aquarius) govern the throat and thyroid, the reproductive and excretory systems, and the heart and circulatory systems. Emphasis in the Fixed signs indicates intractability and stubbornness with a holding back of energy and retaining of toxins. These individuals need to let go of their emotions. *Mutable* signs (Gemini, Virgo, Sagittarius, Pisces) rule the nervous system, respiratory system, digestive system, and lymphatic system. Mutable sign people tend to throw off toxins more readily and often have a faster recovery process. They are adaptable and flexible though often indecisive and wishy-washy.

6. The emphasis of planets in *one sign* or *one house* should be noted. This usually indicates a sensitivity in the corresponding area of the body.

PHYSIOLOGICAL MEANINGS OF THE ASTROLOGICAL SIGNS

Aries/Libra—"balance"—This polarity represents the "I" of Aries and the "we" of Libra. If relationships with one's self and between others is balanced, then the body should be in balance as well. Aries rules the head that takes in oxygen and lets out carbon dioxide. Libra rules the kidneys that eliminate the liquid wastes from the body.

Taurus/Scorpio—"cleansing"—These signs feed the body as well as cleanse and purify by ridding it of waste material—Taurus through the throat and Scorpio through the colon and excretory system. If one takes in too many negative emotions, s/he may need to cleanse her/his body and let go of the desires and strong will of this polarity.

Gemini/Sagittarius—"communication"—Gemini and Sagittarius govern the nervous system and the body's communication system. Gemini rules the arms, hands, shoulders, lungs and nerves, while Sagittarius governs the hips, thighs, sciatic nerve, pancreas and liver. Gemini transmits the messages and Sagittarius distributes them throughout the body. If we are under pressure, nervous or tense, our breathing may become too shallow, and we can develop problems in the area of the lungs; states of anxiety may also lead to problems with the sciatic nerve.

Cancer/Capricorn—"security-oriented"—Cancer and Capricorn provide us with the foundation and structure for our bodies. Capricorn rules the skeletal frame, bones, the teeth, cartilage and skin, while Cancer rules the softer parts, such as the stomach, uterus, and breasts. When something goes awry in our professional work or our domestic or emotional life, it is often our body's structure that gives way with a broken bone or a slipped disc, or one of our sensitive areas develops stomach ulcers or uterine infections.

Leo/Aquarius—"circulation"—Leo and Aquarius, creativity and the expression of it to humanity, govern circulation and oxygenation. Leo rules the heart, the center of the circulatory system, which in Aquarius sends out the energy to all the cells of the body.

Aquarius also rules the ankles; swollen ankles often result from circulatory dysfunction. If we repress our feelings or block our emotions, we tend to have poor circulation (we speak of a "cold" person). Impaired circulation can lead to abnormal heart conditions.

Virgo/Pisces—"digestion and assimilation"—Virgo and Pisces are signs of health and healing; Virgo rules the intestines and the entire digestive system; Pisces governs the duodenum, the first part of the small intestine, which is prone to ulcers. Pisces also rules the lymphatic system that is comprised of cells that attack and neutralize invading bacteria. When we take on too many projects, especially of a mental nature (since Virgo is ruled by the planet Mercury), we have difficulty assimilating our experiences and often develop digestive problems.

Physiological Rulership of Planets

Sun	heart and circulatory system
Moon	fluids, mucous membranes, stomach
Mercury	nervous and respiratory systems
Venus	throat, thyroid gland
Mars	muscles, adrenal glands, blood
Jupiter	liver, pancreas
Saturn	skeletal system, teeth, bones, joints, skin, gall bladder
Uranus	nervous system along with Mercury
Neptune	cerebrospinal fluid, pineal gland, lymphatic system
Pluto	bowels, reproductive system

Physical Symptoms Associated with the Planets

Sun	cardiovascular diseases
Moon	inflammation of mucous membranes, imbalance of body fluids (edema, dehydration), digestive problems
Mercury	neuritis, respiratory ailments, impediments of speech
Venus	throat infections, thyroid imbalance, kidney problems
Mars	swelling and inflammation, fevers, infections, accidents, hemorrhage and blood diseases
Jupiter	liver diseases (hepatitis), pancreatic diseases (hypoglycemia, diabetes), obesity, abnormal growths, tumors
Saturn	arthritis, rheumatism, fractures, spinal ailments, dental

	problems, skin diseases, gallstones
Uranus	cramps, spasm, shock, paralysis, epilepsy, radiation poisoning
Neptune	obscure diseases, hallucinations, poisonings and over-doses, alcoholism and addictions, toxic conditions, schizophrenia
Pluto	destruction of tissue, hidden cell changes, diseases of the reproductive organs

Zodiacal Anatomy

Aries	head, face, eyes, nose
Taurus	neck, throat, mouth, tonsils, vocal cords
Gemini	arms, shoulders, lungs
Cancer	stomach, breasts, diaphragm, uterus
Leo	cardiac region, spleen, heart
Virgo	lower abdominal area, small intestine
Libra	small of back, kidneys, bladder
Scorpio	pelvis, reproductive organs, colon, rectum
Sagittarius	thighs, hips, buttocks, liver, pancreas
Capricorn	knees, bones, gall bladder, teeth, cartilage
Aquarius	calves, ankles, retina of eyes
Pisces	feet, lymphatic system[7]

MEDICAL PALMISTRY

As was explained in the section on Oriental diagnosis, a study of the palms and the nails is an excellent tool in assessing health patterns. The coloring of the hands and nails also provides us with information on the basic vitality and circulation. The condition of particular organs can be determined by individual fingers and certain points on the palm.

NOTES

1. Bernard Jensen, *Iridology Simplified* (Escondido, CA: Iridologists International, 1980), p. 3.
2. Ibid., p. 10.
3. Ibid., p. 13.
4. Ibid., p. 23.
5. Ann Hill, ed., *A Visual Encyclopedia of Unconventional Medicine* (New York: Crown Publishers, Inc., 1978), p. 167.
6. Ibid.
7. Marcia Starck, *Astrology: Key to Holistic Health* (Birmingham, MI: Seekit Pubns., 1982), pp. 8-18.

SPECIFIC DISEASES

If the Western tradition of medicine were a more holistic one, we would not have diseases named and categorized by symptoms. We would have a deeper understanding of imbalance in the body through relating to the elements and the organs as is evidenced in Chinese medicine. For example, a condition of wind in the lungs is very different from excess water or mucus in the lungs, both of which Western medicine refers to as a "cold."

However, in an effort to communicate information in the context of this book, I have categorized symptoms by diseases and recommended treatments accordingly. The treatments are of a general nature since specific supplements and dietary requirements vary from person to person. It is recommended that the reader use these treatments as guidelines and seek out the help of a practitioner utilizing natural therapies (for example, a naturopathic doctor, a homeopathic doctor, an acupuncturist or an herbalist).

AIDS

AIDS (Acquired Immune Deficiency Syndrome) and ARC (Aids-Related Complex) refer to a group of symptoms caused by many viruses including the HIV virus (formerly known as HTLV III, which has 18 different varieties). The other viruses, bacteria, and fungi involved in the opportunistic infections (ARC) include cytomegalovirus, cryptosporidia, Epstein-Barr virus, herpesvirus,

Candida albicans, Pneumocystis carinii, Cryptococcus neoformans, and Mycobacterium avium.

These viruses and bacteria weaken the immune system so that it falls prey to other diseases, the most prevalent of these being cancer in its forms of Kaposi's sarcoma and Pneumocystis carinii pneumonia. In addition to viral particles, nutritional deficiencies, toxic chemicals in the environment and on our food, and emotional stress further deplete our immune system.

The first symptoms of AIDS and ARC include swollen lymph nodes, fatigue, fevers, night sweats, weight loss, and diarrhea.

The biggest mystery concerning AIDS is where the AIDS virus originated and how its first transmission began. For a complete understanding of this, I recommend the books of Dr. Alan Cantwell— *Aids: The Mystery and the Solution* (Aries Rising Press, 1986), and *Aids and the Doctors of Death* (Aries Rising Press, 1988). Dr. Cantwell, a Los Angeles dermatologist and internationally known researcher in the field of cancer microbiology, draws on the work of Dr. Robert Strecker, another Los Angeles dermatologist and researcher, who believes that the origin of the AIDS virus was in the laboratory and relates the first outbreaks of AIDS in both New York and San Francisco to the time immediately following the hepatitis blood tests given to gay men in those cities in 1978 and 1979.

The first outbreaks of AIDS were in the gay community, among IV drug users, and among hemophiliacs who require blood transfusions. AIDS has now reached epidemic proportions where it has infected all social and economic classes throughout the world. The biggest questions are how to cure AIDS and what the meaning of this epidemic is for all of us. Since the virus has so many forms (it is impossible to identify one AIDS virus) and since it mutates one per cent every year, it is difficult to produce a vaccine that accounts for all the species that occur in the course of the disease.

The most helpful treatments for AIDS may be those listed that keep the immune system in balance so that even if one is infected with the HIV virus, symptoms of AIDS do not need to break out. Some of these treatments have also helped to lessen the symptoms once they have begun.

Psychological Factors

It is known that our mental and emotional states as well as levels of stress affect the immune system. The study of the mind/body link to the immune system is termed *psycho-neuro-immunology*. As a result of stress, the thymus shrinks (the thymus gland regulates the immune system) and white blood cells decrease. Depression, fear, and worry increase, and the appetite and sex drive decrease.

Since AIDS is a sexually transmitted disease, many fears arise regarding emotional relationships, and one begins to hold back her/his expressions of love. S/he then feels more alone and constricted. There has also been a stigma in our society regarding the gay population, so the knowledge that one has AIDS is often tied to a gay person's revealing her/his sexual identity. This in itself has been a fear for many and has increased the stress.

Treatments for the Maintenance of a Healthy Immune System

Cleanse the body through colonic irrigations, herbs, and supplements such as aloe vera juice, psyllium seed, and bentonite clay. Juice fasting with vegetable juices, wheat grass juice, vegetable broths, and herb teas is also helpful (see chapter 3). Cleansing the skin through saunas and sweats is important in getting rid of toxins.

Diet

1. Avoid all chemicals and preservatives, caffeine beverages, sugar, chocolate, and cola drinks.

2. Eliminate animal fats in meats and cow's milk products. Yogurts and acidophilus products may be used as well as some goat's milk products.

3. Eliminate wheat and wheat products like pastas and noodles.

4. Eliminate beans as they are difficult to digest.

5. Eliminate highly acidic foods like vinegar, brewer's yeast, tomatoes, cranberries, citrus, soured apples, strawberries, raw spinach, raw green pepper, grapes, and plums.

6. Eliminate shellfish; use fresh fish baked, broiled, or steamed.

7. While doing a cleansing diet, use only fish and yogurt. Later, fertile eggs, tofu or tempeh, and organic liver and poultry may be added.

8. Use lots of cooked whole grains like brown rice, millet, buckwheat, amaranth, barley, rye, oats, and quinoa.

9. Use lots of steamed leafy greens as kale, chard, mustard greens, turnip greens, broccoli, and roots like carrots, potatoes, squashes, and beets.

10. Eat fruit such as bananas, cherries, peaches, apricots, golden delicious apples, pears, berries other than strawberries, cantaloupe or honeydew melons occasionally, on alternate days.

11. Use cold-pressed vegetable oils every other day, especially olive and flaxseed oil.

12. For sweeteners, use barley malt or rice syrups, which are complex carbohydrates. There are cookies and other products available with these in natural food stores.

Homeopathy

In addition to one obtaining her/his constitutional remedy, a few remedies have been found to be helpful for AIDS and ARC:

1. Cyclosprine, which is made from a fungus, suppresses the immune system.

2. Typhoidinum, a remedy made by killing typhoid germs, also has helped the immune system.

(For specific studies on these two remedies, see *Healing AIDS Naturally: Natural Therapies for the Immune System* by Laurence Badgley, M.D., Human Energy Press, San Bruno, CA, 1987.)

Herbs

Many herbs work with the immune system. Chinese herbs have been very potent, particularly astragalus and ligustrum. Consult a practicing Chinese herbalist for a formula. The combination of herbs determines their efficacy.

American herbs used for the immune system include echinacea root, chaparral, and red clover. A formula can be made of echinacea root mixed with sarsparilla root for blood purification. Spearmint may be added to chaparral to make it more pleasant to the palate.

Other Treatments

Acupuncture is very helpful in working with the *chi* energy and in tonifying the spleen, lungs, and kidneys. Body therapies that work with the meridian system like jin shinn and shiatsu should also be incorporated.

All massage and body therapies are nurturing and relaxing. Stress-reduction techniques like biofeedback, visualization, and meditation are important.

Supplements

1. Wheat grass juice contains a high amount of chlorophyll supplying magnesium, potassium, and other minerals. Chlorophyll carries oxygen to body cells. Wheat grass juice also contains vitamin A and the B vitamins. (For more information, see chapter 9 on Nutritional Supplements.)

2. Algae, including blue-green algae, spirulina, and blue-green manna, are high in chlorophyll as well as amino acids and thus supply protein. This is important for those who have little appetite and need a high-energy food source.

3. Mushrooms are a fungus, and certain species contain antiviral materials. In Japan, an extract from the *shitake (Lentinus edodes)* mushroom is being used to treat cancer patients. This extract, called *lentinan,* is given intravenously to patients. In this country, certain supplement companies have *Len shi* capsules, which are extracts of this mushroom.

4. Aloe vera juice is mucilaginous and helps to cleanse the colon, liver, and kidneys. It is an important supplement in clearing out toxins in the body. It also aids digestion and conditions like flatulence. Drinking 1/3 cup of aloe vera juice on an empty stomach early in the day can be very helpful.

5. Acidophilus promotes intestinal bacteria that grow in the colon. Acidophilus cultures are put in yogurt, kefir, and other products. There are some fine strains of acidophilius culture that can be found in powder form in the refrigerators of natural food stores. Using about 1/2 or 1 teaspoon alternate days is important in replacing intestinal bacteria that may have been killed through the use of antibiotics or other chemical drugs. It is also important to use acidophilus after a colonic.

6. Garlic is antiviral and antifungal. It should be used in cooking every other day; fresh garlic is best as it contains the bioflavonoid Quencitin.

Mineral and Vitamin Supplements

1. Trace mineral supplement in powdered form three teaspoons daily.

2. Vitamin C ascorbate in powdered or crystalline form—about 1/2 teaspoon six times daily. (Reduce dose if diarrhea occurs.)

3. Bioflavonoid capsules—1,000 mg six times daily. (One of the bioflavonoids, Quencitin, has strong antiviral properties.)

4. Pantothenic acid—1,000 mg three to four times daily.

5. Beta-carotene—10,000 i.u.'s three to four times daily. (If using carrot juice or algae, less beta-carotene would be needed.)

6. Zinc picollinate—50 mg daily. Zinc is a strong aid to the immune system; it should not be taken at the same time as copper.

7. Potassium/magnesium supplement three to four times daily.

8. Manganese capsules three to four times daily.

9. Iron and B-12 combination three times daily.

10. Co-Enzyme Q-10—20-50 mg daily (see chapter 9).

There are many other supplements that may be helpful, but there is a limit to what the body can assimilate in terms of capsules and tablets. Capsules can be opened and the powder may be taken alone or in some liquid for greater assimilation.

ALCOHOLISM

There is much conflict as to whether alcoholism should be considered a disease. The social and psychological causes of alcoholism are well known; there is less familiarity with the biochemical causes.

Alcoholics tend to be extremely hypoglycemic; alcohol for them acts as a source of energy as sugar does for others. At the same time, it becomes a poison filling the body with toxins and interfering with natural processes. Once the alcoholic is on a nutritional program with enough protein, whole grains and vegetables, as well as supplements of amino acids, pancreas glandular, B vitamins, manganese and magnesium, the craving abates, and the alcoholic can begin to get in touch with the reasons that alcohol was so appealing to her/him.

In addition to nutritional deficiencies, the liver and other organs can be severely damaged through the prolonged use of alcohol. As alcohol is absorbed by the stomach, it goes through the blood stream to the liver. The liver attempts to convert the alcohol to a harmless substance and, in time, the liver becomes extremely toxic.

In his book *Alcoholism and Nutrition* (Univ. of Texas Press, 1958), Dr. Roger Williams speaks of certain genetic tendencies which cause alcoholics to require various nutritional supplements in order to keep their bodies in balance. Dr. Williams found that the amino acid *L-glutamine* was extremely important in reducing the craving for alcohol. Since this compound is tasteless, it can be put in the food of an alcoholic without her/his awareness. Dr. Williams found dramatic results with L-glutamine and also with *vitamin B-3* (niacin). He administered B-3 to 507 confirmed alcoholics and 87 per cent benefited.

Dr. Abram Hoffer, a Canadian physician, also uses massive doses of vitamins to treat alcoholism. He feels that *vitamin C, B-1* (thiamine), and the amino acid *L-cysteine,* which contains sulfur, can be helpful to alcoholics.

Dr. Kenneth Williams of the University of Pittsburgh advises against giving alcoholics coffee (which is often a part of the AA program, along with candy bars). He gives his alcoholic patients lots of B vitamins, plus magnesium and zinc, and keeps them away from caffeine and sugar. This stops anxiety attacks and hypoglycemic symptoms that often push them to drinking.

A study of alcoholics reported them suffering from the following conditions: disorders of the heart muscle, seizures, acute and chronic inflammation of the pancreas, acute and chronic hepatitis, weakening of the muscles, liver disease, infection, bleeding in the stomach and intestines, and delirium tremens. They were all found to be deficient in B vitamins. In experiments with laboratory animals, high doses of B-6 prevented intoxication.

Psychological Characteristics

Alcoholics often come from homes where at least one of the parents has been an alcoholic. They are conditioned to handling their problems through withdrawal into their own world and using alcohol to numb their sensitivity. Then, they are not forced to confront emotional situations that are difficult or relationships with others. Alcoholics usually possess a deep sense of insecurity and anxiety. Generally, they also lack discipline and are impatient. They do not have the ability to endure difficult circumstances for a long period of time. Physical illness, trauma, and emotional depression often lead them to alcohol.

Treatments

Various types of emotional therapy, especially in groups such as AA, are important in helping the alcoholic to feel a part of society and to relate to various like-minded individuals.

Diet

1. Whole grains and whole-grain cereals, preferably twice daily. Whole-grain cereals such as rice cream, buckwheat cream, millet cream, cream of barley, cream of wheat (made from wheat berries), cream of rye (made from rye berries), and oat cream (made from oat berries) should be used in the morning. A different grain can be ground fresh each morning in a small grain-and-seed grinder or a coffee grinder. In the evening, brown rice, buckwheat, millet, or another grain may be used.

2. Plenty of fresh vegetables in salads and soups or steamed and baked.

3. Proteins are important, but nuts and seeds may be difficult to assimilate for those with liver problems. Easy-to-digest proteins include bean curd (tofu), soured milks such as yogurt, kefir, and buttermilk, fresh fish, and organic poultry from non-chemical sources. Organic liver (calf or beef) from non-chemical sources is also important. Heavier meats such as beef, lamb, and pork are difficult to digest as are shellfish; they deplete the pancreatic enzymes.

4. A maximum of one portion of fruit or fruit juice every other day in order to minimize the amount of sugar and acids. Citrus fruits, strawberries, and soured apples are not good. In addition, vinegar, nutritional yeast, raw spinach, rhubarb, raw green pepper, cranberries, and tomatoes should be avoided.

5. Fats used should be natural, unsaturated oils, especially cold-pressed olive oil on salads or vegetables every other day.

6. No sugar should be used and little honey. Barley malt syrup or rice syrup may be used instead since they are complex carbohydrates.

7. No salt and little soy sauce. All other spices and saltless vegetable seasonings may be used.

8. No coffee, tea, or other beverages containing caffeine such as cola drinks and cocoa. Herb teas, vegetable juices, and mineral water may be used instead.

Supplements

1. Aloe vera juice is very important for cleansing the liver as well as the colon and kidneys. Drink one-half cup every other day on an empty stomach for the first month or two; then one-fourth cup.

2. To cleanse the liver and gall bladder, two tablespoons cold-

pressed olive oil or flaxseed oil plus the juice from half a lemon on arising three mornings a week.

3. Liquid lecithin—two tablespoons once every other day after a meal (days that olive oil isn't used).

4. Liquid chlorophyll—two or three tablespoons twice a day in half a glass of water cleanses the liver and is a high source of magnesium.

5. High-potency acidophilus (such as maxidophilus) to restore intestinal bacteria—1/2 tablespoon on alternate days for one month.

6. Multivitamin and mineral capsule three times daily.

7. Free-form amino acid capsule three times daily.

8. B vitamins, non-yeast base, three times daily.

9. Zinc picollinate or chelate three times daily.

10. Bioflavonoid capsules three times daily. Vitamin C is often too acid for the body.

11. Vitamin A tablet (beta-carotene) every day.

12. A pancreas glandular three times daily is important in keeping up blood sugar.

Herbs

1. Dandelion root tea is helpful for the pancreas and liver—two cups every other day.

2. Echinacea root to cleanse the blood and build up the immune system—one cup every other day for two months; can be mixed with dandelion root.

3. Other herbs that act as liver tonics are Oregon grape root, golden seal, and wild yam. Also, Chinese herbs such as *bupleurum* are excellent in formulas for the liver.

4. Herbs that are strong nutritional sources include alfalfa, nettles, parsley, dandelion leaves, yellow dock, kelp, and sea vegetables.

Other Treatments

1. Colonic irrigations and short juice fasts to cleanse the colon and liver are very important.

2. Acupuncture treatments have proved most beneficial in stimulating the liver, pancreas, and other organs.

ALLERGIES

Allergies are the most common physical ailments and are becoming more and more widespread with the increase of chemical substances in our environment and in our food. A new branch of medicine has evolved in the alternative health field which calls itself *clinical ecology*. It deals with testing for food allergies and other substances in the environment to which an individual is particularly sensitive.

Clinical ecologists use *subcutaneous* (under the skin) injections and *sublingual* (under the tongue) drops for testing. They test for only one substance at a time so they can observe all patient reactions, including heart rate. They also test with much more varied concentrations of extracts than traditional allergists. When they create an allergic reaction, they continue testing with different concentrates until they find one that eliminates the reaction. This is called the *neutralizing dose* and is given to the patient to self-administer either sublingually or subcutaneously when there is a reaction to the offending substance. This allows people to control their environment and, in time, diminish their own treatment.

Chronic food allergies are affecting about 60 per cent of the population, but most people who have them aren't even aware of them. Many people have symptoms all the time (like headaches and tiredness) that they never relate to allergies. Severe symptoms like dizziness and various neurological and emotional traits, such as temper tantrums, irritability, nervousness, anxiety, and depression, are also related to allergies. Thyroid, hormonal, and blood sugar imbalances are caused by allergies as well.

The body adapts to the allergens just as it adapts to the toxins in cigarettes through a reaction known as the "specific adaptation response." After a certain amount of time, the food wears off and the craving for it begins again, just as in addictive states. The most common food addictions are sugar, chocolate (which also contains a lot of caffeine), coffee, tea, and cola beverages. These are the ones recognized the most easily. Other common allergies include cow's milk products (many people are allergic to the lactose in cow's milk); wheat; eggs; citrus fruits; tomatoes; strawberries; spinach, rhubarb, and other foods high in oxalic acid; nutritional yeast (also very acidic); vinegar; raw green pepper; cranberries; and peanuts (due to the aflatoxins or mold found on the peanuts). People often crave very acidic foods such as lemons, soured apples, and cranberry juice when their bodies are already extremely acidic. What they usually need is some cooked whole grains and vegetables for balance.

Allergic conditions are related to emotional states; during periods of stress and increased emotional sensitivity, our bodies react by becoming more sensitive to foods and other allergens in our environment. If we can begin to get a handle on the roots of the emotional situation, we can lessen the intensity of the allergic reaction.

One client of mine was having extreme allergies—not just to foods, but to most substances in her environment. She couldn't even find a bed that was made of a material that didn't affect her sinuses— she was sleeping on a mat which brought her near the dust on the floor to which she was allergic. When we began doing some deep therapeutic work on some of her emotional problems and childhood traumas, the allergies lessened and she regained her physical health by avoiding certain key foods that triggered allergic responses.

Dealing with allergies is a complex physiological process because it involves the immune system, the liver, the pancreas and blood sugar, the spleen, and the lymphatic system.

The liver produces an enzyme called *histaminase* which serves as a natural antihistamine. If the liver is congested with fats or accumulated toxins, it cannot produce histaminase. Avoiding food additives in canned or packaged foods, artificial coloring, chemically grown or sprayed food, refined foods, alcohol, sugar, coffee and tea will help to keep the liver free of toxins. Frequent juice fasts with a colonic irrigation or high enema are helpful as well as taking two tablespoons of cold-pressed olive oil or flaxseed oil with the juice of one-half lemon several mornings a week. This will serve to detoxify the liver and promote the bile flow as well. An herbal tea made from Oregon grape root also aids in promoting the flow of bile.

Many people with allergies have difficulty assimilating proteins and starches and lack digestive enzymes, especially pancreatic enzymes. It is often necessary for them to take a pancreatic glandular supplement to aid the pancreas and a good digestive enzyme after meals, especially the meals where they consume protein and carbohydrates. Specific digestive problems can also be helped by using aloe vera juice.

In allergic individuals, the adrenal glands are usually depleted. This involves not only the energy level but the production of hormones. The adrenal cortex releases a natural cortisone to destroy white blood cells and thus inhibit inflammation in addition to emitting the hormone aldosterone which fights stress and prevents fatigue. An adrenal glandular supplement can be helpful. Even better is the amino acid L-phenylalanine, which is needed to produce adrenaline and noradrenaline, also known as epinephrine and norepinephrine (see chapter 9 on Nutritional Supplements). Pantothenic acid, one of the B-complex vitamins, is also important in stimulating the adrenal glands and in increasing the production of cortisone. Certain herbs, especially Siberian ginseng, fo-ti tien, and gotu-kola, help to activate the adrenals.

The spleen is a reservoir for the blood and contains a high number of erythrocytes, or red blood cells. In times of exertion and emotional stress, when the oxygen content of the blood needs to be increased, the spleen releases its store of red cells into the blood stream. The spleen also keeps the blood free from wastes and infecting organisms. It contains lymphatic tissue in which lymphocytes are manufactured and thus is important in cleansing the body through the lymph system. The Chinese herb astragalus strengthens the spleen. Colonic irrigations help to cleanse the lymph system as do herbs like echinacea root.

Treatments

1. The most important treatment is to cleanse the colon and detoxify the liver. The first step is through colonic irrigations, high enemas, and short juice fasts. When the colon is cleansed, assimilation of foods is increased and excess mucus is eliminated. Cleansing the colon stimulates the liver to produce more bile and the pancreas to produce more enzymes. In addition, aloe vera juice should be taken every other day (preferably on an empty stomach), and several mornings a week two tablespoons of cold-pressed olive oil or flaxseed oil with the juice of half a lemon (adding garlic and cayenne are optional) should be taken. This helps to decongest the liver and promote a better flow of bile.

2. Eliminate all refined and packaged foods and any foods containing preservatives and chemicals. Avoid all foods that produce excess mucus in the body (sugars, chocolate, cow's milk products, wheat) and foods that are common sources of allergies (citrus, strawberries, tomatoes, yeast, vinegar, raw spinach, raw green pepper, and cranberries).

3. Acupuncture and other Oriental therapies like jin shinn, acupressure and shiatsu are extremely effective in balancing the spleen and pancreas as well as in decongesting the liver, lungs, and other organs.

4. Homeopathic remedies are helpful in controlling allergic reactions.

5. Biofeedback, autogenics, and other meditative techniques enable one to gain control of the nervous system and limit the intensity of the allergic reaction.

6. Certain *herbs* are helpful for allergies. Comfrey and slippery elm are healing to the mucous membranes. Marshmallow root stimulates the adrenals and acts specifically on respiratory allergies. Mullein and yerba santa are also good for the respiratory system as are the Chinese herbs ephedra and magnolia flowers. Astragalus strengthens the spleen. Dandelion root is good for the liver and pancreas. Oregon grape root promotes the flow of bile. For skin allergies, salves containing comfrey ointment, golden seal, and myrrh are healing.

Supplements

1. Aloe vera juice—four to six tablespoons every other day on an empty stomach.

2. A good trace mineral made from organic sea vegetables three times a day. Allergic individuals tend to lack iron, magnesium, zinc, and often calcium and manganese.

3. Liquid chlorophyll—two tablespoons in half a glass of spring water two times daily.

4. Free-form amino acid capsules two or three times daily.

5. Pantothenic acid—three tablets (500-1,000 mg) daily.

6. A zinc tablet for the immune system three times daily.

7. Bioflavonoid complex three times daily.

8. Vitamin A (beta-carotene) one or two times daily.

9. A digestive enzyme two or three times a day after meals.

10. Manganese capsules three times daily.

11. Some form of potassium, such as potassium/magnesium capsules or potassium/calcium/magnesium capsules, three times daily.

Special Foods

1. Foods high in iron, such as wheat grass juice, dulse, organic

calves' liver, beets, and red cabbage.

2. Foods high in vitamin A such as carrot juice and yellow and orange vegetables.

3. Green leafy vegetables high in vitamin C, calcium, and magnesium.

4. Local bee pollen is often helpful for allergies. Be careful of Spanish bee pollen which is sprayed.

ALZHEIMER'S DISEASE

Alzheimer's disease is a form of senility which is characterized by physical atrophy and shrinking of the brain. There is no atherosclerosis or blockage of the arteries such as occurs in the cardiovascular type of senility.

Both forms of senility produce memory loss, disorientation, and personality changes.

Once Alzheimer's disease begins, it is difficult to reverse the process, although certain nutrients such as choline (which produces acetylcholine, the neurotransmitter that plays a central role in memory and intelligence) may prove helpful.

There seems to be a predisposition within some families to Alzheimer's. One-third of all Alzheimer cases are familial in origin. These same families have a higher than normal incidence of Down's syndrome and leukemia. These familial cases come on as early as 40, while non-familial cases occur after age 60 or 70.

To date, it has not been shown that Alzheimer's disease has a single causative factor. It could be that a slow-acting virus is at work in the brain. Other possible causative agents include oxygen deprivation and exposure to toxic metals. Alzheimer's may also be caused by a lack of brain glucose.

Studies have shown that aluminum, a toxic metal, may be important in Alzheimer's disease. Aluminum causes nerve-cell damage in the brain and interferes with neurochemicals involved in the transmission of impulses. Aluminum can attack the DNA of nerve cells and cripple essential functions.

In 1980 a Yale scientist published a study showing that elderly individuals with high aluminum levels had a greater incidence of nervous system problems, including poor memory and impaired visual/motor coordination. The increase of Alzheimer's disease seems to parallel the increased use of aluminum in our society.

Treatments

1. Acupuncture treatments can help keep the natural flow of *chi* energy through the meridians to all the organs.

2. Body therapies such as shiatsu, acupressure, and jin shinn maintain the energy flow to the various organs.

3. Chelation therapy may help to release toxic substances from the blood (see Arteriosclerosis).

4. Homeopathy—finding the correct constitutional remedy can be beneficial.

5. Blue-green algae has proved helpful for many with Alzheimer's (see article by Victor Kallman[1]) as have treatments with hydrogen peroxide which help to oxygenate the blood.

Diet

1. Totally avoid all chemicals and processed foods, caffeine, and alcohol.

2. Drink lots of fresh vegetable juices made from carrots, turnips, celery, cucumber, parsley, and beets.

3. Eliminate animal products such as meat and dairy products (except some soured-milk products like yogurt and goat's milk yogurt).

4. Eat lots of steamed green leafy vegetables and sea vegetables for minerals.

5. Eat whole grains, particularly buckwheat, millet, barley, oats, rye, and brown rice.

6. Proteins may include fresh fish (not shellfish), a few fertile eggs a week, some goat's milk yogurt or cheese, tofu, and a small amount of nuts or nut butters.

Supplements

1. Liquid lecithin (a source of choline)—two tablespoons two to three times daily.

2. Aloe vera juice—four tablespoons on alternate days on an empty stomach to cleanse the colon, liver, and kidneys.

3. Liquid chlorophyll—three tablespoons in one-half glass of water three times a day to cleanse the liver and for magnesium.

4. Multivitamin/mineral capsule three times daily.

5. Bioflavonoids—three 1,000 mg tablets daily.

6. Vitamin C ascorbate in crystalline form—one tablespoon three times daily.

7. Zinc capsules—two or three daily.

8. Manganese capsules—three times daily.

9. Pantothenic acid—1,000 mg two times daily.

10. B complex (non-yeast base)—1,000 mg three times daily.

11. Potassium, such as KM (a liquid blood-purifying formula) or potassium/magnesium capsules, three times daily.

12. B-12 (preferably in liquid form)—100 mcg three times daily. (B-12 injections would be very helpful.)

13. GH-3 (anti-aging nutrient developed by Dr. Ana Aslan in Romania)—liquid or tablets three times daily for three weeks, and then stop for two weeks.

14. Evening primrose capsules if GH-3 is not being used—two or three daily.

ARTERIOSCLEROSIS

Arteriosclerosis, or hardening of the arteries, is a forerunner of heart disease and strokes (cerebral vascular accidents) and is one of the leading causes of death in this country. There are two types of arteriosclerosis: arteriosclerosis proper in which the hardening is the result of mineral deposits in the middle layer of the artery wall, and *atherosclerosis* in which fatty substances collect in the inner lining of the arteries to form atheromatous plaque. The plaque encroaches upon the passageways and gradually obstructs the flow of blood. Atherosclerosis is by far the more common and more serious.

If the coronary arteries which supply blood to the heart muscle are partly blocked, the result may be *angina pectoris,* a pain or feeling of tightness in the chest. Sometimes the lining of an affected artery can cause the blood to clot as it flows past. The blood flow may be obstructed or the clot may break away from the artery wall and be carried through the blood stream until it lodges and blocks the flow of blood elsewhere. More frequently, an atheromatous plaque is the site of the formation of a blood clot. If it occurs in the coronary arteries, it can cause a *coronary occlusion* or *thrombosis* (heart attack). If the arteries supplying the brain are blocked, a *cerebral vascular accident* or stroke can occur. In the arteries leading to the legs, a blockage or *peripheral thrombosis* can cut off circulation to the affected limb.

Arteriosclerosis often arises in connection with other diseases. People suffering from diabetes tend to develop the disease earlier than non-diabetics. (Diabetics are often overweight.) Hypertension, hyperthyroidism, and certain disorders of the metabolism such as gout may lead to arteriosclerosis.

As personality types, those with arteriosclerosis often have difficulty relating to others emotionally and "opening up their heart." They have been hurt in some deep manner during their lives and tend to close down and protect their feelings by closing up. They are often very compulsive and need to achieve a lot in their work to fulfill a tendency toward insecurity. They drive themselves very hard and often appear detached and distant to others.

Treatments

1. Emotional therapies that work with releasing old patterns of hurt and sensitivity and opening up to relationships.

2. Cleansing of the body and juice fasting is important. Many with arteriosclerosis have diets high in hydrogenated fats and saturated fats found in meat and dairy products. It is important for them to cleanse their colons and do short vegetable juice fasts with herb teas and soup broths (only a small amount of fruit juice).

3. Exercise is extremely important, especially vigorous outdoor exercise such as swimming, running, and hiking. Also, aerobic exercise classes and dance are good. Sedentary activities contribute much to arteriosclerosis.

4. *Diet:* Avoid all sugars, refined products, and preservatives. Avoid all meats except occasionally organic poultry or organic liver. Eliminate shellfish, dairy products (except soured-milk products such as yogurt and kefir) and wheat products. Substitute rye bread, corn bread, millet bread, rice crackers and other grains. Up to four *fertile* eggs a week may be eaten. Eat steamed and raw vegetables, fresh fruit (but not more than once a day), whole grains, nuts and seeds, fish, tofu (bean curd), and yogurt. Cold-pressed vegetable oils, especially olive oil and flaxseed oil, should be used. Barley malt syrup and honey on occasion may be used as sweeteners.

5. Be careful of environmental sources of metal poisoning such as aluminum and copper cooking utensils, lead cans, and city water with added chemicals in it. Toxic metals entering the body can be deposited on the walls of the aorta and arteries.

6. *Chelation therapy,* or chemoendarterectomy, is based on the

principle that every cell of the body is dependent on essential nutrients which are brought to it by the circulation of the blood. Every cell is also dependent on the same circulation to take away the toxic products of metabolism. Any process that interferes with this flow will upset the balance in the cell and change its ability to function properly.

The circulatory system has a built-in safety mechanism to withstand a certain amount of obstruction. The flow through the average blood vessel to the organ it supplies is greater than is needed. This margin permits younger people to function without symptoms, even though the process of arteriosclerosis has produced a narrowing of the arteries.

Chelation (the word *chelate* comes from the Greek *chele*, "to claw") refers to the way certain chemicals and proteins can bind metallic ions which are positively charged to a negatively charged chelating agent. Most metals have a positive charge of two; the chelating agent has a negative charge of two which can combine with the positive one of the metal and hold it in its grip. This chelate has different properties from the metal alone and is sensitive to changes in temperature, acidity, and other chemicals in the body.

Chelation occurs as a process in nature—the transportation of iron in and out of cells is handled by a chelating process. The iron in hemoglobin which carries oxygen is an example of a chelated metal. In the plant world, chlorophyll, which converts carbon dioxide and water into starch, is a chelate of magnesium.

An example of the chelation process would be the removal of inorganic calcium from the body. Calcium is deposited on the walls of the blood vessels and heart valves, around tendons, joints, and ligaments, in the skin and kidneys. By chelating the inorganic calcium, calcification can be reduced over a period of time. Calcium is not the only material present in the linings of the blood vessels. When it is chelated out, the remaining material containing fatty substance, other minerals, and cholesterol is dissolved, metabolized by the liver and excreted via the intestinal tract. The diameter of the blood vessels is greatly increased, and more blood can flow to the organs and tissues of the body.

Herbs

Hawthorn berries are especially helpful; other herbs which are good for the heart include lily of the valley, yarrow, motherwort, garlic, onion, mistletoe, borage, lavender, and lemon balm. Cayenne, red clover, Chinese cinnamon, and ginger root (boiled as a tea) aid circulation. Red clover is also a blood purifier as are golden seal, chaparral, and echinacea root.

Supplements

1. Liquid lecithin—about two tablespoons every other day after meals. Lecithin helps reduce cholesterol and deposits in the arteries.

2. Vitamin C—from 1,000 to 3,000 mg daily in crystalline or powered form. Vitamin C helps conversion of cholesterol into bile oxide.

3. Bioflavonoid complex—three times daily.

4. Liquid chlorophyll—about two tablespoons in half a glass of spring water twice a day for magnesium.

5. A multivitamin/mineral complex three times daily.

6. B-complex made from a non-yeast base three times daily.

7. Vitamin E (dry form, not oil-based)—600 to 1,000 i.u.'s daily.

8. Free-form amino acid capsules three times daily.

ARTHRITIS

Arthritis is characterized by inflammation of the joints and connective tissue. Rheumatism is a general term for arthritis and applied to almost any pain in the joints or muscles. In arthritis, the joints become inflamed, enlarged, and swollen. The cartilage loses its elasticity, becoming dry and brittle, and the ligaments and muscles which surround the joint may also become inflamed, losing tone and flexibility. Swelling and pain often increase during motion.

There are various types of arthritis with *rheumatoid arthritis* and *osteoarthritis* the most widespread. In rheumatoid arthritis, the most painful and crippling form, one or more joints often become swollen and inflamed. If the disease progresses, there is degeneration of the joint with possible deformities and immobility. Osteoarthritis is much less crippling because it does not cause the two bone surfaces to fuse and immobilize the joint.

Other common types of arthritis include *lupus* (systemic lupus erythematosus), a disease of the connective tissue producing changes in the structure and function of the skin joints and internal organs; it affects seven times as many women as men. *Spondylitis* (ankylosing spondylitis) is caused by an inflammation of the joints of one or more vertebrae. *Gout*, resulting from a defect in body chemistry, leads to high blood levels of uric acid and forms needle-like crystals in the joint. *Bursitis* is the inflammation of a *bursa*, a sac-like structure resembling a joint located between the skin and bone.

People who take on a lot of responsibilities and carry a heavy load have arthritic tendencies. Often they feel very guilty, do not like what they are doing, and yet maintain that they are the only one who can do the job or take care of the situation.

Most arthritis sufferers tend to be emotionally reserved; they have difficulty expressing anger and turn their aggression inward. Their anger often manifests as pain. Often they have had a difficult childhood with one extremely authoritarian parent. Their emotional suppression may have led to anxiety during adolescence, and they often had strong sexual inhibitions.

There is also a tendency to be self-sacrificing as well—desiring to serve others out of a strong sense of responsibility, yet experiencing frustration when they do it, guilt when they don't.

Sometimes a catalyst such as a death in the family, a move, a change of occupation, or some added responsibility brings on the condition. Once individuals have arthritis, it becomes more difficult to express their emotions. Feelings of inferiority increase as well as dependency on others due to their limited mobility.

Two clients of mine are good examples of this. One is a woman in her mid-forties who has bad arthritis in her hands and fingers. She works 12 hours a day in an office in order to support both her teen-age son and her mother who is living with her. She was very resentful of her mother's living with her, but claimed she was the only one of the brothers and sisters who could take care of her. She had some treatments for her arthritis, but it wasn't until she finally asked for help from other members of the family that her arthritic condition was somewhat alleviated.

The second is a very creative lady who works in directing and writing scripts for TV and theater. In her early forties she got lupus. In addition to supporting her teen-age daughter (who was going to a private school and to college), she was also sending money to her mother. The pressure of these financial obligations made her very anxious about her work, and she no longer enjoyed it. She conferred with a doctor who uses alternative healing methods and finally gave up the idea of supporting her mother. Her condition has greatly improved.

Among the physiological causes of arthritis are toxicity in the blood stream and faulty removal of wastes. Uric acid and cholesterol can build up in the blood stream. Most arthritic patients are constipated (another holding back), and this leads to accumulation of toxins in the body. Stress periods produce adrenal exhaustion as well as the malfunctioning of other glands of the endocrine system. When the glands are no longer able to produce sufficient cortisone and other hormones, a severe hormonal imbalance results. This imbalance, combined with toxins from the system and a weakened nervous system, affects the structure of various tissues.

Treatments

1. The most important treatment for arthritis is cleansing. To get rid of toxic wastes and strengthen the immune system, colonic irrigations and high enemas are important as well as cleansing of the skin through saunas and steam baths.

2. Exercises for the joints and limbs are necessary to increase body mobility and loosen the muscles. Swimming is an excellent form of exercise for the arthritic patient since water is very relaxing. Yoga exercises are also good because they work with the breath and relaxation.

3. Physical therapies that break up old patterns of body armoring and crystallization help. Feldenkrais exercises are a good way of reprogramming the body and giving it new awareness.

4. Techniques that help the nervous system to relax, such as meditation, autogenics, and biofeedback, are beneficial.

5. Acupuncture is helpful in relieving pain, working with the immune system, and stimulating the adrenal glands to produce a natural type of cortisone.

6. Occasional liquid fasts with vegetable juices, soup broths, and herb teas will aid the cleansing process. These should be done only a few days at a time with very little fruit juice because arthritic patients tend to have a very acidic system and often low blood sugar as well.

7. Devil's claw is the most important *herb* in treating arthritis. Herbs such as comfrey and comfrey root, borage, alfalfa, wintergreen, sarsaparilla root, and oat straw are also helpful. Wintergreen

and willow contain salicylic acid, which aids in relieving pain.

8. Soaking afflicted limbs in a hot Epsom salts solution (one-half pound of Epsom salts in a large basin) is helpful. Also, rubbing a mixture of peanut oil and jojoba oil on sore joints every other day aids in dissolving some of the crystallized material. Castor oil packs, made by heating the castor oil and dipping a flannel cloth in it, can be applied to the affected area.

Diet

Emphasize cooked whole grains, steamed vegetables, fish, organic poultry, soured-milk products such as yogurt and kefir, and a few fertile eggs a week. No other cow's milk products should be used. Rye breads, millet breads, and rice crackers should be used instead of wheat bread. Strongly acidic foods such as sour apples, apple juice, strawberries, tomatoes, raw spinach, rhubarb, cranberries, vinegar, nutritional yeast, and citrus should be avoided. Fruit should be kept to a minimum with about one portion every other day.

Refined products, coffee, teas, alcohol, and sugars should be eliminated. Barley malt syrup or rice syrup can be used for sweetening with some honey.

Supplements

1. Aloe vera juice—four to six tablespoons on alternate mornings.
2. A multivitamin/mineral three times daily.
3. Liquid chlorophyll—two or three tablespoons two times a day in half a glass of water.
4. A manganese tablet or capsule three times daily.
5. Bioflavonoid complex three times daily.
6. Pantothenic acid (1,000-2,000 mg) three times daily.
7. Adrenal glandular supplement two to three times a day.
8. A free-form amino acid capsule two or three times daily.
9. Zinc two times daily.
10. PABA capsules (550 mg) three times daily.

ASTHMA

Asthma is an extreme allergic reaction that involves tightness in the chest and labored breathing. Muscle fibers surrounding the bronchial tubes tighten up after an encounter with air pollutants, dust, mold, pet dander, food, or drugs. The lining of the lungs becomes swollen and inflamed and produces a sticky mucus that is often coughed up.

Fear of an asthma attack and not being able to breathe makes the asthmatic extremely nervous, and s/he tends to tighten up her/his chest even more. Relaxation techniques and deep breathing are important tools in controlling asthma.

The lungs are related to the element Air or Metal in the Chinese system. An excess of Air or Metal indicates mental energy which needs to be balanced with the physical (Fire), emotional (Water), and practical, grounding disciplines (Earth). Emotionally, the lungs are related to grief and worry.

There are many emotional causes involved in asthma. Fear of being separated from or losing the mother at an early age is a major cause. Since the respiratory function is so related to the mother, the act of breathing on one's own is a first step in becoming independent. When there is fear of doing this, breathing becomes labored and difficult. The conflict is between the need to be independent and the dependency on the mother. When they are emotionally upset, extremely sensitive children may react to the presence of various allergens in their environment.

Asthmatic children tend to have difficulty adapting to new surroundings and events. This kind of change may catalyze an asthma attack.

In general, asthmatics tend to be compulsive in their behavior. They are not adaptable and need to plan for changes months ahead. They hold on to a lot of grief and anguish from childhood, which tends to congest the lung and chest area.

Treatments

1. The major treatment for asthmatics is for them to get in touch with their hidden fears and anxieties. Once they can bring these to conscious awareness, the sources for provocation of attacks diminish. Unburdening the pain and grief from childhood is also important.

2. Relaxation techniques such as meditation, biofeedback, and autogenics are very helpful in learning to control the breath and other bodily processes.

3. Yoga exercises or other exercises that loosen up the body

as well as strengthen muscles and deepen breathing are very important.

4. Ridding the lungs of excess mucus is necessary. The lungs are related to the colon or large intestine through the meridian system of the body. Colonics loosen up old mucus in the large intestine and enable one to breathe and assimilate food better.

5. Certain *herbs* work to expel excess mucus from the lungs and cleanse the lymph system. Horehound, elecampane root, and osha root may be simmered individually and used as teas. Slippery elm, marshmallow root and comfrey root are other herbs which may be simmered that are soothing to the mucous membranes. Coltsfoot, mullein, and yerba santa are helpful to the respiratory system. Lobelia is good for wheezing. The Chinese herb ephedra is excellent in combination with Chinese licorice and ginger.

6. Eliminate any foods that are the source of allergens, especially sugar, refined carbohydrates, cow's milk products, and wheat which form excess mucus in the lungs and colon.

Supplements

1. Aloe vera juice—four to six tablespoons every other day on an empty stomach to cleanse the lungs and colon.

2. Free-form amino acids or L-phenylalanine—three capsules daily for adrenal glands and energy.

3. Multivitamin/mineral capsules three times daily.

4. Liquid chlorophyll—two to three tablespoons in half a glass of spring water two times daily.

5. A manganese capsule three times daily.

6. Zinc—three tablets or capsules for the immune system.

7. Pantothenic acid—1,000 mg three times daily.

8. Vitamin B complex three times daily.

9. Bioflavonoids three times daily.

10. Some form of potassium, such as potassium/magnesium capsules, three times daily.

BLADDER INFECTIONS

Bladder infections are related to urinary tract infections and are more common in women than in men. This is because anatomically a woman's urethra is only 1-1/2 inches long, so bacteria can easily reach the bladder. These bacteria are most often the Escherichia coli, normal inhabitants of the bowel. Since a woman's urethra and rectum are close together, this also makes women more susceptible (many women wipe from back to front, increasing the risk).

Physical causes of urinary tract infections include holding back urination due to time circumstances, unhygienic places or garments that are difficult to remove. Pantyhose, tight jeans, and synthetic underwear in fabrics that don't breathe (nylon and acrylic) increase the warm, moist environment these bacteria thrive on.

Physiologically, the bladder is related to elimination and cleansing and to relationships. Holding on to old fears and emotional patterns, not "letting go," leads to blockage and subsequent infections of the bladder and kidneys. In Chinese medicine, the bladder and kidney are related to the Water element and the emotion of fear. Crying is another form of purification and emotional release related to Water. One who is unable to shed tears often has problems in the bladder and kidney area.

Treatments

There has been much misunderstanding about the acid/alkaline balance in the body, and many books and practitioners recommend increasing the body's acidity with cranberry juice and vitamin C to discourage the growth of bacteria. In fact, when the bladder and kidneys are not functioning properly, the body tends to be overly acid and there is a strong lack of potassium. The use of certain herbs as well as more alkaline foods and supplements seem to help this imbalance.

1. Certain diuretic *herbs* increase urination. The best ones are dandelion leaf, uva ursi, nettles, buchu, corn silk, couch grass, cleavers, and alfalfa. In some cases juniper berries work very well. Put 1-1/2 teaspoons of the berries in 1-1/2 cups of water and simmer for 5-10 minutes. Drink two cups every other day.

2. A poultice made of cottage cheese (dry curd) over the crotch area helps stop the stinging and burning and draws out inflammation. One teaspoon of cottage cheese should be used and the poultice should be changed several times a day.

3. The diet should include plenty of fresh vegetables, sea vegetables high in the trace minerals, as well as whole grains, fresh fish, and soured-milk products which are helpful in controlling the bac-

teria. Buckwheat and buckwheat sprouts are high in rutin, a supplement that is essential for proper functioning of the bladder and kidney. Fruit and fruit juice should be eliminated.

Supplements
    1. Multivitamin/mineral capsules three times daily.
    2. Potassium/magnesium capsules three times a day.
    3. Zinc capsules or tablets three times daily.
    4. Bioflavonoid complex three times daily (contains rutin).
    5. Vitamin A is particularly helpful for bladder infections but must be used in its dry form as beta-carotene (not in its oil form from fish liver oil). Take three times daily.
    6. Vitamins B-3, B-6, and B-12 are important either as individual supplements or in a B complex with a non-yeast base. Take three times daily.

BRONCHITIS

Bronchitis is an inflammation of the bronchial tubes which carries air from the mouth to the lungs. It often develops as a result of a cold or respiratory infection which causes the mucous lining of the bronchial tubes to swell and overflow. In an attempt to expel mucus from the lungs, the body develops a cough. The cough is a way of getting rid of the poisons which have started this problem.

Bronchitis can be exacerbated by cold, damp weather and the eating of heavy mucus foods such as sugar, refined carbohydrates, cow's milk products, and wheat. Since the lungs are related to the colon in Chinese medicine, digestive problems and conditions of blockage in the colon need to be worked with as well.

Psychologically, the lungs correspond to grief and worry. The excessive coughing is often an attempt to cough up the grief and held-back emotions. Since the lungs relate to the element Air, there is a need to balance out this element by cutting back on mental activities and adding more physical and emotional ones such as singing and dancing. Mucus represents the Water element and symbolizes excess emotions that are trapped in the chest area.

Treatments
    1. Ridding the lungs of excess mucus by cleansing the digestive

tract through colonic irrigations and enemas is most important.

2. Eliminate all foods mentioned previously that form excess mucus.

3. Certain *herbs* help to expel mucus and can be soothing to the bronchials as well. Aloe vera juice is important in cleansing the lungs and colon. Other herbs are osha root, horehound, elecampane root and wild cherry bark. Slippery elm, comfrey, marshmallow root, and borage are soothing to the bronchioles. Coltsfoot and mullein are excellent as well. Lobelia is helpful for bronchial spasms. The Chinese herb ephedra (*ma huang*) contains ephedrine and is also beneficial.

4. A cough syrup made from herbs such as wild cherry bark, slippery elm and horehound with a bit of honey is recommended. (See bibliography for books where such formulas are contained.)

5. Yoga exercises and breathing techniques are most essential. Slowing down the breath can ease up the coughing and promote greater relaxation.

6. Massage work that relaxes the body and stimulates the lymphatic system is most helpful.

Supplements

1. Liquid chlorophyll—two or three tablespoons daily in one-half glass of water provide magnesium to relax the nervous system.

2. Aloe vera juice—four to six tablespoons alternate mornings.

3. A trace mineral or multivitamin/mineral tablet or capsule three times daily.

4. Vitamin C—too much may be too acidic; try two tablespoons of a powdered ascorbate twice daily.

5. Bioflavonoid capsules three times daily.

6. Vitamin B complex in a non-yeast base two or three times daily (1,000 mg).

7. Pantothenic acid—1,000 mg daily.

8. PABA three times daily (use 550 or 1,000 mg tablets).

9. Vitamin A in its form as beta-carotene two or three times daily.

10. Zinc capsules or tablets three times daily.

BURNS

Burns can destroy human tissue and be extremely painful and cause victims a good deal of shock. The nervous system needs to be treated in addition to tending to the burned area.

First-degree burns are red, discolored, and somewhat painful, but do not involve breakage of the skin.

Second-degree burns show skin breakage and are accompanied by swelling, blisters and damage to nerve endings.

Third-degree burns involve destruction of skin surface and tissue.

Burns often occur as a result of moving too fast or holding a lot of anger within, "feeling burned." They teach us to slow down and become calm and centered; we also learn how to deal with the issues that are burning up inside us.

Treatments

1. Reduce heat from burned areas by immersing in cool water.

2. Apply immediately secretions from the aloe plant (break a piece of the stem and rub juice on the burn); aloe vera gel; comfrey or plantain leaves ground up into a poultice; the oil from vitamin E capsules; clay poultices; or bicarbonate of soda mixed with water. These will help with relieving pain and speed up healing.

3. A homeopathic remedy is helpful. Cantharis is the remedy most often used though aconite may be used where there is great pain and shock accompanying the burn. Nettle salve is also used in homeopathy.

Supplements

1. Vitamin E taken internally is helpful—800-1,000 i.u.'s in the dry form, not the oil-based capsules, three times daily.

2. Vitamin C in large doses helps burns to heal—about 1,000 mg daily on alternate days (in ascorbate form).

3. Bioflavonoid capsules—1,000 mg three times daily.

4. Vitamin A is important in preventing infection—10,000 mg as beta-carotene twice daily.

5. For shock and the balancing of the nervous system, two or three tablespoons of liquid chlorophyll twice daily and magnesium tablets three times daily for a few days.

6. Vitamin B complex (non-yeast base)—1,000 mg three times daily.

CANCER

Cancer is a family of diseases that is characterized by uncontrolled growth of cells. There are three basic types of cancer: carcinomas, sarcomas, and leukemia-like cancers.

Carcinomas are the most common cancers; they are malignant tumors that occur in the epithelial cells that cover tissues and body cavities and in glandular organs such as the breast. Cancers of the lungs, stomach, mouth, and prostate and gastrointestinal cancers would be classified as carcinomas.[2] *Sarcomas* are less common, but highly malignant. They form in connective tissues, muscle, bone and cartilage.[3] *Leukemia-like cancers* include: (a) leukemia, which results from the overproduction of white blood cells, followed by their underproduction; (b) lymphomas, tumors in lymphoid tissue which cause the overproduction of lymphoid cells (cells found in bone marrow from which all blood cells are thought to arise); and (c) multiple myelomas, a bone-marrow tumor, which is the rarest form of cancer that causes the overproduction of plasma cells.[4]

An adult who has cancer will usually have a carcinoma, while young children most often have leukemia. Cell mutation may be caused by chemical damage to cell membranes or by damaged DNA. A precancerous cell is a mutated cell that may lead to a full-fledged cancer unless the mutated cells are recognized by the immune system and destroyed. The cell membrane is the protective outer skin of a cell that is responsible for the transport of nutrients into the cell and the removal of waste products. The cell membrane also contains sensors for detecting the proximity of neighboring cells and controls the production of more cells. If the cell membrane is damaged, uncontrolled growth may result.

There are many explanations for the changes in the physiology of a cell. Emotional states and traumatic conditions certainly have the power to change cellular structure. Those who strongly advocate this belief have worked with meditation and visualization exercises to balance cells. Others believe that an invading virus or bacteria is responsible for cellular change and depletes the immune system as well. Still others emphasize the environmental causes of cancer—pollution in air and water and increased amounts of radiation to which we are all subject.

While many conditions of physiological imbalance may lead to the growth of cancer cells, emotional situations often trigger and exacerbate these conditions. A trauma, death of a loved one, divorce, a move to a new locality, or loss of a job can lead to strong physiological changes in the body. When one has not been dealing with her/his emotions or processing them on a daily basis, many feelings get "stuffed under the rug" and begin to gnaw away at the subconscious.

Psychological Characteristics

Cancer patients tend to have a lot of repressed emotions, especially anger and hostility. In Chinese medicine, the liver is related to anger, and in cancerous conditions the liver is extremely congested. Traditional Chinese medicine relates cancer to "heat in the blood," whereas Western herbal medicine would phrase it as "toxic blood" or "toxic liver." There is a strong need to cleanse the liver thereby increasing the bile flow as well.

Many of those with cancer are extremely sensitive, vulnerable human beings. They often see themselves as victims and easily take on the worries and anxieties of those around them. They have difficulty speaking up for themselves and are often dealing with issues like self-esteem and self-empowerment.

Treatments

1. The most important treatment is to begin to make changes and adaptations in one's life style. One needs to see clearly the stresses and emotional anxieties in her/his life and begin to deal with and resolve these issues.

2. Visualization techniques introduced by Drs. Carl and Stephanie Simonton (see their book *Getting Well Again* [Bantam, 1981]) are very helpful in achieving a healthy integration of mind and body.

3. A complete physiological cleansing will rid the body of toxic material, get each organ functioning properly, and build up the immune system. Colonic irrigations and enemas are most helpful. There are many variations of these treatments; wheat grass implants after an enema should also be done. Coffee enemas have been used successfully (see Dr. Max Gerson's *A Cancer Therapy: Results of 50 Cases* [Totality Books, 1977]). The number of colonics and enemas weekly depends on the individual in terms of need and toleration. In addition, a juice fast of a few days to several weeks is advisable. The fast should include predominantly vegetable juices (especially

beet juice), soup broths, herb teas, and a small amount of fruit juice such as black cherry or prune. The juice from organic liver has also been used, especially for those with leukemia and those needing large amounts of iron.

4. After the juice fast and cleansing, some foods may be gradually reintroduced into the diet. These should include raw and cooked vegetables, sea vegetables, a small amount of fruit (every other day), and cooked whole grains (except wheat, which is highly mucus-forming). Vegetable oils should be taken, especially flaxseed oil and cold-pressed olive oil, which are very important for the liver and gall bladder. In two months' time, some protein may be introduced—tofu (soybean curd), baked or broiled fish, soured-milk products such as yogurt and kefir (especially those made from goat's milk), and sometimes up to four fertile eggs weekly. Nuts and nut butters are difficult to digest when the liver is not functioning properly and should be used sparingly. If eaten, they should be soaked first; almonds are often used.

5. Herbal teas are important in cleansing the blood, decongesting the lymph system, and rebuilding the immune system. The best *herbs* to drink are chaparral (if the taste is unappealing, spearmint or peppermint may be added), red clover, echinacea root, golden seal, yarrow, and violet. A combination of chaparral and red clover is excellent. Simmer three teaspoons of chaparral and two teaspoons of red clover in four cups of water until it is reduced to three cups. Drink three cups on alternate days for several weeks. Echinacea root may be substituted for the chaparral, which can also be used in capsules, but these are less effective. The herb thyme, sprinkled on food, is good for the thymus gland. The Chinese herb astragalus is also good for the immune system.

Making herbal poultices and applying them to the affected area is another excellent remedy. A ginger root poultice draws out toxins and increases the circulation. Grate a small piece of ginger root and put in a tea ball or cheesecloth. Simmer in a large pot of water 15 or 20 minutes. When ready, soak a cloth in the tea and apply to affected parts of the body, short of scalding. Cover with a dry towel and keep re-applying until area turns red. Other poultices that are also helpful are comfrey leaves, plantain leaves or violet leaves. The leaves may be steeped in hot water, wrapped in cheesecloth, and applied with a cloth or towel.

6. Acupuncture treatments are extremely helpful in revitaliz-

ing organs, restoring the body to its normal metabolism, and increasing energy.

7. Bodywork is important for circulation and energy flow. Especially helpful is lymphatic massage for cleansing the lymph system. Shiatsu, jin shinn, and other types of Oriental bodywork stimulate meridians which go to each organ and increase energy.

8. Homeopathic remedies can balance the metabolism and increase the vital force. Each person needs to be treated individually with the remedy which is best suited to her/his constitution.

9. Flower essences are very important in balancing out emotional states such as depression and anxiety and may be used in conjunction with other therapies.

Supplements

1. Aloe vera juice—about 1/4 to 1/2 cup upon arising on alternate days.

2. Two tablespoons cold-pressed olive oil or flaxseed oil with juice of half a lemon on alternative mornings.

3. Liquid lecithin—two tablespoons after a meal twice daily on alternate days.

4. Free-form amino acid capsules—three daily.

5. Pancreas glandular supplement—two or three tablets daily.

6. Thymus glandular—three tablets daily.

7. A multiple digestive enzyme (including pancreatic enzymes, ox bile, papain, and pepsin)—one after each meal.

8. Liquid chlorophyll (if not drinking parsley, celery, or another green drink)—two or three tablespoons in half a glass of spring water three times daily.

9. Wheat grass juice—1/2 oz. on alternate days.

10. Vitamin C (powdered in ascorbate form)—about 2,000 mg daily.

11. Bioflavonoid capsules—1,000 mg three times daily.

12. Vitamin A (from beta-carotene)—10,000 i.u.'s twice daily.

13. Vitamin E (dry form)—800-1,000 i.u.'s twice daily.

14. Vitamin B complex (non-yeast base)—1,000 mg, three tablets or capsules daily.

15. Zinc picollinate—three capsules daily.

16. Potassium/magnesium capsules—three daily.

CANDIDA

Candida albicans is a micro-organism or yeast fungus which is found in various parts of the body such as the intestinal tract, the vaginal canal, rectum, and other warm, moist areas. It is thought that overuse of antibiotics and other immuno-suppressant drugs contribute to candida growth because they destroy the "friendly bacteria" in the intestines which normally control fungus. The yeast fungi invade and colonize the body's cells and organs, releasing toxic chemicals into the blood and causing vaginitis, rectal itching, chronic diarrhea or constipation, bladder infections, headaches, acne, mental confusion, anxiety, and nervousness.

Food allergies, hypoglycemia, and an extremely acid body—all of these accompany candida. A diet high in sweets, fruit, and acid foods, such as tomatoes, green pepper, spinach, and vinegar, exacerbates the condition and is often a causative factor as well.

Psychological Characteristics

Psychologically, emotional and sensitive individuals seem to be candidates for candida. Artists, psychics, those who work in healing and counseling, tend to have more acid bodies which are receptive to the growth of the candida fungus. It is important for them to learn to protect themselves from pulling in the emotions of others and to learn to clear themselves after working with others.

Treatments

The basic treatment procedure for candida usually involves three steps: (1) eliminating all antibiotics and drugs from the system, (2) changing the diet to deprive the yeast of food upon which it flourishes, and (3) strengthening the body's immune system.

Two drugs, Nystatin (which has several side effects) and Caprisan, a form of caprillac acid made from coconut oil, are being used.

However, it is best to work with natural treatments that cleanse the body and build up the immune system. Recommended are the following:

1. Colonic irrigations are the most important treatment to cleanse the intestinal tract and control yeast growth. They should be taken monthly in the first phases of the condition.

2. For women whose vaginal area is affected, douching with

acidophilus is helpful—four tablespoons to one quart of warm water—as well as inserting acidophilus capsules into the vagina.

3. Various *herbs* are helpful. Garlic is a standard blood purifier and should be included in the diet every other day. Black walnut is a strong antifungal herb used both internally and externally in an alcohol solution. Pau d'arco (also called *taheebo*) is a Brazilian herb that works with the immune system and is a blood purifier. Echinacea root is also a strong blood purifier that builds the immune system. Marshmallow root stimulates the immune system and soothes the mucous linings of the intestine. Dandelion root is helpful in toning the liver and pancreas. To increase adrenal energy, which is often depleted from the immuno-suppressant drugs, Siberian ginseng, fo-ti (the Chinese herb of longevity) and gotu-kola are helpful.

4. Certain homeopathic remedies have been useful and have helped the body rebalance.

5. Acupuncture treatments have worked to stimulate the organs and build up the immune system.

Diet

1. Eliminate all chemical additives and preservatives as well as canned and packaged foods.

2. Eliminate yeast-based foods such as B-complex vitamins, alcoholic beverages, mushrooms, certain cheeses, vinegar, cider, and nutritional yeast.

3. Eliminate highly acidic foods such as citrus, sour apples, grapes, plums, cranberries, strawberries, tomatoes, raw green pepper, and raw spinach. These tend to make the body more acidic; coffee and chocolate, besides being high in caffeine, are two other very acidic foods.

4. Cow's milk products, such as cheese, butter, and cottage cheese, are sources of allergies. Use yogurts and soured-milk products since they contain lactic acid which is helpful to the growth of "friendly intestinal bacteria."

5. Eliminate meats, except organic poultry and organic liver.

6. Eliminate shellfish, a strong source of food allergies.

7. Eliminate salt and all foods high in sodium, such as soy sauce, miso soup, salad dressings, and canned soups.

8. Prepare plenty of cooked vegetables, particularly leafy greens, high in minerals.

9. Include fresh vegetable juices as a source of vitamins and minerals.

10. Include sea vegetables, such as dulse, kombu, wakame, and alaria, as high sources of minerals.

11. Eat whole grains, especially at breakfast, as a source of B vitamins and as a way to keep blood sugar up throughout the day. Use brown rice, buckwheat, barley, millet, rye, oats, amaranth, and cornmeal. Avoid wheat as it tends to be mucus-forming. Many candida diets eliminate most grains because of possible mold. If the grain is bought in a good health food store, it is generally safe. Test it out, if necessary, with radiesthesia or muscle testing.

Supplements

1. Free-form amino acid capsules—three daily to balance blood sugar.

2. Potassium/magnesium capsules—three daily.

3. Powdered trace minerals from sea vegetables—two to three teaspoons daily, or three tablets or capsules.

4. Zinc picollinate or chelated zinc—three daily.

5. Evening primrose oil capsules—two or three daily for the immune system.

6. Pantothenic acid—500-1,000 mg two or three times daily.

7. B-12, preferably in liquid form on alternate days.

8. Bioflavonoid capsules—1,000 mg three times daily. Beware of using too much vitamin C as it acidifies the body even if it is buffered.

CHRONIC FATIGUE SYNDROME

Chronic Fatigue Syndrome, or Epstein-Barr virus, has been steadily increasing among the population since 1983 when it was first diagnosed. Its symptoms are that of a chronic mononucleosis. The Epstein-Barr virus is a herpes virus which is, in fact, the cause of infectious mononucleosis. Like all herpes viruses, it is latent and deep in the B cells of the immune system. The cells are responsible for producing antibodies which circulate in the body, destroying invading viruses and bacteria.

Among CEBV patients (Chronic Epstein-Barr Virus), elevated antibodies to the Epstein-Barr virus are found, indicating that the virus is multiplying. The only known cause of CEBV is a virus called "human B lymphotropic virus," or HBLV, because of its affinity for B cells. HBLV in combination with the EB virus can be devastating to the immune system. The EB virus is a "transforming" virus, which means that it incorporates its own genetic material into a cell's DNA, transforming the cell into a different unit altogether.

Chemical pollutants and toxins have been known to exacerbate the virus and increase the intensity of symptoms.

CEBV often starts like a flu with fever, weakness, and extreme exhaustion. In time, its symptoms include metabolic disturbances resulting in weight loss and gain; cognitive function problems, including impaired reasoning, spatial disorientation and amnesia-like episodes; chest pain and shortness of breath; joint pain; fevers; swollen glands; ringing in the ears; swollen feet and hands; numbness and tingling in legs and arms; rashes and herpes-like lesions; hair loss; miscarriages in women and impotence in men.

Many of those with CEBV have had to leave their jobs and give up careers because they have been unable to read, write, or think clearly.

Psychological Studies

CEBV symptoms seem to come after a prolonged period of stress. Women are hit more than men, particularly women in their thirties and forties. Many of the women studied have been over-achievers, Type A personalities working long and hard hours. They haven't been aware of their stressful lives until after becoming ill with CEBV symptoms. What they have had to learn is to do the absolutely essential things and cut down their daily chores. Dealing with CEBV has often catalyzed people to pursue a more inner spiritual path. More research is necessary to uncover other common psychological patterns.

Treatments

1. Injections of B-12 and folic acid have helped the nervous system and energy level.

2. Acupuncture treatments several times a week combined with Chinese herbal therapy have proved helpful to many with CEBV.

3. Homeopathy—certain remedies have been very beneficial in controlling the symptoms of CEBV.

Supplements

    1. An antioxidant multivitamin/mineral after meals four times daily.

    2. Blue-green algae or liquid chlorophyll for detoxifying the liver and as a source of magnesium three times daily.

    3. Bioflavonoid capsules—six daily after meals, two or three times a day.

    4. Potassium/magnesium capsules—six daily after meals, two or three times a day.

    5. Manganese capsules—extremely important for the nervous system—one capsule after meals three times daily.

    6. Pantothenic acid—1,000 mg three times daily after meals for stress and to help the adrenal cortex.

    7. Thymus glandular—three times daily after meals for the immune system.

    8. A digestive enzyme including pancreatin and bile to break down foods and help the pancreas—one or two after meals.

Herbs

    Blood purifiers such as chaparral, echinacea root, sarsaparilla root, red clover, burdock root, and gentian should be considered. Chaparral may be mixed with one of the mints to make it more palatable. Adrenal stimulants such as gotu-kola, fo-ti, or ginseng may also be helpful.

Diet

    1. Eliminate all processed foods, sugars, and caffeine products.

    2. Eliminate meat except organic calves' liver, beef liver, chicken livers, turkey, or lean chicken.

    3. Eliminate foods such as chocolate, vinegar, cranberries, tomatoes, green pepper, spinach, citrus fruits, strawberries, watermelon, plums, and grapes.

    4. Eliminate dairy products such as milk, butter, and cheese. Substitute acidophilus products such as yogurt, kefir, acidophilus cottage cheese, and kefir cheese.

    5. Eliminate shellfish, but include fresh fish—baked, broiled, or steamed.

    6. Eliminate wheat. Substitute other grains such as rye, rice, millet, buckwheat, barley, amaranth, and oats as cereals or as bread or crackers.

7. Prepare lots of steamed vegetables, especially leafy greens such as kale, chard, collard greens, mustard greens, and bok choy.

8. Eat whole grains and whole-grain cereals in the morning and one other time during the day.

9. Use plenty of fresh vegetable juice such as carrot-celery, parsley, cucumber, or beet. Liver juice is also excellent for its iron and B-12.

10. Eat root vegetables such as beets, turnips, rutabagas, potatoes and squashes.

11. Eat proteins such as yogurt, fresh fish, fertile eggs, tofu, and organic liver if it is appealing.

12. Eat small amounts of fruit, perhaps on alternate days, such as bananas, peaches, cherries, baked apples or pears, golden delicious apples, cantaloupe or honeydew melons, blueberries or blackberries.

CIRCULATION PROBLEMS

Poor circulation results from blockages in the arteries like arteriosclerosis and atherosclerosis where the arteries cannot carry as much blood to the heart and the lymphatic system is congested and cannot properly rid the body of carbon dioxide and waste material. When not enough oxygen reaches the lungs, the body reacts by lowered temperature.

Psychologically, poor circulation (cold hands and feet and being cold much of the time) may correspond to a feeling of detachment from others and keeping the heart closed. Those with poor circulation often tend to distance themselves from others and do not allow themselves to experience their emotions.

Treatments
1. Therapeutically working with causes of emotional detachment and separation.

2. Plenty of exercise, especially aerobic-type exercises that stimulate the heart. This may be aerobic dancing, swimming, jogging, and other sports where the heart is actively increasing its potential. *Be careful of these exercises if you have a heart condition.*

3. Acupuncture treatments are particularly helpful in stimulating circulation and working with the triple burner, the organs that

increase warmth and fire.

4. Bodywork such as shiatsu, acupressure, and jin shinn, which stimulate the meridians and facilitate the flow of energy to all organs.

Diet

Emphasize cooked foods which promote body warmth—cooked whole-grain cereals in the morning, especially from buckwheat, millet and barley; root vegetables such as potatoes, squashes, yams, rutabagas, and beets; spices such as cayenne, ginger, curry powder, coriander, turmeric, cinnamon, and mustard. Juicing ginger root with vegetables is also helpful. Avoid cow's milk products and wheat (which tend to form excess mucus and block arteries), red meat, shellfish, all refined products and sugar, and too many fruits and fruit juices, which are cooling to the body. Avoid food eaten cold—warm it up to room temperature at least.

Herbs

Make herb teas from ginger root (simmer a piece of root with two cups of water for 10-15 minutes), Chinese cinnamon (one tablespoon of bark per 1-1/2 cups water), and red clover blossoms. Fo-ti tien, a Chinese herb for vitality, is also warming to the body and may be simmered as the others. There are a multitude of Chinese herbs which increase body heat.

Use warming spices in cooking such as cayenne, curry, and ginger. Garlic is excellent for poor circulation. For cold feet, sprinkle cayenne in the socks and take foot baths with mustard powder.

Supplements

1. Flaxseed oil—two tablespoons on alternate days help to unclog arteries.

2. Niacin or B-3—100 mg on alternate days causes flushing which increases circulation. This can be an uncomfortable feeling, so beware of taking too much niacin.

3. Three teaspoons powdered or three tablets or capsules. Those with poor circulation tend to be low in iron and zinc.

4. Liquid chlorophyll as a source of magnesium. Magnesium is the most important mineral in maintaining the health of the heart. Take two to three tablespoons two times daily in half a glass of spring water.

5. Vitamin E—800-1,000 i.u.'s in dry form three times daily.

6. Bioflavonoid complex—1,000 mg daily. It contains rutin which is helpful to circulation.

7. Octacosanol (see chapter 9)—two super-strength capsules (5,000 mg) daily. If using this, you do not need vitamin E.

8. Magnesium capsules (preferably with potassium or calcium)—three times daily.

COLDS

Colds are catalyzed by viruses that are even tinier than bacteria. The virus is a scavenger which invades the cells when the cells themselves are not in top functioning order. It generally moves into the area of the nose and throat, and the body reacts by forming mucus to rinse away the invader and by increasing the body's temperature.

Causes of a cold can be excessive fatigue, overindulgence in food or drink, improper exposure to the elements, worry, and various types of stress.

Psychologically, a cold is often a time to stop and slow down, to rest and handle certain issues that one may have been avoiding.

Treatments

1. Most physiological treatments for colds are preventative—these include rest, exercise, proper nutrition, and staying warm in cold weather. The Japanese sleep with a hot water bottle on the kidneys at the small of the back. During the winter, it is especially important to get plenty of fresh air and do deep breathing exercises to keep the lungs open.

2. The most important preventative measure for colds and flus is to take time out from one's daily routine for relaxation and centering. Yoga, meditation, tai chi, and exercise classes can be helpful.

3. At the first sign of a cold, a liquid fast with hot herbal teas, soup broths, and vegetable juices should be initiated. In addition, an enema or colon irrigation should be taken to clear out the mucus and detoxify the body.

4. Saunas and steam baths are excellent for cleansing the body and breaking up mucus in the lungs and chest.

5. Bodywork and massage, especially lymphatic massage,

stimulate the meridians and organs of the body and improve circulation.

6. Putting hot oils and liniments on the chest will break up inflammation there and promote body warmth.

7. Avoid heavy mucus-forming foods such as cow's milk products and wheat; also food such as red meat, shellfish, pasta, beans and other carbohydrates. Include fresh vegetables (mostly cooked), a small amount of fruit, cooked whole grains, bean curd, eggs (a few a week), fresh fish, and nuts and seeds.

8. Drinking *herb* teas such as elecampane root, horehound and marshmallow roots (roots need to be simmered for ten minutes with one teaspoon of the root to 1-1/2 cups of water) will help break up congestion and cleanse the lymph system. The Chinese herb ephedra (*ma huang*) is excellent. Other good herbs to use as teas for the lungs are slippery elm, comfrey, mullein, coltsfoot, and yerba santa. Herbs such as cayenne (sprinkled on food) and teas made from red clover blossoms, ginger root, and Chinese cinnamon (cassia bark) are warming to the body and stimulate circulation. Garlic and onions are also good; garlic purifies the blood and onions stimulate the circulatory system.

Supplements

1. Homeopathic remedies like Euphrasia, Allium cepa, and Allium ceva alleviate colds. (See bibliography on chapter 13 for books on homeopathic first aid.)

2. Vitamin C—a powdered ascorbate form that can be put in juice or water during a liquid fast. The amount varies from person to person, depending on how acid one's body is.

3. Bioflavonoid capsules—1,000 mg four times daily.

4. Vitamin A—when there is an accompanying infection, use 10,000-20,000 i.u.'s of beta-carotene three times a day; if no infection, use twice daily.

5. Vitamin B complex (in non-yeast base)—500 mg tablets three times a day.

6. Liquid chlorophyll—two or three tablespoons in half a glass of spring water two times daily.

7. Trace minerals or multivitamin/mineral capsules four times a day.

8. Aloe vera juice—1/4 to 1/2 cup on alternate mornings to cleanse lungs and colon.

9. Two tablespoons cold-pressed olive oil or flaxseed oil with the juice of half a lemon on alternate mornings to cleanse the liver (garlic and cayenne optional).

COLITIS

Colitis is an inflammation of the lining of the colon. It is often referred to as mucous colitis, spastic colitis, or irritable bowel syndrome. Spasms occur in the lower portion of the bowel, commonly accompanied by cramps in the upper stomach. Frequently, there is constipation, often alternated with diarrhea. As the condition worsens, mucus is often secreted. Ulcerative colitis is more serious than mucous colitis; it produces diarrhea, loss of weight, and sometimes anemia.

Colitis often results from poor dietary habits: grabbing meals "on the go," not relaxing during meals, and eating quick snacks and junk foods. It can also be caused by overuse of laxatives.

Psychological Characteristics

In colitis, there is an excess of the Air element, indicating an overuse of the mental function. There needs to be more physical exercise and more involvement with others on an emotional, feeling level (singing and dancing). Those who have a tendency to colitis have similar personality traits to those who tend towards ulcers. They worry a lot, store much tension in their bodies, and tend to be "workaholics," often with strong demands on themselves for perfection.

Treatments

1. Dealing with psychological problems and alleviating unnecessary anxieties and worries is most important.

2. Relaxation techniques such as meditation, biofeedback, and autogenics are very helpful in treating colitis.

3. Massage treatments that work on loosening up the colon area.

4. Increasing exercise—especially exercise that involves deep breathing, such as yoga and tai chi.

Herbs

1. Relaxing nervine herb teas such as vervain, catnip, and spearmint are good; hops and scullcap may be used in the evening.

2. Herbs that aid digestion, such as peppermint, spearmint, wintergreen, and papaya leaf, are beneficial.

3. Drink herb teas that are mucilaginous and healing to the colon, such as slippery elm, comfrey, borage, and mullein.

Diet

Pay careful attention to diet. Avoid tobacco, alcohol, coffee, tea, any stimulants, refined carbohydrates, foods with chemical additives, and sugars. Avoid acidic foods such as vinegar, nutritional yeast, tomatoes, raw spinach, raw green pepper, cranberries, strawberries, sour apples and pears (golden delicious apples are best or baked apples and pears), grapes, watermelon, plums, and citrus. Eat fruit only a few times a week, preferably bananas, peaches, papaya, cherries, apricots, baked apples, or pears. Eliminate fruit juices.

Use easy-to-digest whole-grain cereals in the morning, such as rice cream, millet cream, and buckwheat cream. Emphasize steamed and baked vegetables with salads a few times a week. Avoid fried and sautéed foods. Broil or bake fish and organic poultry. Include soured-milk products such as yogurt or kefir.

Eat in a relaxed, quiet atmosphere, chewing each mouthful of food carefully.

Supplements

1. Aloe vera juice—four to six tablespoons on an empty stomach on alternate mornings. This will help with both diarrhea and constipation.

2. High-potency powdered acidophilus—1/2 teaspoon daily for about three weeks; repeat every other month for a week or two.

3. Liquid chlorophyll (for magnesium)—two or three times daily in half a glass of spring water.

4. Manganese (chelated or capsules)—three times daily.

5. Vitamin B complex (non-yeast base)—500 mg three times daily.

6. Trace minerals (preferably in powdered form for digestion) or multivitamin and minerals—three times daily.

7. Pantothenic acid—500-1,000 mg three times daily.

8. Vitamin A as beta-carotene—one or two tablets daily.
9. Bioflavonoid complex—1,000 mg three times daily.

CONSTIPATION

Constipation refers to conditions where there are infrequent bowel movements or hard, small stools which sometimes can be difficult to pass. This indicates that food is not being properly digested and assimilated and that nutrients are not reaching the cells. Constipation results when there is insufficient exercise, a poor diet with little roughage, use of chemical drugs, and states of tension, worry, and anxiety. It is a symptom of many diseases and often is accompanied by fatigue and lack of energy (indicating that energy is not being dispersed into the system). Constipation can often result in hemorrhoids or hernia from too much straining.

Physiological causes of constipation may involve poor peristalisis (the contraction and relaxation of muscle fibers in the alimentary canal) or a blockage in the colon due to a tumor, cyst, or other growth. Constipation also results from a lack of bile production, which indicates a poorly functioning liver and gall bladder. Herbs and foods that increase bile production and cleanse the liver can be very helpful for this condition.

Psychologically, those who tend to hold back feelings and emotions, who restrain themselves from expressing anger and hostility, and who cannot honestly confront people are more prone to constipation.

Treatments
1. Exercise of all types is the most important treatment for constipation. Swimming and yoga exercises that work directly with the solar plexus area are excellent. Various forms of dance, such as belly dancing, Polynesian dance, and African dance, utilize abdominal muscles and make this area of the body more fluid and loose. There are many exercises and stretches to strengthen abdominal muscles and bring energy into this central region.

2. Colonic irrigation and enemas work well for cleaning the colon and rectum and relieving constipation. Colonic irrigations may be taken alternative months with enemas in between. Taking an enema with olive or flaxseed oil can be very helpful.

3. Various types of bodywork and massage are helpful for constipation as they stimulate the organism involved in the digestive process. Also, many individuals who suffer from chronic constipation have very tight bodies that need to be loosened.

Herbs

Certain herbs are mucilaginous and help to soften the bowel, enabling it to pass through the rectum more easily. The juice from the aloe vera plant as well as teas from flaxseeds, slippery elm, and comfrey are excellent for their mucilaginous quality. Slippery elm may also be used in powdered form and added to cereals and juices. Liver herbs such as Oregon grape and wild yam stimulate bile flow.

Diet

Diet plays an important part here. The traditional dietary treatment has been to add bran to the morning meal, but this is not necessarily the best suggestion. Bran comes from wheat and produces a certain amount of mucus in the system; many people are also allergic to wheat. Eating cooked whole-grain cereals in the morning is most helpful. Also include mucilaginous foods such as ground flaxseeds or ground chia seeds (one or two teaspoons added to cooked grains or sprinkled on salads or vegetables). Okra is an excellent vegetable to add to the diet.

Fermented foods are also important since they help to nurture and grow good intestinal bacteria. Yogurt, kefir, buttermilk, and other products contain acidophilus; sauerkraut and kim chee (an Oriental-type pickle that is fermented with hot spices added) have proved beneficial. Certain spices bring heat to the body, and these serve to stimulate digestion and increase bile flow. Ginger root, grated on foods, juiced with vegetable juices, or drunk as a tea, is one of these. Cayenne, curry powder, turmeric, coriander, and cinnamon are also effective in stimulating digestive juices and enzymes. Cold-pressed olive oil used on salads several times a week increases bile. It may be taken two mornings a week upon arising with the juice of half a lemon to flush the liver.

Avoid foods which tend to form a lot of mucus in the colon. These include sugar, refined carbohydrates, and dairy products, especially butter, cheese, and milk (soured-milk foods such as yogurt and kefir are better). Beans are difficult to digest and cause fermentation and gas in the colon. Pasta, noodles, tortillas and other heavy carbohydrates also tend to create blockages in the colon. Red meats are difficult to break down and digest and should be avoided.

Some foods stimulate bile production, especially liver (organic), lecithin, eggs (fertile), beets and beet juice, cold-pressed olive oil, and flaxseed oil.

Supplements

1. Aloe vera juice—four to six tablespoons every other morning upon arising.

2. Two tablespoons of cold-pressed olive oil or flaxseed oil plus the juice of half a lemon upon arising two mornings a week.

3. Liquid lecithin—one or two tablespoons after a meal on alternate days (use on days when olive oil is not being taken).

4. Liquid chlorophyll—two or three tablespoons one or two times daily as a source of magnesium. It helps to relax the stomach and colon.

5. Trace minerals—two or three teaspoons of powdered, or three tablets. The need for iron is particularly high in those who tend to be constipated and have a low bile production.

6. Digestive enzymes including pancreatic enzymes, ox bile, pepsin and papain after each meal.

7. Vitamin B complex (non-yeast) base—500 mg three times daily.

8. Bioflavonoid complex tablets—1,000 mg three times daily.

DIABETES

Diabetes is a malfunctioning of the metabolic system characterized by the body's inability to utilize carbohydrates. Carbohydrates are generally broken down in the form of glucose, the energy source for the body. The hormone insulin, produced in the pancreas, is essential for the conversion of glucose into energy. It is secreted directly into the blood stream. When there is not enough insulin, blood sugar rises because insulin is essential for transporting glucose into the cells. As blood sugar levels increase, the kidneys eliminate sugar into the urine. The high level of sugar in the blood makes one particularly susceptible to infection.

The physiological causes of diabetes are many. Obesity is one important factor; excessive eating and consumption of alcoholic beverages are others. Certain types of diabetes are thought to be hereditary as well.

Psychologically, the diabetic is often a very bitter person. Circumstances in life have made her/him adopt this pattern, and the body compensates by producing an increased amount of sugar. Symptoms of diabetes often become manifest during a period of stress. Under conditions of stress there is an increased release of adrenalin and cortin. Adrenalin raises the blood sugar, and cortin causes the liver to make more glycogen, which is converted into glucose, thereby raising blood sugar.

Treatments

If treatment includes proper exercise, a balanced alkaline diet, and other important herbs and supplements, the diabetic may be able to forego insulin injections.

1. Exercise is the most important factor in stimulating the metabolism and determining insulin needs. All types of exercise is helpful—aerobic exercise, swimming, jogging, dance—in addition to some yoga or tai chi for centering and balancing body organs.

2. Cleansing the liver is a prime concern. Two tablespoons cold-pressed olive oil should be added to the juice of half a lemon and taken several mornings a week on an empty stomach. This helps flush out the liver and aids the bile flow. On alternate mornings, aloe vera juice (about 6 T.) should be used.

3. Colonic irrigations and enemas are necessary for aiding the digestion and assimilation of foods. These will also help the liver and pancreas. A wheat grass implant (1 oz. of wheat grass in an enema bag without water) after the colonic or enema is also helpful. Retain 10 minutes or longer.

4. Acupuncture treatments stimulate the pancreas to produce insulin and enzymes. They also help to keep the vital energy flowing.

5. Body therapies such as shiatsu, jin shinn, and acupressure also work with the pancreas and help balance other organs as well.

Herbs

Herbs are most important in regulating blood sugar and in increasing insulin.

1. Agrimony, Oregon grape root, and wild yam are good herbs for the liver and stimulate bile production. As teas, use 1 teaspoon

root per 1-1/2 cups water and simmer 10-15 minutes.

2. Dandelion root tea (same proportions) is an excellent tea for the pancreas and liver; it helps to balance blood sugar and maintain energy throughout the day.

3. String bean pod tea substitutes for insulin. Skins of the pods of green beans contain silica and hormone substances closely related to insulin. Drink one cup on alternate days.

4. Other helpful herbs are those high in natural minerals such as alfalfa, nettle leaves, comfrey, borage, raspberry leaf, and plantain.

Diet

Dietary emphasis should be alkaline. Diabetics tend to over-acidity. Carbohydrates should be complex carbohydrates such as whole grains and beans that break down slowly in the system.

1. Absolutely avoid alcohol, tobacco, coffee, black teas, sugar, salt, refined carbohydrates, and preservatives.

2. Milk products should be avoided (except for yogurt and soured milk).

3. Avoid wheat.

4. Avoid citrus fruits (except for lemons used with olive oil), strawberries, soured apples and apple juice (apples should be baked), watermelon, plums, tomatoes, cranberries, green peppers, vinegar, and nutritional yeast.

5. Winter squash and carrots may be eaten on occasion since they are high in sugar. Avoid beets, sweet potatoes, and yams.

6. Eat a maximum of two to three portions of fruit a week (papaya, peaches or nectarines, baked apples or pears, golden delicious apples, cantaloupe or blueberries).

7. Honey should be avoided. Use barley malt or rice syrup (complex carbohydrates) if necessary.

8. Use non-sodium vegetable seasonings.

9. Plenty of whole grains should be eaten, especially buckwheat, millet, barley, brown rice, amaranth, rye, and oats. A cooked whole-grain cereal is important in the morning because it takes eight hours to break down and will maintain energy throughout the day.

10. Eat fresh vegetables, particularly steamed, twice daily, supplemented by soups and salads. Use plenty of greens since they are rich in chlorophyll.

11. Proteins that may be eaten are tofu (bean curd), soured-milk products, fertile eggs (up to four a week), fresh fish (no shellfish), organic poultry and liver, and occasionally soaked nuts. (Nuts are difficult to assimilate due to bile production.)

12. Use cold-pressed olive oil every other day on salads and vegetables.

13. Jerusalem artichokes and string beans are high in insulin.

Supplements

1. Liquid lecithin—two tablespoons after two meals on alternate days (helps with the liver and bile production).

2. Liquid chlorophyll—two to three tablespoons twice daily in half a glass of spring water.

3. A multivitamin/mineral three times daily.

4. Manganese in chelated or aspartate form three times daily.

5. Zinc picollinate or chelated three times daily.

6. Potassium/magnesium capsules—three daily.

7. Bioflavonoid complex—1,000 mg three times daily.

8. Pantothenic acid—500-1,000 mg three times daily.

9. Vitamin E in dry form—800-1,000 i.u.'s two times after meals on alternate days.

10. Pancreas glandular supplement—three daily.

11. A multiple digestive enzyme (with pancreatin, ox bile, pepsin, and papain)—one after each meal.

12. Free-form amino acid capsules—three daily. May be alternated monthly with the pancreatic glandular (one the first month and the other the second month).

DIARRHEA

Diarrhea may result from minor causes such as food poisoning, bacterial infection, and emotional stress or as a result of major illness such as ulcerative colitis, cancer, or dysentery. In either case, the intestines are not absorbing the nutrients the body requires and large amounts of vitamins and minerals are being washed away. Dehydration through fluid loss can also become a problem in the long run.

Chronic diarrhea often is a result of nervousness and anxiety; those who experience it need to stabilize their emotions and work with calming and centering therapies. Individuals who give a lot of themselves, constantly "pouring out" their emotions, often suffer from diarrhea. They need to learn to focus more and balance out their emotional life.

Treatments

1. Colonic irrigations and enemas are helpful in ridding the body of bacteria that are causing the diarrhea. They also bring some liquid back into the intestinal tract and help prevent dehydration. Raspberry leaf or blackberry leaf tea in the enema bag is good. (Make up one quart tea by steeping a few tablespoons of the herb in boiling water; add room temperature spring or distilled water to fill up the rest of the bag.)

2. A liquid fast of two or three days with vegetable juices, vegetable broths and herb teas is helpful in getting rid of bacteria. No fruit juice should be used, but, if it is desired, a small amount of papaya juice may be included.

3. Acupuncture and Oriental body work such as jin shinn, shiatsu, and polarity therapy help to rebalance organs and restore the vital force.

4. Certain homeopathic remedies are effective in destroying intestinal bacteria and other micro-organisms.

Diet

Easy-to-digest foods should be gradually added. Ground-up grains made into rice cream, buckwheat cream, barley cream, and millet cream are especially good. Steamed vegetables and vegetable soups are excellent. Avoid salads and raw vegetables. Soured-milk products such as yogurt, kefir, kefir cheese, and sour cream are most helpful for replacing intestinal bacteria. Tofu (bean curd) is another easy-to-digest protein, as are poached or soft-boiled eggs (fertile). Avoid fruit and fruit juice as it is too acidic. Nuts and seeds are difficult to digest, so it is best to wait about a week before reintroducing them into the diet. Soaked nuts would be best.

Herbs

Herb teas can be very beneficial for diarrhea. Raspberry leaf, comfrey, borage, plantain, nettles, and alfalfa help to replace minerals that have been lost.

Golden seal leaf and papaya leaf are good teas for digestion as are peppermint, spearmint, and wintergreen. Chewing a clove of garlic or adding it to vegetable juices or food is an excellent remedy for intestinal bacteria.

A poultice of comfrey or plantain leaves can relax and soothe intestinal muscles.

Supplements

1. Aloe vera juice—four to six tablespoons daily helps to cleanse intestines of bacteria and micro-organisms.

2. High potency acidophilus—1/2 teaspoon upon arising for one to three weeks, depending on severity of diarrhea.

3. Liquid chlorophyll (to replace magnesium)—two to three tablespoons two times daily.

4. Trace minerals (preferably powdered from sea vegetables)—two to three teaspoons or several tablets or capsules.

5. Potassium/magnesium capsules three times daily to replace potassium.

6. Vitamin B (non-yeast base)—500-1,000 mg three times daily.

7. Bioflavonoid capsules—500-1,000 mg three times daily.

8. Vitamin A (dry form as beta-carotene)—10,000 i.u.'s alternate days.

9. Digestive enzymes—one after meals.

DIGESTIVE DISORDERS

Digestive disorders (flatulence, indigestion, intestinal cramps) result from overeating, poor food combinations, eating too fast, eating while emotionally upset, and excess tension and anxiety. If one does not take the time to sit and relax at meals or eats hurriedly at her/his desk, indigestion becomes quite common.

Often digestive complaints indicate some issues in one's life that one is not assimilating or digesting. This is because we don't always take the time to slow down and process our feelings and emotional concerns.

Much indigestion results from dietary habits where large meals are eaten at one sitting with many different types of foods. Especially difficult for digestion is the habit of eating raw vegetable salads before the main course protein. Protein needs hydrochloric acid for digestion, and when salads are eaten beforehand they leave little hydrochloric acid for the protein foods. If salads are eaten at the same meal with protein and cooked food, they should be eaten with the protein or afterward.

Fruit should never be eaten with a meal, nor should desserts. Since fruit often has an acidic reaction on the body (as do sweets and desserts), it should be taken separately several hours after a meal. Liquids also should not be drunk with a meal as they wash away the digestive enzymes. At least half an hour should elapse before drinking water or herb tea.

Treatments

1. Exercise before meals is most beneficial in relaxing the body and stimulating digestive enzymes. At least 15 minutes of yoga exercise, stretches, tai chi, or other exercise will both relax the body and calm the mind.

2. Eat meals in a quiet atmosphere without television or telephone interruption. Don't eat when tense or emotionally upset. Eat a small amount of food several times a day (only one or two foods at a time) to promote digestion.

3. Juice fasts and liquid broths and soups are helpful in giving the digestive system a rest. Fast one day a week on liquids.

4. Colonic irrigations and enemas help to cleanse the system and get rid of old fecal material as well as bacteria that may be causing gas.

Diet

Avoid heavy, starchy foods such as tortillas, beans, and pasta. Use whole grains (ground in the morning) and whole-grain breads without wheat (which causes excess mucus in the system). Avoid heavy proteins such as red meats and shellfish. Eat poultry and organic liver occasionally. Fish, broiled or baked, may be eaten a couple of times a week. Avoid cheeses, milk, butter; substitute soured-milk products such as yogurt, kefir, and buttermilk, which are easier to digest and aid the growth of intestinal bacteria. Avoid sugars and desserts. Use barley malt syrup and rice syrup or honey occasionally.

Use mostly cooked vegetables—steamed, baked, or in soups. Sautéed vegetables are difficult to digest as are too many raw vegetables. Eat simple salads with only a few foods at a time such as lettuce, sprouts, cucumber, grated carrots, or zucchini. Avoid tomatoes, raw green peppers, and radishes. Do not put nuts, seeds or bean sprouts on salads. Eliminate citrus fruits, soured apples, strawberries, cranberries, vinegar, and nutritional yeast. These increase body acidity. Eliminate coffee and black teas. Use herbal teas that aid digestion. Include fermented foods such as sauerkraut, sour bread and soured vegetables.

Herbs

Garlic is an excellent remedy for gas. It rids the intestines of putrefyng bacteria.

Teas that aid digestion by increasing the mucilage in intestinal linings are flaxseed, slippery elm, comfrey, and borage. Teas that are beneficial after meals include peppermint, spearmint, wintergreen, and papaya leaf. A tea made from ground dill seed, anise seeds, and fennel seeds (two teaspoons dill and fennel seeds, one teaspoon anise seeds, with three cups of water immersed for 10 minutes) is very helpful for digestive problems.

Adding thyme, dill weed, fennel, basil, and oregano (one at a time) to foods is a good digestive aid.

Supplements

1. If additional hydrochloride is needed, use the juice of half a lemon in 1/2 cup boiling water after meals or one tablet of betaine hydrochloride.

2. Comfrey pepsin tablets—one or two daily to settle the stomach and to stimulate digestive enzymes.

3. Multiple digestive enzymes after meals—should include pancreatin, pepsin, ox bile, papain, and bromelain.

4. Aloe vera juice—four to six tablespoons (on empty stomach) daily will help to get rid of flatulence and putrefying intestinal bacteria.

5. High-potency acidophilus—1/2 teaspoon powdered acidophilus or 2 teaspoons liquid every other day may be needed for a few weeks (alternate with aloe vera juice).

6. Liquid chlorophyll—two to three tablespoons, two times daily in half a glass of spring water.

7. Trace minerals—two teaspoons powdered or several tablets daily.

8. Potassium/magnesium capsules three times daily.

9. B vitamins daily (non-yeast base)—500 mg two to three

times daily.

10. Bioflavonoid capsules—1,000 mg three times daily.

EAR PROBLEMS

The ears are an extremely sensitive part of the body. When there is difficulty with the ears or impaired hearing, we need to consider what it is we may not want to hear at that time. Many young people have developed hearing problems because of their need to shut out information that would be too painful for them.

An earache may be an infection of the middle ear. It is usually a result of fluid in the Eustachian tubes after a cold or flu. The ear may sometimes become inflamed with accompanying fever and pains.

The most helpful treatments for earaches are keeping the ear warm with hot water bottles and a heating pad and keeping it clean and free of wax. There are several natural treatments which are beneficial.

Treatments

1. A poultice for the ear may be made by boiling one clove of garlic in one-half cup water until soft. The cooled garlic clove may be placed on the outside of the ear, covered with a piece of clean cotton, and held in place by tape.

2. Make a tea of mullein flowers using one teaspoon to one-half cup boiling water. Mix one tablespoon of this with one tablespoon olive oil and let stand for a few hours. Use one drop of this liquid in each ear a few times a week.

3. A few drops of garlic oil in each ear help clear infections. Grind up a clove of garlic and place it in a half pint of olive or flaxseed oil. Allow the garlic to sit in the oil for at least half a day. Then, strain off the garlic and place the oil in the ear.

4. To clean ears of wax, hydrogen peroxide can be used. One should lie on her/his side with the ear up and place a medicine dropper full of hydrogen peroxide in the ear. Allow it to fizz for a few moments and then shake the residue. A piece of cotton dipped into a warm mixture of glycerin and witch hazel and then inserted into the ear will also work.

5. Massaging certain parts of the ear and around the neck can be helpful.

6. Particular homeopathic remedies are beneficial for ear infections.

Supplements
1. Vitamin A in its dry form as beta-carotene—10,000 i.u.'s two or three times daily when there is a sign of infection; later, one time daily.
2. Bioflavonoid complex—1,000 mg three times daily.
3. Vitamin C in its ascorbate form—about 1,000 mg daily or less, depending on individual need. Later, use on alternating days.
4. A good source of magnesium such as liquid chlorophyll is very important since the ears are sensitive instruments connected with balance and the nervous system. Two to three tablespoons liquid chlorophyll two times daily.
5. Manganese tablets or capsules two or three times daily. Manganese is most important for the nervous system and the conduction of electrical impulses.
6. Vitamin B-12 is also important for the nervous system, and usually lacking; liquid B-12 may be used daily.

ECZEMA

Eczema is a skin rash which may develop on any part of the body. It may result from allergies, excess toxins in the body, as well as emotional and nervous disorders. The symptoms of redness and itchiness, which occur often, indicate withheld anger and resentment.

Treatment
Eliminate toxic materials through juice fasting and colon cleansing. Three to four days of fasting with vegetable juices and broths followed by a colonic irrigation is the first step in getting rid of eczema.

Diet
Eliminating any processed foods, chemical additives, sugars, coffee, and dairy products (which often cause allergic reactions and build up excess mucus in the system) is necessary. Yogurt and soured-milk products may be included in the diet, as well as goat's

milk products on occasion. Eliminate wheat and substitute all other grains and rye breads in addition to soy, corn, and millet breads. Cut down the acidity in the diet by eating less fruit (perhaps one portion on alternate days), and eliminate soured apples, strawberries, tomatoes, vinegar, nutritional yeast, cranberries, and raw spinach, which are all highly acidic. One may substitute golden delicious apples or baked apples or pears, bananas, peaches, cherries, and melons, except for watermelon. Grapes and plums are acidic. Eliminate shellfish, which contain many allergens, but substitute broiled and baked fish. Eliminate meat except for organic poultry and calves' liver.

Herbs

1. Dandelion leaf tea or dandelion greens in salads help to rebuild cells.

2. Make a blood-purifying tea from 1/2 oz. saffron, 1 oz. burdock root or dock root, and 2 oz. red clover. Add these to one pint boiling water. Simmer for 15 minutes and strain. Drink two cups daily.

3. Golden seal powder in capsules or as a tea is a good blood purifier.

4. Comfrey ointment, myrrh and golden seal ointments, and golden seal powder may be used externally.

Supplements

1. PABA—550 or 1,000 mg three times daily.

2. A good trace mineral, made from sea vegetables preferably, two or three times a day, or a multivitamin/mineral three times daily.

3. Potassium/magnesium supplement three times daily.

4. Pantothenic acid—500 mg two times daily.

5. Bioflavonoid complex—1,000 mg three times daily.

6. Vitamin A (as beta-carotene)—10,000 i.u.'s two times daily.

7. Vitamin E (in dry form)—800-1,000 i.u.'s two times daily.

EPILEPSY

Epilepsy is a nervous-system disorder which gives rise to convulsive seizures as a result of a disturbance of brain-wave impulses.

There may be a momentary or prolonged loss of consciousness and involuntary convulsive movements. In petit mal seizures, there is twitching around the eyes or mouth with a loss of consciousness of only a few seconds. In grand mal seizures, the patient falls unconscious with foaming at the mouth and shaking limbs. S/he may even hurt her/himself during the seizure. Seizures last from a few seconds to a few minutes, and the frequency of seizures varies with individual patients.

Epileptics usually have a very sensitive nervous system from birth. They may have suffered an injury to the brain or head area. They seem to be extremely deficient in magnesium and manganese and some of the B vitamins. Providing these nutrients often clears up the symptoms.

On an emotional level, epileptics often have some very deep-seated frustrations and desires that they have not been able to express. Sometimes it is emotions such as rage and anger that have been there as root patterns from other lifetimes and from childhood. Helping them to get in touch with these emotions is an important part of their therapy.

Treatments

Homeopathic magnesium remedies, such as magnesium phosphate (200x) or magnesium chloride (200x) several times a month, are very helpful. Other remedies found for individuals and used as constitutional remedies are also beneficial.

Diet

1. Avoid all sources of chemical additives and foods that cause allergic reactions like chocolate, peanuts, citrus fruits, strawberries, tomatoes, cow's milk products (yogurt and soured milks are often okay), wheat, and shellfish.

2. Avoid all stimulants such as coffee, black tea, and cola drinks.

3. Eat plenty of green leafy vegetables high in calcium and magnesium.

4. If one eats meat, organic calves' liver and beef liver provide a good source of B-12, which is difficult to obtain from other foods. B-12 supplements may also be used.

5. Whole grains like buckwheat, millet, brown rice, rye, barley, oats, and amaranth are high in B-complex vitamins.

6. Sea vegetables like dulse, wakame, kombu, hijiki and nori are high in minerals needed for the nervous system.

Herbs

1. The nervine herbs vervain, hops, catnip, wood betony, chamomile, and spearmint should be drunk often.

2. Herbs high in calcium, magnesium and potassium like comfrey leaves, borage, raspberry leaves, alfalfa, and plantain should be used daily.

3. Tea made from lobelia a few times a week relaxes the nervous system and brain waves.

4. Avoid peppermint, yerba maté, and other stimulant herbs.

Supplements

1. Liquid chlorophyll—two to three tablespoons in half a glass of water a few times a day help to balance magnesium and relax the nervous system.

2. A potassium/magnesium supplement four to five times a day is extremely important.

3. A multivitamin mineral providing all the minerals three times a day.

4. A chelated manganese tablet or manganese aspartate four to five times daily.

5. Pantothenic acid—1,000 mg three times daily.

6. B complex (non-yeast base)—500-1,000 mg three to four times daily.

7. Octacosanol, made from wheat-germ oil, is an important supplement in getting oxygen to the lungs and brain area. Two per day (if possible, in the super-strength 5,000 mcg).

8. Bioflavonoid complex—1,000 mg three times daily.

EYE PROBLEMS

Problems related to the eyes often have to do with what one does not want to see in her/his life. Many sensitive individuals experience visual problems when there is something in their environment that is difficult to handle. They do not want to see the truth of the situation, so they develop physical problems with the eyes.

In general, near-sighted people live more for the here and now, while far-sighted people forego certain pleasures and possessions to accumulate security in the future. Near-sighted people often want to do things now; far-sighted people may tend to procrastinate.

The two eyes represent the female/male relationship or the mother/father relationship. When the emotional natures of the parents are difficult, the child may develop astigmatism and have difficulty focusing her/his eyes.

Eye exercises can be very helpful for eye problems. The Bates System of eye exercise has been invaluable. These exercises include sunning the eyes outdoors, palming to relax the eyes, blinking and using a candle or flame for focusing.

Treatment for eye infections
1. A poultice of violet leaves helps swelling and soreness of the eyes. Use one teaspoon of the leaves to one cup boiling water. Steep for five minutes and use strained leaves in a poultice for 15 minutes.

2. Washing the eyes with a solution of eyebright tea helps eye inflammations and infections. Make a solution by steeping one teaspoon of tea in one cup water.

3. A poultice of grated potatoes is also very helpful for the eyes.

Supplements for eye infections
1. Vitamin A in dry form as beta-carotene—10,000 i.u.'s two or three times daily.

2. Bioflavonoid complex—1,000 mg three times daily. Rutin is particularly important for the eyes since it helps to decrease capillary tension.

3. Vitamin C (in ascorbate form)—1,000 mg daily for infection.

4. Vitamin B-2 (about 100 mg) on alternate days helps with night blindness. Other B vitamins may be helpful as long as they are not in a yeast base.

5. A good trace mineral in powdered form or tablets or a multivitamin/mineral three times a day.

6. Liquid chlorophyll—two to three tablespoons two times daily for magnesium and relaxation.

Cataracts and Glaucoma
With cataracts and glaucoma, it is also important to acknowledge what it is that we have not wanted to see in our lives. When a

cataract forms, the crystalline lens of the eye becomes clouded or opaque. Vision is diminished as opacity increases. Surgical treatment, which is often performed, involves the removal of the crystalline lens.

In glaucoma there is an increase of pressure inside the eye which interferes with vision. This is due to a disturbance in the production and drainage of fluid that fills the interior of the eye in front of the lens. Too much fluid may be produced or the normal amount may not drain properly. The eye drops that are usually prescribed constrict the pupil to allow more space for the fluid; they also help the fluid to flow through the walls of the canal. Unfortunately, these drops have many side effects. They distort the vision for the first 30 to 40 minutes after they are taken, and they also make it difficult to perceive colors clearly.

Treatments for cataract and glaucoma

1. Stress-controlling techniques such as autogenics, biofeedback, and visualization have been helpful in working with glaucoma.

2. In terms of diet, research has shown that the use of animal fats in meat, butter, cream, cheese, and eggs, which contribute to cholesterol buildup in the arteries, is an important factor in the formation of cataracts. A diet low in animal products and high in grains, vegetables, fruits, nuts, seeds, and fish may be helpful.

3. The supplements listed above are also helpful.

GALL BLADDER PROBLEMS

The gall bladder is one of the body's containers, providing a storage area for the bile. When the liver is congested and not functioning properly, the gall bladder is usually involved. Many individuals who develop gall bladder problems are overweight and tend to overeat, especially foods high in animal fat. Those who develop gallstones may be very crystallized in their thinking, needing to break up old patterns in terms of ideas and awareness. Some of these individuals are also very bitter.

Over 90 per cent of gallstones are composed of cholesterol. Clinical studies also show that the phospholipid concentration in the bile of those with gallstones is low. Using lecithin in the diet (especially in its liquid form) as well as olive oil and flaxseed oil (on salads and vegetables) keeps the cholesterol dispersed and prevents the formation of gallstones.

Treatments

1. To remove gallstones, a juice fast of several days is helpful, followed by a colonic irrigation or olive oil enema (3 T. olive oil to 1 qt. water) if colonics are not available. The following morning take half a pint of olive oil and lie on your right side for two hours. Repeat once if necessary. This should help gallstones pass out of the system.

2. In general, first thing in the morning, take two tablespoons of cold-pressed olive oil with the juice of half a lemon on an empty stomach. This should be done two or three times a week.

3. A ginger root compress on the gall bladder area is extremely helpful in inflammatory conditions and for relieving pain and congestion. Grate up fresh ginger root until there is enough for two small balls. Place in tea balls or cheesecloth and boil in two quarts of water for 15-20 minutes. Soak a cloth in this tea and apply as hot as possible to abdominal area. Cover with a dry towel and repeat several times.

4. A castor oil pack is also helpful on the abdominal area. Heat three to four tablespoons castor oil and dip in flannel cloth. Place cloth on affected area and cover with a plastic sheet. A towel and electric heating pad may also be placed over it.

5. For acute gall bladder conditions, make a coffee enema. Use one cup of strong coffee added to one pint warm water. Try to retain this for 10 minutes, or as long as possible. It helps the bile flow and relaxes the liver and gall bladder.

Diet

1. Eliminate meat, animal fats, margarine, and commercial oils.

2. Eliminate cow's milk products like butter, cheese, cream, and milk (yogurt and soured-milk products may be used on occasion).

3. Eliminate heavy carbohydrates like pasta, noodles, and beans.

4. Use cold-pressed vegetable oils, especially olive oil, almond, and sunflower; they stimulate bile production and contain the fat-digesting enzyme lipase.

5. Beet juice and beet soup promote bile flow as does peach

juice, peaches, pear juice, baked pears, radishes, and daikon radish. Poached and raw eggs are also helpful to bile flow; about four eggs weekly.

Herbs

Certain herbs like Oregon grape root, wild yam, and dandelion root are helpful to the gall bladder. Simmer 1 teaspoon root to 1-1/2 cup water for 10-15 minutes, and drink several times a week.

Supplements

1. Aloe vera juice—about four to six tablespoons alternate mornings on an empty stomach cleanse the liver and gall bladder.

2. Liquid chlorophyll—three tablespoons in half a glass of water twice a day (a good source of magnesium and a liver cleanser).

3. Liquid lecithin—two tablespoons after a meal alternate days. (Granular lecithin may be used as a substitute, but it is not as good.)

4. Digestive enzymes after meals.

5. Choline—500 mg alternate days for fat intake.

6. Inositol—500 mg on alternate days for cholesterol intake.

7. Biotin—25 mg on alternate days.

8. B-12 (with liver concentrate if possible)—50 mcg daily. This stimulates iron production, which is essential to bile flow.

9. Multivitamin minerals three times a day.

10. Bioflavonoid complex—500-1,000 mg three times a day.

11. Two tablespoons cold-pressed olive oil on food alternate days (when liquid lecitihin is not used).

HEADACHES

There are many types of headaches but, in general, they are caused by some congestion in the system and tension. Foods to which one is allergic often cause headaches. Also, when one eats too quickly or doesn't allow enough time for digestion, a headache results. Pressure in the temples and forehead usually indicates tension in the stomach, and throbbing pain results from congestion in the liver, spleen, or digestive tract. When an internal organ is congested, it will send signals to the brain which are interpreted as pain in the head rather than pain from that organ.

Muscle tension causes headaches; the muscles of the scalp contract, causing tiny spasms in the veins and stricture of blood flow. The circulation of blood is cut off to the surrounding tissue, the oxygen level drops, and pain is the outcome. Migraines are more serious and usually result because the blood vessels in the neck and brain dilate from a closing down of the central blood vessels in other parts of the head.

Many people who are "heads" of organizations or large families or who bear a lot of responsibility often have headaches. This is from the tension and pressure they carry in their lives.

Treatments

1. Getting enough sleep and rest; learning to relax the body at any time of the day by closing the eyes, doing some deep breathing, and feeling the energy flow to all parts of the body.

2. Eating regular meals and taking time to digest is important since low blood sugar is often the cause of headaches.

3. Exercise is essential for getting oxygen circulating to all parts of the body. Yoga and tai chi can be most helpful if practiced daily.

4. Massaging the head and rubbing certain acupressure points is an excellent quick treatment for headaches. If headaches are chronic, there may be some vertebrae out of place in the spine. In this case, a chiropractic adjustment can provide much relief.

5. Certain homeopathic remedies, particularly magnesium remedies and the cell salts Mag Phos and Kali Phos, are excellent for relieving headaches. Kali Phos relaxes the head and brain. The magnesium level in the body is low where there is tension, pain or spasm.

Herbs

1. At the sign of a headache, one or two of the nervine herbs—vervain, spearmint, catnip, chamomile, or hops—can be helpful.

2. Drinking herb teas high in calcium and magnesium like comfrey, borage, raspberry leaf, plantain, alfalfa, and nettles facilitates relaxation and relief of tightness in the body.

Supplements

1. Liquid chlorophyll—two or three tablespoons twice daily in half a glass of water. Chlorophyll contains the magnesium ion and is a high source of this mineral.

2. Potassium/magnesium capsules—three or four daily.

3. A multivitamin mineral—three or four daily.

4. B-12 supplement—100 mcg daily.

5. Pantothenic acid—500-1,000 mg three times daily for tension.

6. Bioflavonoid complex—1,000 mg three times daily. Rutin helps the circulation, thereby bringing more oxygen to the head.

HEART DISEASE

Heart diseases include many disorders such as aneurysms, atherosclerosis, hypertension, and heart attacks. An *aneurysm* is a blood-filled sac formed by a pouching in an arterial or venous wall. Aneurysms may occur in any major blood vessel. *Atherosclerosis* is a form of arteriosclerosis, which includes many diseases of the arterial wall. In this disorder, an artery becomes thickened with soft fatty deposits called *atheromatous plaques*. As atheromas grow, they may impede blood flow in affected arteries and damage the tissues they supply. Atherosclerosis is a slow, progressive disease which may start in childhood, producing no symptoms for many years. The most common disease affecting the heart and blood vessels is *hypertension*. Primary or essential hypertension is elevated blood pressure that cannot be attributed to any particular organic cause. Secondary hypertension is caused by disorders such as arteriosclerosis, kidney disease, and adrenal hypersecretion.

The term "heart attack" includes myocardial infarctions—formation of dead cells in the heart muscle due to interruption of the blood supply to the area; and coronary occlusions—the closing off of a coronary artery, which may occur when the artery is plugged by a blood clot within the vessel or when fatty deposits in the wall of the vessel clog the artery.

Factors which contribute to heart disease include high blood cholesterol, high blood pressure, cigarette smoking, obesity, and lack of exercise. According to recent research, high blood cholesterol or serum cholesterol is not determined by the amount of cholesterol in the diet but rather by the factors which alter the synthesis or excretion of cholesterol. A reduction in cholesterol breakdown is known to result from exposure to high levels of *atmospheric carbon monoxide*, which accounts for the importance attached to cigarette smoking and pollution. *Cigarette smoking*, through the effects of nicotine, stimulates the adrenal gland to oversecrete aldosterone, epinephrine and norepinephrine, which in turn cause constriction of blood vessels. *Overweight people* develop extra capillaries to nourish fat tissue. The heart, therefore, has to work harder to pump the blood through more veins. *Exercise* strengthens the smooth muscle of blood vessels and enables them to assist in general circulation. Exercise also increases cardiac efficiency and output.

Immediate physiological causes of heart disease are inadequate coronary blood supply, anatomical disorders, and faulty electrical conduction in the heart.

There are many emotional factors involved in heart disease— holding back or restraining feelings is a major one. Sudden traumas or life changes often bring these feelings to the surface and the heart literally "breaks open." Since the heart is the seat of love, the circulation system carries this love, through the blood, to all other parts of the body. To withhold love for someone is to create a block in the circulation system. Sometimes one puts up a "block" to guard her/ his own privacy or protect her/himself from the outside world. Also, a very sensitive individual may have to become "hardhearted" in her/his work or business to do things that are not part of her/his character. This type of action also puts extreme pressure on the heart.

In their book *Type A Behavior and Your Heart* (Fawcett, 1981), Meyer Friedman and Ray Rosenmann have catalogued the cardiovascular personality type. The Type A personality strives to accomplish too much and to participate in too many events in an allotted time segment. They constantly create deadlines and are unable to relax and enjoy themselves. Because of these deadlines, they don't have time to think problems through and, therefore, fall into stereotyped thinking and judgments. They also tend to be extremely impatient and are strongly competitive in their work. On the surface, they appear to have confidence and self-assurance, but they actually experience a deep sense of insecurity. They also possess an easily aroused hostility, which is usually kept under control. As a group, they show a higher serum cholesterol, a higher serum fat, smoke more cigarettes, eat more foods high in cholesterol, and suffer more from high blood pressure. When physiological tests were administered, blood fat and hormone abnormalities were indicated.

Treatments

1. Long-term psychological and spiritual therapies which put one in touch with old emotional blocks.

2. Increased physical exercise. Sedentary activities contribute to the formation of arteriosclerosis.

3. Activities like yoga, tai chi, and meditation which slow down the nervous system.

Diet

1. Avoid the tendency to overeat.

2. Avoid alcohol, coffee, black tea, stimulants, sugar, and chemical and processed foods.

3. Eliminate salt and foods containing high amounts of sodium like soy sauce, miso soup, and processed and packaged foods. Use non-sodium vegetable seasonings.

4. Eliminate animal products like red meats, butter and cow's milk products (yogurt and soured milks are okay occasionally).

5. Use non-hydrogenated cold-pressed vegetable oils such as olive, sesame, soy, and safflower. These help break down high serum cholesterol and are a good source of vitamin F.

6. Include lots of steamed green vegetables high in calcium and magnesium.

7. Include whole grains and cereals high in B-complex vitamins.

Herbs

1. Herbs high in calcium and magnesium like borage, comfrey, and raspberry leaf should be drunk as teas.

2. Use herbs that increase circulation like cayenne (one teaspoon on salad or soup several times a week), red clover tea, ginger root tea, and Chinese cinnamon tea.

3. Hawthorn berry, lily of the valley and motherwort are good heart tonics and may be appropriate.

Supplements

1. Lecithin, especially in its liquid form, helps in dissolving fatty deposits in the tissues and arteries—two tablespoons daily.

2. Vitamin F (unsaturated fatty acids), available in capsules and also cold-pressed vegetable oils or evening primrose oil—twice daily.

3. Liquid chlorophyll—two to three tablespoons twice daily for magnesium.

4. Trace minerals containing calcium, potassium, iron, and other important minerals, preferably in powdered form for assimilation, three times daily.

5. Octacosanol—two to three capsules on alternate days assists in getting more oxygen to the heart.

6. Vitamin E—600-1,000 i.u.'s daily in dry form (alternate with octacosanol).

7. Bioflavonoid complex—1,000 mg three times daily. Rutin strengthens artery walls and makes the capillaries more supple.

8. Vitamin C in ascorbate form—1,000 mg daily—helps in converting cholesterol to bile acids; also good for the connective tissue.

9. Vitamin B complex (non-yeast base) three times daily.

10. Potassium/magnesium capsules three times daily.

11. A manganese capsule or tablet three to four times daily for the nervous system.

12. Pantothenic acid—1,000 mg two to three times a day for stress.

HEMORRHOIDS

Hemorrhoids are a protrusion of the mucous membrane of the rectum. They bleed sometimes and are usually quite painful. They are often called "piles" and are varicose veins of the rectal wall. Constipation is a contributory cause of hemorrhoids, so it is important to deal with this condition first (see Constipation).

Hemorrhoids, like constipation, are often a result of held-back emotions and repressed sexual energy. These feelings need to be dealt with and released in order to clear up the condition.

On a physiological basis, there are many soothing natural ways to treat hemorrhoids.

Treatments
1. Sitz baths and water treatments are two of the oldest remedies. Fill a bathtub with six to eight inches of hot water. Sit in the tub with knees drawn up so that only the sitz bones or lower part of the body is covered by water. Sit in hot water for 5 minutes, then fill with cold water and sit in that for 5-10 seconds. This can be repeated

once or twice and done several times a week.

2. Suppositories made from garlic or peeled raw potato have brought much relief.

3. Putting a garlic clove in the rectum before bed is also helpful.

4. Pollen suppositories (Cernitory) have been effective in bringing relief. These have been used in Sweden and other European countries and are now available in the U.S.

5. Vitamin E or wheat-germ oil rubbed directly on the hemorrhoids until the oil is absorbed is soothing.

6. Two ounces of olive oil injected into the rectal area in a syringe or an olive oil enema (3 T. to 1 qt. water) is very effective.

7. Exercise is especially important. Sedentary activities contribute to constipation and hemorrhoids. Yoga postures are particularly good since they stretch muscles and internal viscera.

Herbs

1. Aloe vera juice—four to six tablespoons on alternate days, drunk on an empty stomach, relieves constipation and is soothing to the mucous lining.

2. Drink a mixture of slippery elm and flaxseed—1 t. each to 1-1/2 cup of water and simmer.

3. Collinsonia root—as tea, tablets or capsules, taken alternate days for a few weeks.

4. Adding ground flaxseeds or chia seeds to morning cereal or vegetables provides extra mucilage.

Homeopathy

Certain remedies chosen individually are helpful in working with the release of old patterns and letting go of emotions in addition to the physiological symptoms.

Diet

Follow diet for Constipation. Include lots of fresh and cooked vegetables, especially okra, daikon radish and beets. A large quantity of cooked whole grains is necessary to provide bulk and roughage in the diet.

Supplements

1. Bioflavonoid complex—1,000 mg three times daily. Rutin helps to rebuild blood vessel walls.

2. A calcium/magnesium supplement—three capsules daily. Calcium is also important in building blood vessel walls.

3. B complex (non-yeast base)—1,000 mg, three capsules daily.

4. Liquid lecithin—two tablespoons alternate days after meals helps the bile flow and soothes the intestinal walls.

5. A multivitamin mineral three times daily.

6. Vitamin E in dry form—400-600 i.u.'s alternate days.

HERPES

Herpes simplex virus is found in two forms: herpes simplex virus type 1 (HSV-1) and herpes simplex virus type 2 (HSV-2). Type 1 mostly affects the upper regions of the body, especially the head and neck. Its major symptoms are clusters of small red lumps around the lips that turn into painful blisters called cold sores or fever blisters. Type 2 affects the lower regions of the body in which there may be lesions around the genitals, buttocks, and thighs. Both varieties can be transmitted through sexual contact.

Herpes does not respond to antibiotics. When one contracts the herpesvirus, there may be no symptoms at first. Later, blisters can develop on the external genital organs; sometimes women develop blisters on the vagina or cervix which go unnoticed until they rupture and develop into open sores. The lymph glands in the groin may also become swollen and painful.

An initial outbreak of herpes usually lasts about 12 days after which the virus enters a latent stage. In some cases, no additional outbreaks may occur. In others, symptoms may return several times a month. An outbreak of genital herpes can have severe consequences during pregnancy and childbirth.

Physiologically, those who suffer repeated outbreaks of herpes tend to have a highly acidic body. They need to rebalance physically through a diet high in whole grains, cooked vegetables, and proteins (as fish, soured-milk products, and tofu) with few animal products. There is a strong need to cut back on fruit (eating it about once every other day) and other acid foods like tomatoes, spinach, vinegar, and nutritional yeast. Most sweeteners and salty foods like soy sauce, miso soup, packaged soups and salad dressings that have salt added should also be eliminated from the diet.

Psychologically, these individuals tend to be very emotional and sensitive. Often they have problems with their mate and dealing with their sexuality. Constant outbreaks on the genital area is one way to avoid confronting this issue.

Treatments

1. External treatments include a hot sitz bath. Fill a tub almost half full with hot water and sit in it for 10-15 minutes. The hot water causes a loosening of fat and mucus deposits in the pelvic area.

2. Women with herpes may find a douche helpful. Add two tablespoons acidophilus to the douche, which helps to balance the pH in the vaginal area.

Herbs

1. External application of aloe vera gel, golden seal ointment and myrrh can be very helpful.

2. Drink herb teas that cleanse the immune system and are purifying to the blood, such as Chinese astragalus root, pau d'arco (a Brazilian herb that is an excellent blood purifier and liver cleanser), echinacea root, sassafras, and red clover.

Diet

1. Avoid processed foods, sugar, and stimulants like coffee, chocolate, and cola drinks.

2. Eliminate citrus fruits, sour apples, strawberries, grapes, watermelon, tomatoes, raw spinach, cranberries, vinegar, and nutritional yeast. Eat fruit no more than once every other day—baked apples and pears, bananas, papaya, cherries, peaches, berries (except strawberries), and melons (except watermelon).

3. Eliminate salt and foods high in sodium.

4. Eliminate animal products—meat (organic poultry would be fine on occasion) and cow's milk products (soured milks like yogurt are okay a few times a week).

5. Eat plenty of whole grains.

6. Eat a lot of cooked vegetables. Salads should be steamed rather than raw.

7. Eat proteins like fish, tofu (bean curd), and soured-milk products.

Supplements

1. Aloe vera juice (cleanses the colon and liver)—four to six ta-

blespoons on alternate days on an empty stomach.

2. Evening primrose oil capsules—two to three daily for the immune system.

3. A multivitamin mineral three times daily.

4. Potassium/magnesium supplement three times daily.

5. B-complex capsule or tablet three times daily.

6. Pantothenic acid—500 mg three times daily.

7. Vitamin E in dry form—400-800 i.u.'s on alternate days.

8. Bioflavonoid complex—1,000 mg daily.

9. Be careful when using vitamin C, especially if it is not being taken in its form as ascorbate. It can make the body too acid!

HYPOGLYCEMIA

Hypoglycemia, or low blood sugar, is the most common disease syndrome in our country today. Physiologically, it is a metabolic disease related to malfunctioning of the pancreas. Within the pancreas are cells known as the islands of Langerhans which produce insulin. Insulin is a hormone that keeps the sugar level balanced in the blood stream. When too little insulin is present, the sugar in the blood increases, known as diabetes or hyperglycemia. When the insulin absorbs too much sugar, low blood sugar, or hypoglycemia, results.

After a meal, the adrenal glands (cortical hormones) monitor the liver, determining how much sugar to release to satisfy the energy requirements of the body. The pancreas produces the insulin needed. When sugar is ingested into the blood in the form of food, the pancreas injects more insulin than is required, creating a condition known as *hyperinsulinism*, a large amount of blood sugar absorbed in a short amount of time. This, in turn, leaves the blood sugar lower; the adrenals become exhausted in trying to bring the sugar back to normal; and one turns to caffeine and other stimulants which activate the adrenal glands to induce the liver to break down glycogen and convert it into glucose, or blood sugar.

Hypoglycemia is also related to food allergies, which often bring on the symptoms of hypoglycemia. Eliminating certain foods can be helpful in controlling blood sugar.

Symptoms of hypoglycemia include fatigue, headaches, dizziness, depression, indigestion, irritability, poor memory, lack of confidence, and anxiety.

There are many emotional factors involved in hypoglycemia. Since the pancreas is located near the solar plexus, those individuals who tend to be highly sensitive pull in energy in this area of the body. When they are under stress or in an emotional state, it affects the pancreas and the blood sugar drops, giving them symptoms of physical weakness as well as depression and irritability.

Treatments

1. Working with stress-reduction techniques like biofeedback, autogenics, and other meditative techniques helps one to be aware of states of imbalance in both the psyche and the body and to balance them accordingly.

2. Colon irrigations are important in aiding assimilation and digestion so that the enzymes work to break down foods properly.

3. Acupuncture treatments as well as jin shinn, shiatsu, and other Oriental types of massage balance the meridians of the body and enable the metabolism to work better.

Diet

1. Avoid sugar in all forms. Honey is not especially good, except occasionally. Use barley malt or rice syrup as they are complex carbohydrates and provide slower assimilation.

2. Avoid all processed and refined foods, as well as all chemical additives.

3. Avoid coffee and caffeine substances like tea, cocoa, chocolate, and cola beverages.

4. Avoid salt and foods high in sodium such as soy sauce, miso soup, and salad dressings.

5. Eliminate cow's milk products except for soured milks like yogurt, kefir, and acidophilus cottage cheese.

6. Cut down fruit and fruit juice to one time every other day to keep sugars lower. Eliminate citrus fruit, strawberries, soured apples, watermelon, grapes, tomatoes, vinegar, nutritional yeast, raw spinach, raw green pepper, and cranberries, all highly acidic foods.

7. Eliminate wheat; use other breads like rye, millet, corn, rice cakes, and rye crackers. Incorporate all other grains into the diet like buckwheat (not a wheat), barley, oats, and brown rice.

8. Eliminate shellfish; use fresh fish, baked or broiled.

9. Eliminate red meats since they contain high amounts of uric

acid. Use organic poultry, calves' liver, and chicken liver.

10. Eliminate heavy carbohydrates like pasta, tortillas, and most beans (aduki beans are the easiest to digest) since they are difficult to metabolize. Use mung bean noodles, rice noodles, and buck-wheat noodles.

11. Eat cooked whole-grain cereals in the morning since they take eight hours to break down and keep the blood sugar up most of the day.

12. Eat frequent small meals throughout the day.

Herbs

1. Dandelion root (one or two cups alternate days) is a good herb for the pancreas and liver that helps to normalize blood sugar.

2. Parsley juice or tea is helpful in rebuilding the adrenal glands, which become depleted when blood sugar is low.

Supplements

1. Free-form amino acid capsules help to regulate the blood sugar—about three daily.

2. Enzymes including pancreatin, bile, lipase, papain, and bromelain should be taken after each meal.

3. A multivitamin mineral three times daily.

4. Potassium/magnesium capsules three times daily.

5. A manganese capsule or tablet three times daily, especially if allergies are involved.

6. Pantothenic acid—1,000 mg three times daily.

7. Bioflavonoid complex—1,000 mg three times daily.

8. Flower remedies work to balance emotional states and re-plenish adrenal energy.

INSECT BITES AND STINGS

Insects that bite and sting can be divided into two classes—those that bite to protect themselves (bees, wasps, ants, spiders), and those that bite to eat us (mosquitoes, fleas, ticks, bedbugs, lice).

Fleas and Flies

1. Rue tea and thyme tea repel fleas; use one teaspoon rue to one cup water and steep. This can be sprayed into the room or on

plants.

2. Hanging pennyroyal or eucalyptus leaves in the room or wearing them in pouches repels fleas and flies.

3. Placing bay leaves in containers of grains or flour keeps out insects.

Mosquitoes

1. Rub pennyroyal, eucalyptus, or citronella oil on the body to repel mosquitoes.

2. Crush up pennyroyal or eucalyptus leaves and wear in a pouch on the body.

3. Take plenty of B vitamins, especially B-1 and B-12. Some magnesium daily in the form of liquid chlorophyll (2-3 T. in 1/2 glass of spring water) is also helpful.

4. On bites, use a mud compress, cornstarch poultice, or moistened plantain leaves.

5. The homeopathic remedy Euphrasia (30x potency) is good for swollen or inflamed bites.

Stinging Insects (Bees, Wasps, Hornets, Yellow Jackets)

1. Brush the insect away; do not pull it off or it may inject more venom. Suck out the venom; this will lessen swelling and somewhat alleviate an allergic reaction.

2. Take homeopathic Apis Mel (30x) or Ledum (30x) to reduce swelling.

3. Externally, put mud, a drop of honey (from the hive, if possible), a paste of moist baking soda, wheat-germ oil, oil from vitamin E capsules, crushed plantain leaves, or raw potato on the sting. These all work to relieve the swelling and pain.

Lice

The eggs attach themselves to the base of the hair follicles and are difficult to remove.

1. Clean hair with water and green soap and cut off as much as possible.

2. Use the following mixture: 2 T. oil of rue and 8 oz. beer with 1 qt. tobacco water (water in which a handful of tobacco has been infused). Wash with this mixture twice daily for one week. Wait and apply it again in two weeks.

3. Pennyroyal oil applied to the body helps get rid of lice.

4. An ointment of the fruit and leaves of wormwood mixed with lanolin in the blender may be applied to the body.

Spiders
Bicarbonate of soda applied to spider bites relieves swelling and itchiness.

Scabies
Wash affected parts with green soap. Make tea of two teaspoons juniper berries to one pint water. Drink two cups daily, and bathe in it.

KIDNEY AND BLADDER PROBLEMS

The kidneys and bladder cleanse wastes from the blood system and eliminate them in the urine. Without proper intake of liquids, the kidney becomes clogged because it cannot excrete these toxins. When the toxic residue remains in the body, it can cause lower back pain and inflammation of the kidneys.

If the kidneys are not functioning properly, edema or swelling of the body, particularly around the ankles, often occurs. This retention of water may be related to the holding back of emotions. When one is having problems in relationships and not eliminating emotions, kidney and bladder problems often result.

An example of this is a woman who had lost one kidney, was on a dialysis machine, and was in danger of losing her second kidney. When she realized that her relationships with her husband and two sons had been extremely difficult and related this to her kidney problems, she experienced great healing.

Treatments
1. A ginger root compress applied to the kidney and bladder area. Grate fresh ginger root and put in tea balls or cheesecloth in two quarts of water. Make a strong ginger root tea and apply a hot compress to lower back area.

2. A poultice of dry-curd cottage cheese on the crotch area stops stinging and burning of the kidneys and draws out the inflammation. Use one teaspoon cottage cheese, and change several times a day.

Herbs

1. Dandelion leaf is an excellent diuretic. Drink two cups daily for water retention and kidney cleansing. Cleavers, nettles, and alfalfa are also helpful drunk as teas.

2. For kidney infections, take pipsissewa tincture twice daily.

3. Juniper berry tea (1 t. berries to 1 cup water) increases urination and is soothing to the urinary tract.

Diet

1. Eliminate all refined and processed foods, sugars, coffee, and black tea.

2. Eliminate salt and all foods high in sodium like soy sauce, miso soup, packaged soups, and bottled salad dressings. The intake of high amounts of sodium increases body acidity and the loss of potassium. When the kidneys are not functioning properly, there is a sodium/potassium imbalance.

3. Eliminate all red meat since it has a high content of uric acid.

4. Cut down fruit to alternate days, and eliminate citrus fruits, strawberries, sour apples, grapes, plums, and watermelon.

5. Other strongly acidic foods to eliminate are tomatoes, raw spinach and raw green peppers, vinegar, nutritional yeast, and cranberries. The old myth about cranberry juice being good for kidney infections is, in fact, untrue. Cranberry juice makes the body more acidic (it contains benzoic acid and contributes to the susceptibility to yeast and other infections).

6. Eliminate cow's milk products, except for the soured milks—yogurt, kefir, acidophilus cottage cheese, etc.

7. Eliminate wheat—use all other whole grains and whole-grain cereals and breads.

8. Include asparagus, a good diuretic; parsley and parsley juice, which is very cleansing to the kidneys; and garlic, a good blood purifier.

Supplements

1. Bioflavonoid complex containing rutin—1,000 mg three times daily.

2. Vitamin A (as beta-carotene)—10,000 i.u.'s twice daily.

3. Potassium capsules or potassium/magnesium capsules three times daily.

4. A good source of magnesium like liquid chlorophyll—two

or three tablespoons in half a glass of water alternate days.

5. A multivitamin mineral three times daily.

6. Zinc chelate or picollinate—two or three times daily.

7. Evening primrose oil—three capsules daily for kidney or bladder infections.

Homeopathy

Certain remedies are very helpful for kidney and bladder problems and should be chosen according to the individual.

Flower Remedies

Flower essences work well in dealing with emotional causes.

MENOPAUSE

Menopause refers to hormonal changes which occur for most women between the ages of 40 and 50. (However, it is not unusual for these changes to occur after 50 and, in some cases, before the age of 40.) Menopausal symptoms may include hot flashes, disturbances in calcium metabolism, nervousness, irritability, depression, general restlessness and insomnia. When hormonal balance is maintained, the time of menopause can be a healthy, relaxed, and balanced life phase.

Hormonal balance is related to blood sugar. When blood sugar levels are normal, few of the uncomfortable symptoms associated with menopause result. In order to keep blood sugar levels and metabolism normal, it is important to maintain good digestion and a balanced diet with few sweets and acid foods. This also involves periodic cleansing of the colon and liver.

Psychologically, dealing with the idea of aging and understanding that aging need not imply physical deterioration is most important. Women who believe that menopause is the entrance into a new cycle of creativity and freedom and look forward to this time have little problems with physical symptoms.

Treatments

1. Physical exercise, especially exercises like yoga that help to balance internal organs, is important. Various forms of aerobics as aerobic dance, walking, jogging, swimming, and other sports main-

tain muscle tone and improve circulation.

2. Regular cleansing of the colon with short vegetable juice fasts followed by a colonic or high enema will help to achieve a normal metabolism.

3. Obtaining one's correct constitutional homeopathic remedy can be extremely helpful in adjusting to hormonal changes. See a homeopathic practitioner.

4. Various *herbs* help in the estrogen/progesterone balance. They may be used individually or in combination with other female toning herbs. Herbs that are especially beneficial are sarsaparilla root (simmered as a tea), squawvine (steeped as a tea), and dong quai (this may be simmered as a root or taken in tablets or capsules). A good toner for the female organs like raspberry leaf or blessed thistle is important to drink on alternate days.

5. Proper body alignment is essential at this time. Adjustments and cranial work are helpful to good body alignment; cranial work also balances and relaxes the nervous system.

6. Massage treatments and various body therapies, in addition to being relaxing, aid the circulation and keep organs toned.

Diet

1. Avoid all refined and processed foods.

2. Avoid stimulants to the nervous system like coffee, black tea, cola drinks, and cocoa.

3. Avoid heavy animal proteins such as red meat, cheese, and butter. Use fresh fish (not shellfish), organic poultry and liver, and soured-milk products like yogurt and kefir.

4. Avoid sugar and sweet foods. Try substituting barley malt or rice syrup for honey since they are complex carbohydrates and take longer to break down.

5. Avoid citrus fruits, strawberries, sour apples, plums, grapes, watermelon, tomatoes, raw spinach, raw green pepper, yeast, vinegar, and cranberries.

6. Use plenty of good whole grains (oats, rye, amaranth, buckwheat cream, rice cream) as cereals in the morning and brown rice, buckwheat, millet, and barley during the day.

7. Eat lots of steamed vegetables, especially the greens like kale, bok choy, mustard greens, collard greens, chard, and turnip greens. These are especially high in calcium, magnesium and potassium.

8. Eat fresh vegetable salads and vegetable juices. Emphasize carrot, turnip, celery and parsley as a juice combination and lots of greens and sprouts in salads.

9. Incorporate iron-rich foods such as dulse (a sea vegetable that may be steamed with vegetables or put in soups), beets, red cabbage, prune and fig juice, cherries and cherry juice.

Supplements

1. Liquid chlorophyll—two to three tablespoons twice daily when no other green juices are taken. This supplies the required magnesium.

2. Calcium/magnesium supplement or potassium/magnesium supplement—three times daily. (There is a special supplement called Osteo-Novum made by Cardiovascular Research Company that has all three minerals and vitamin D.)

3. A good trace mineral containing zinc, selenium, manganese, iron—three times daily. A powdered supplement from sea vegetables is best.

4. B-6—100 mg three times daily on alternate days.

5. B-12 in liquid form, if possible, with iron added. Two or three doses; alternate with B-6.

6. Vitamin E in dry form—600-1,000 i.u.'s, two or three doses alternate days.

7. Bioflavonoid capsules—1,000 mg three times daily.

8. GH-3 tablets from Romania (used as an anti-aging supplement to balance hormones) or evening primrose oil capsules. GH-3 is used alternate days for three weeks (two tablets a day) and then stopped for two weeks. Three capsules of evening primrose oil should be taken on alternate days for a month or two and then stopped for a few weeks. These may not be needed if dong quai or sarsparilla root teas are used.

9. Free-form amino acid capsules are often needed for blood sugar—three daily.

10. If allergies are present or any kind of stress, use pantothenic acid—1,000 mg two or three times a day.

MENSTRUAL PROBLEMS

Many women experience difficulties, such as cramps, headaches, breast tenderness, water retention, low blood sugar, depression, anxiety, and tension, prior to menstruation. This is due to hormonal and metabolic changes at this time which lower the levels of calcium, magnesium, potassium, and some of the B vitamins, particularly B-6. These symptoms are generally referred to as PMS, premenstrual syndrome, but other problems may occur, such as excessive bleeding (menorrhagia) or missed cycles (amenorrhea).

In Native American society and other tribal societies, women were in touch with their cycles and actually looked forward to their menses as a time to go within themselves, to spend time in the Moon Lodge and become more aware of dreams and intuitive states. Because physical vitality can be lower during this time, it is a good time for reflection and inner processes. In modern Western society, women still go on with their normal activities, working in buildings with uncomfortable chairs, fluorescent lights and little air; taking care of children; cooking and cleaning house. Many of the symptoms referred to as PMS are a reaction to having to maintain these routines when one is feeling physically less vital and more sensitive. They are also a reaction to many bad experiences women have had with their menses from childhood (discomfort, pain, excessive bleeding) and a basic attitude of dreading this time of the month. In addition, many women have a lot of sexual fears and fears concerning pregnancy that surface shortly before menstruation begins.

If a woman can have some time to herself during her menses to pay attention to her inner processes, the following treatments will help the hormonal and metabolic changes.

Treatments

1. Regular exercise, especially yoga postures, keep the lower back flexible and energize internal organs.

2. Bodywork and massage is very nurturing and helpful in balancing meridians and *chi* energy.

3. Frequent cleansing like colonic irrigations and high enemas promote good digestion and assimilation of nutrients. This is important for the functioning of the metabolic system.

4. Meditation and other therapies that relax the nervous system are helpful throughout the month.

5. Hydrotherapy in the form of warm hip baths promotes circulation in the lower parts of the body.

6. Certain homeopathic remedies may be helpful on an individual constitutional basis.

7. Individual flower essences are excellent at this time.

Herbs

1. Raspberry leaf tea is a good hormonal balance for all types of problems. It should be drunk alternate days.

2. Blessed thistle and squawvine teas also help to balance the hormonal system; use as teas alternate days in combination with raspberry leaf.

3. Dong quai is an important herb for amenorrhea and other menstrual problems; it should be drunk as a tea, often in combination with other herbs. (Consult a good Chinese herbalist for specific ones.)

4. Sarsaparilla root is high in progesterone; it is also a good blood purifier and should be drunk alternate days as a tea.

5. Tansy promotes menstrual flow.

Diet

1. Emphasize foods high in calcium and magnesium like leafy green vegetables and herbs, carrot and turnip juices, yogurt and soured-milk products.

2. Include lots of whole grains for B vitamins, especially in the morning with whole-grain cereals.

3. During the menses, iron-rich foods like beets and beet juice, dulse (a sea vegetable), red cabbage, figs and prunes, and nettle leaf tea should be incorporated into the diet in large amounts (also organic calves' liver and beef liver for non-vegetarians).

4. Cook with sea vegetables because they are high in trace minerals.

Supplements

1. GH-3 tablets, an anti-aging hormonal formula originated by Dr. Ana Aslan in Romania, are excellent for hormonal balance. They may be used for three weeks (two every other day) and then stopped for two weeks.

2. If GH-3 tablets are not used, evening primrose oil capsules should be used—three daily for several weeks and then stopped for a couple weeks.

3. Vitamin B-6—100 mg three times daily, alternate days.

4. Vitamin B-12 (preferably in liquid form) or 50 mcg tablets three times daily, alternate days (alternate with B-6).

5. Potassium/magnesium capsules or calcium/magnesium/potassium capsules—three daily.

6. A multivitamin mineral or trace minerals—three daily.

7. Bioflavonoid complex—1,000 mg three times daily.

8. Vitamin E—600-800 i.u.'s, two to three, alternate days. (Not necessary if using evening primrose oil capsules.)

9. Manganese helps the nervous system and hormonal balance—three times daily.

MIGRAINE

Migraine refers to severe headaches which usually occur on one side of the head and are sometimes accompanied by nausea, vomiting, or changes in vision.

Physiologically, migraines are caused by the constriction and dilatation of cerebral arteries. Allergies (foods, pollen and other inhalants, and chemical pollutants) have been shown to be causative agents for these types of headaches. Hypoglycemia or low blood sugar may also contribute to migraines.

Psychologically, migraines are caused by emotional disturbances, tension, and anxiety. Those who are heads of groups, organizations, and large families feel a certain responsibility; they often manifest tension in the area of the head. People who tend to hold back emotion may develop blockages to the cerebral arteries from time to time in a migraine attack.

Treatments

1. Emotional and psychological therapies to deal with the repression of emotions.

2. Regular exercise where the whole body gets a workout, especially if one is sitting a lot during the day.

3. Breathing exercises like yoga breathing which bring more air to the lungs and aid circulation to cerebral arteries.

4. Acupressure, shiatsu, and other massage techniques that relax the body, particularly the shoulder, neck, and head area.

5. Nervine *herb* teas like vervain, hops, scullcap, chamomile, spearmint, and catnip relax the nervous system.

6. Cranial work which balances the cerebrospinal fluid and nourishes the nervous system.

Diet

1. Avoid all sugars, sweeteners, foods containing caffeine, and foods containing chemicals and preservatives (that means most canned and packaged food).

2. Avoid common sources of allergies like cow's milk products (the soured milks like yogurt may or may not be okay) and wheat products.

3. Avoid other foods that may cause allergic reactions such as citrus fruit, strawberries, sour apples, cranberries, watermelon, grapes, plums, tomatoes, raw spinach and green pepper, yeast, and vinegar.

4. Avoid red meats and use only organic poultry or liver.

5. Avoid shellfish, and be sure fish is from fresh, unpolluted waters.

6. Avoid salt (use non-sodium vegetable seasonings), soy sauce, and miso soup.

7. Use whole grains that are sources of B vitamins like buckwheat, brown rice, millet, barley, rye, oats, amaranth, and corn at least once a day, preferably as a breakfast cereal.

8. Use plenty of green leafy steamed vegetables high in calcium and magnesium.

9. Eat small frequent meals.

Supplements

1. Pantothenic acid—1,000 mg three times daily.

2. B-complex vitamin (non-yeast base)—1,000 mg three times daily.

3. Multivitamin mineral capsules—three daily.

4. Liquid chlorophyll—two or three tablespoons twice daily as a source of magnesium when no other green vegetable juices are taken.

5. Calcium/magnesium or potassium/magnesium capsules—three daily.

6. Manganese capsules—three to six daily.

7. Free-form amino acids to help blood sugar balance—three capsules daily.

8. Bioflavonoid capsules—1,000 mg three times daily.

MULTIPLE SCLEROSIS

Multiple sclerosis, a disease of the nervous system, attacks the brain and spinal cord. Many conditions may result from this, such as visual disturbances, tremor and shaking of the limbs, faulty speech, impaired balance, loss of bladder and bowel control, and paralysis in specific areas. Though MS, as it is called, is a chronic condition, there are cycles where it improves.

Psychologically, MS may be related to inflexibility. Those individuals who have MS are often inflexible and rigid. They need to let go of their tight control and learn to flow more with the universal energy.

Treatments

1. Psychological and spiritual therapies to deal with changes in life style and emotional problems.

2. Physical therapy like exercise, massage, and other bodywork to relax muscles and increase the circulation to the limbs affected.

3. Cranial adjustment which helps to balance cerebrospinal fluid and nerve endings.

4. Hydrotherapy like hot mineral baths and hot and cold showers to stimulate and relax the nervous system.

5. Cleansing the colon through the use of aloe vera juice, colonics, and high enemas allows the body to break down foods for better assimilation of nutrients.

Diet

1. Eliminate all refined and processed foods, foods with chemical additives, sugars, and caffeine-containing foods.

2. Eliminate salt, soy sauce, miso, and other foods high in sodium.

3. Eliminate highly acidic foods such as strawberries, cranberries, citrus fruits, sour apples, tomatoes, plums, grapes, raw green pepper and raw spinach, yeast, and vinegar.

4. Eliminate red meats and cow's milk products, except for soured milks like yogurt.

5. Eliminate wheat, shellfish, and peanuts; all cause highly allergic reactions.

6. Include cereal germ oils like wheat-germ oil which is a

source of arachidonic acid, a fatty acid important in helping MS.

7. Include fermented foods like sauerkraut and pickles which are high in lactic acid.

8. Eat plenty of steamed vegetables, especially the green leafy ones high in magnesium and calcium.

9. Include foods high in iron like beets, the sea vegetable dulse, prune and fig juice, and blackstrap molasses.

10. Include plenty of whole grains for B vitamins.

Supplements

1. Lecithin (in liquid form if possible)—two tablespoons twice daily, alternate days.

2. Liquid chlorophyll (as a source of magnesium)—three or four tablespoons twice daily if no other green juice is also being taken.

3. Pantothenic acid—1,000 mg three times daily.

4. B-12 (preferable in liquid form)—two times daily, alternate days.

5. B complex (non-yeast base)—1,000 mg three times daily.

6. B-3 (niacin)—100 mg on alternate days.

7. B-13 (orotic acid) on alternate days.

8. A multivitamin mineral four times daily.

9. Potassium/magnesium or calcium/magnesium capsules—six daily.

10. A manganese capsule or chelated manganese—three to six daily.

11. Free-form amino acid capsules—three daily.

12. Octacosanol (made from wheat-germ oil, a good source of arachidonic acid)—super-strength—three on alternate days.

13. Evening primrose oil capsules—three daily, alternating with octacosanol.

NEURALGIA AND NEURITIS

Neuralgia and neuritis (when pain is the chief symptom it is referred to as neuralgia; when inflammation, paralysis and other symptoms result, the term neuritis is used) attack the peripheral nerves, the nerves that link the brain and spinal cord with the muscles, skin, organs, and other parts of the body. The causes of neuritis include toxemia where certain substances like lead, arsenic, and mercury may produce a generalized poisoning of the peripheral nerves with tenderness, pain, and paralysis of the limbs. Other causes may include alcoholism; vitamin-deficiency diseases as beri-beri; some viral and bacterial infections like diphtheria, syphilis, and mumps; as well as extreme tension and anxiety conditions.

Some attacks of neuritis begin with a fever; neuritis caused by lead or alcohol poisoning, however, comes on very slowly over weeks or months.

Psychologically, paralysis of certain nerves may result from fear, resistance and anxiety states. When there are fears and held-back energy, the circulation to certain areas of the body is impeded and may eventually result in paralysis of those nerves.

Treatments

1. Cleansing the body of toxic substances is most important; in extreme cases of toxemia, chelation therapy may be necessary; in other cases, frequent colonics and high enemas to cleanse the colon and saunas to cleanse the skin are advisable.

2. Acupuncture works well to get the vital force (*chi* energy) flowing to the organs.

3. Shiatsu, acupressure, and other types of massage therapy help to break up toxins and increase circulation to various organs.

4. Cranial work nourishes the nervous system and keeps the cerebrospinal fluid flowing to all the nerve endings.

5. Certain *herbs* work well to increase circulation within the body. Chinese herbs like Chinese cinnamon and ginger root are helpful as are blood-purifying herbs like chaparral, echinacea root, and red clover.

Diet

1. Avoid all chemical additives and preservatives, sugars, sweeteners, and caffeine-containing foods.

2. Avoid salt, soy sauce and foods high in sodium.

3. Avoid red meats and use only organic poultry and liver.

4. Avoid shellfish and use only fish from unpolluted waters.

5. Avoid highly acid foods such as cranberries, strawberries, citrus fruits, tomatoes, raw spinach, raw green pepper, yeast, and vinegar.

6. Include steamed and raw vegetables, especially green leafy

vegetables.

7. Include sea vegetables rich in minerals like dulse, wakame, kobu, and nori.

8. Include whole grains like brown rice, millet, barley, buckwheat, oats, and rye.

9. Drink fresh vegetable juices, particularly carrot-celery (celery is helpful to the nervous system) and carrot-parsley (parsley is high in magnesium and vitamin A).

Supplements

1. Aloe vera juice—four to six tablespoons on alternate days to cleanse the colon and liver.

2. Olive oil and lemon—two teaspoons cold-pressed olive oil with the juice of half a lemon on alternate mornings upon arising to clean the liver.

3. Liquid chlorophyll—three tablespoons twice daily (unless some fresh green vegetable juice is taken).

4. Pantothenic acid—1,000 mg three times daily.

5. B complex (non-yeast base)—1,000 mg three times daily.

6. Niacin—100 mg on alternate days.

7. A trace mineral (preferably in powdered form) or multivitamin mineral three times daily.

8. Potassium/magnesium capsules or calcium/magnesium capsules—six daily.

9. Manganese capsules—three to six daily.

10. Free-form amino acid capsules—three daily.

11. Bioflavonoid capsules—1,000 mg three times daily.

OSTEOPOROSIS

Osteoporosis is a metabolic bone disease which leads to thinning of the skeleton and inadequate calcium absorption into the bone. It is often a process of aging and seems to affect women more than men. Causes of osteoporosis are diminished physical activity, hormonal changes which lead to lack of estrogens or androgens, low intake of calcium, and the body's inability to absorb nutrients.

Symptoms of osteoporosis include frequent fractures and the collapse of the vertebrae without compression of the spinal cord.

Psychologically, the bony frame is what holds us up; often hurt pride, feeling underrated, lacking confidence, and the inability to stand up for oneself contribute to the process of osteoporosis.

Treatments

1. Plenty of exercise is important in preventing osteoporosis as well as in treating it. Regular daily exercise like walking, swimming, and jogging, as well as yoga exercises which work with the spine should be incorporated.

2. Colonic irrigations are extremely important since regular cleansing of the colon helps food to assimilate.

3. *Herbs* that contain high mineral content should be drunk as teas. Horsetail grass and shave grass are extremely high in silica, which is most important for calcium absorption. Other herb teas to include are oatstraw (calcium), alfalfa (all minerals), nettle leaves (iron), plantain (potassium), comfrey (calcium and magnesium), borage (calcium and magnesium), and raspberry leaf (magnesium).

Diet

1. Eliminate all chemical additives, food preservatives, sugars, sweeteners (except barley malt syrup and rice syrup), coffee, tea, chocolate, and caffeine drinks.

2. Include sea vegetables like dulse, kombu, wakame, arame, and nori, which are high in trace minerals.

3. Include plenty of cooked and steamed vegetables, especially green leafy vegetables, high in calcium and magnesium.

4. Include raw vegetable juices as carrot-turnip-parsley, carrot-turnip-celery, carrot-beet, carrot-cucumber, and other green vegetable juices.

5. Eat foods high in lactic acid like yogurt, kefir, soured-milk products, sauerkraut, and pickles.

6. Include plenty of whole grains, especially oats which are high in calcium, but also buckwheat, millet, rye, brown rice, barley, and amaranth. Avoid wheat as it tends to form a lot of mucus and is a source of food allergies.

7. Include fresh fish but avoid shellfish.

8. Eat fresh organic poultry and organic liver if desired, but avoid red meats and all non-organic meats.

9. Avoid salt and products high in sodium like soy sauce and miso soup.

Supplements

1. A good trace mineral, preferably powdered from sea vegetables—three teaspoons daily—or a multivitamin mineral three times daily.

2. Potassium/magnesium/calcium supplement—four daily. Osteo-Novum, made by Cardiovascular Research Co., contains all these minerals plus vitamin D.

3. Silica capsules—three daily.

4. Liquid chlorophyll (important as a source of magnesium)—two or three tablespoons three times daily when not using any green vegetable juice or other magnesium sources.

5. Digestive enzymes—one after each meal for assimilation.

6. Evening primrose oil capsules for hormonal balance—three daily for three months, then stop two months.

7. Vitamin E—600-1,000 i.u.'s twice daily alternate days in dry form.

8. B complex (non-yeast base)—1,000 mg three times daily.

9. Bioflavonoid complex—1,000 mg four times daily.

10. Pantothenic acid—1,000 mg three times daily.

PARKINSON'S DISEASE

Parkinson's disease is a progressive disease of the brain characterized by stiffness of muscles and tremors. Movements may become slower at first; then there is a loss of mobility in the facial area.

Parkinson's is caused by damage to several areas of the brain. This may be a result of a viral infection, carbon monoxide poisoning, or, in later life, cerebral arteriosclerosis.

Psychologically, there is often frustration involved and a rigidity of ideas that needs to be broken up.

Treatments

1. Physical therapies that work with muscular structure are important. Deep bodywork like rolfing, bioenergetics, and related therapies helps to break up crystallization in the psyche as well as in the body.

2. Regular daily exercise to increase circulation to the brain and heart should be done. Yoga and stretching exercises should also be incorporated into the regimen.

3. Cleansing of the colon to promote assimilation of nutrients should be performed periodically.

4. Homeopathic remedies are important in aiding the nervous system and brain. Consult a homeopathic practitioner to find the correct constitutional remedy.

5. *Herbs* that relax the nervous system like vervain, hops, scullcap, chamomile, catnip, and spearmint are beneficial; also, herbs that increase circulation such as ginger root, Chinese cinnamon, red clover blossoms, and cayenne.

Diet

1. Avoid all foods containing caffeine like coffee, black tea, chocolate, and cola drinks as well as all sugars and sweeteners, chemicals, and preservatives.

2. Include whole grains high in B complex such as buckwheat, millet, barley, brown rice, oats, rye, and amaranth.

3. Include green leafy vegetables high in calcium and magnesium.

4. Include raw vegetable juices, especially green vegetables which contain chlorophyll and, therefore, magnesium.

5. Include plenty of sea vegetables like dulse, wakame, kombu, and nori to obtain large amounts of minerals.

6. Include fresh fish (high in minerals) but not shellfish.

7. Eliminate cow's milk products like cheese and butter, but include soured milks like yogurt and kefir.

8. Eliminate salt and high-sodium foods like soy sauce.

9. Eliminate red meats but include organic poultry and organic liver.

Supplements

1. B-complex vitamin (non-yeast base)—1,000 mg three times daily.

2. B-6—500 mg three times every other day (alternate with B-12).

3. B-12 (liquid with iron, if possible)—three doses alternate days.

4. B-15—three times alternate days.

5. Liquid chlorophyll—three tablespoons three times daily if no green juice is taken.

6. Potassium/magnesium/calcium capsules—three daily.

7. Pantothenic acid—1,000 mg three times daily.

8. Trace minerals, preferably powdered from sea vegetables—three teaspoons daily—or a multivitamin mineral—three daily.

9. Manganese capsules or chelated manganese—six daily.

10. Bioflavonoid capsules—1,000 mg four times daily.

11. Co-Enzyme Q-10—30 mg two to three times alternate days.

PROSTATE PROBLEMS

The prostate is a reproductive organ in the male, located under the bladder and surrounding the urethra. It secretes a thin, slightly alkaline fluid that flows through ducts into the urethra. This fluid is secreted continuously, and the excess passes from the body into the urine. The rate of secretion increases during sexual stimulation, and the fluid helps to transport sperm cells as they move from the testicles to the urethra.

Enlargement of the prostate occurs often in men over the age of 50. Because of its position around the urethra, enlargement interferes with the passage of urine from the bladder. Urination becomes difficult, and the bladder never completely feels empty. If the prostate is markedly enlarged, chronic constipation may result as well.

Sexual excitation without orgasm or ejaculation can frequently lead to an enlarged prostate. Psychologically, guilt about sex or fears of aging may bring about prostate problems.

Treatments

1. Exercise is most important; walking, swimming, jogging, and other forms of exercise should be done daily. Certain yoga postures have been found to benefit prostate problems and can be done to prevent them from occurring. One good exercise is to lie flat on the back, pull the knees up as far as possible, then press the soles of the feet together. Holding the soles pressed together, the legs should be lowered as far as possible with a forceful movement.

2. Hot sitz baths with chamomile added can be very soothing. Fill the tub with six inches of hot water and wrap chamomile in cheesecloth or other material so that it infuses into the water. This can be done daily.

3. Natural remedies include bee pollen or pollen extract. In Sweden, a particular mixture known as Cernitory is used, which is

available in limited amounts in the U.S. If using Cernitory, take two pills alternate days; if using loose bee pollen, take two teaspoons alternate days.

4. Another natural remedy is pumpkin seeds, which are especially high in iron and also contain phosphorus, protein, the B vitamins and some other factor which seems to benefit the prostate. These, however, can be difficult to digest, so just a small handful alternate days should be used.

5. *Herbs* that are helpful for the prostate are juniper berries (simmer 1 t. berries in 1-1/2 cups water, and drink 2 cups alternate days) and echinacea root (simmer 1 t. root in 1-1/2 cups water and drink 2 cups alternate days for enlargement of prostate). Ginseng is helpful in replenishing male hormones.

Diet

1. Avoid alcohol, coffee and caffeine beverages, sugar, salt and foods high in sodium, chocolate, chemicals, and preservatives.

2. Avoid cow's milk products like milk, cheese, butter, and cottage cheese. Use soured milks like yogurt and kefir and goat's milk products instead.

3. Avoid wheat as it is another source of mucus buildup in the system; use rye breads and crackers, rice cakes, oats, barley, buckwheat, brown rice, millet, amaranth, and corn.

4. Eliminate red meats; use organic poultry and liver.

5. Eliminate shellfish; use fresh fish from unpolluted waters.

6. Eat plenty of fresh steamed vegetables, especially green leafy ones high in minerals.

7. Use fresh vegetable juices such as carrot-celery, carrot-turnip-parsley and especially carrot-cucumber (cucumbers are good for the male hormones).

8. Use cold-pressed vegetable oils like flaxseed oil, olive oil, sesame oil, soy oil, and sunflower oil since they are high in vitamin F or essential fatty acids.

9. Cook sea vegetables like dulse, nori, wakame, and kombu which are high in zinc and trace minerals.

Supplements

1. Trace minerals, preferably powdered from sea vegetables—two to three teaspoons daily or two to three tablets daily—or a multivitamin mineral—three capsules daily.

2. Zinc capsules or chelated zinc—three daily.

3. Potassium/magnesium capsules—three daily.

4. Liquid chlorophyll—two tablespoons twice daily for magnesium.

5. Liquid lecithin for essential fatty acids—two tablespoons alternate days.

6. Vitamin F—three capsules, alternate days.

7. Vitamin E—600-800 i.u.'s in dry form two times on alternate days (not necessary if using octacosanol).

8. Octacosanol capsules (made from wheat-germ oil)—two on alternate days.

9. Bioflavonoids—1,000 mg three times every day.

PSORIASIS

Psoriasis is a chronic skin disease characterized by bright red patches covered with silvery scales. These lesions may appear on the elbows, scalp, back of arms and legs, palms of hands and soles of feet. Psoriasis often occurs in conjunction with rheumatoid arthritis, suggesting it is an immune system disease and related to allergies.

Acute attacks of psoriasis occur during times of extreme stress and anxiety, while the chronic condition may always be present to some degree. Individuals who have a fear of being touched and are not happy with their bodies often get psoriasis and other skin conditions.

Treatments

1. Cleansing is of primary importance in ridding the body of toxins which break out on the skin. The colon should be cleansed through colonic irrigations and high enemas; the liver, through liver flushes (2 T. cold-pressed olive oil with half a squeezed lemon twice a week); the skin, through dry brush massages and saunas; and the kidneys, with various herbs. In all skin diseases the kidneys play an important part.

2. Soaking in baths with sea salt (1/2 cup) and baking soda (1/2 cup) are helpful to cleanse the skin and the aura as well. They draw out certain toxic minerals. If one is able, swimming in salt water is also excellent.

3. Plenty of invigorating exercise in the fresh air helps to elimi-

nate toxins from the body.

4. *Herbs* are important internally for cleansing and purifying the blood. Aloe vera juice cleanses the colon and kidneys as well. Teas made from chaparral, echinacea root, pau d'arco, red clover blossoms, burdock, sarsaparilla root, sassafras, and golden seal are beneficial. For external use, salves made from golden seal, calendula flowers, marigold flowers, and myrrh work well. For redness and swelling, fomentations or compresses from comfrey, plantain, dandelion leaves and periwinkle are excellent. They may be kept on the area 20-30 minutes.

5. Various homeopathic remedies are excellent. Kali Sulph (potassium sulfate), Kali Mur (potassium chloride), and other potassium remedies are often used.

Diet

Psoriasis and other skin diseases are based on allergies, so it is important to eliminate certain foods.

1. All canned and packaged food, foods with preservatives and chemicals, caffeine-based substances like cola drinks and coffee, chocolate and sugars should be eliminated.

2. Salt and salty foods like soy sauce are bad for the kidneys and imbalance the sodium/potassium level.

3. Extremely acid foods like tomatoes, citrus fruits, vinegar, yeast, raw spinach and green pepper, cranberries, strawberries, and soured apples should be eliminated. Fruit should be eaten every other day and consist of bananas, peaches, golden delicious apples, papayas, berries, and cantaloupe. Plums and grapes are also acidic.

4. Shellfish are a major cause of allergies; fresh fish from unpolluted waters may be included.

5. Cow's milk products like butter, milk, and cheese should be eliminated. Yogurt and soured milks may be included a couple of times a week.

6. Wheat and wheat products should be eliminated.

7. Beef, pork, lamb, and all fatty and non-organic meats should be cut out. Organic poultry and liver may be had on occasion.

8. Plenty of steamed and raw vegetables should be eaten.

9. Whole grains, especially buckwheat (which is a good source of rutin), should be included.

10. Cold-pressed oils as flaxseed oil, olive oil, and sunflower oil are good sources of vitamin F.

Supplements

1. Liquid chlorophyll—two to three tablespoons twice daily in half a glass of water to provide magnesium.

2. Liquid lecithin—two tablespoons alternate days after a meal.

3. Trace minerals (preferably powdered sea vegetables)—three teaspoons daily—or a multivitamin mineral three times daily.

4. A potassium supplement or potassium/magnesium capsules—three times daily.

5. Zinc picollinate or chelate—three times daily for the immune system.

6. A manganese capsule or tablet—three times daily.

7. Bioflavonoid capsules—-1,000 mg three times daily (contains rutin).

8. Vitamin A from beta-carotene—two times alternate days.

9. Vitamin E in dry form—600-800 i.u.'s. three times alternate days.

10. Pantothenic acid—1,000 mg three times daily.

11. PABA is excellent for skin conditions—1,000 mg three times daily.

SCIATICA

Sciatica is a condition of inflammation along the sciatic nerve, which runs from the lower spine down through the pelvis and thighs and continues on to the heels. Any degree of injury along this nerve or related nerves may cause it to throb in pain. Sciatica is often caused by a mild arthritic inflammation of the lower spine; however, slipped discs, dislocation of hips, or pelvic fractures can be responsible. Sometimes certain muscles of the legs may become partly paralyzed as a result, causing immobility. True sciatic neuritis, however, is comparatively rare. It can be caused by certain toxic substances such as lead and alcohol.

Emotionally, sciatic conditions occur when there is a lot of worry and also when there are some rigid patterns that are difficult to give up in one's life.

Treatments

1. Acupuncture treatments are often helpful for sciatic conditions in relieving pain and pressure along the nerves.

2. Massage therapies like shiatsu, acupressure, and other types of massage are important on a weekly basis.

3. Cranial work is essential for sciatica since it helps to balance the cerebrospinal fluid which goes to the nerve endings.

4. Applying pieces of flannel with heated peanut oil or olive oil to affected areas helps to ease the pain.

5. *Herbs* that help internally are nervine teas like chamomile, scullcap, spearmint, vervain, and catnip. Herbs that are high in magnesium and calcium like borage, comfrey, raspberry leaf and alfalfa are also beneficial. Externally, liniments made from mustard, wintergreen, and eucalyptus are soothing to afflicted areas.

6. Hot baths and water jets on painful spots are very soothing.

7. Exercises and yoga postures that stretch the spine and relax muscles should be done twice daily.

Diet

1. Avoid all preservatives, caffeine foods, and sugar.

2. Avoid citrus fruits, tomatoes, vinegar, yeast, cranberries, soured apples, and strawberries, and keep fruit to a minimum.

3. Eat lots of whole grains rich in B vitamins, especially millet, buckwheat, barley, oats, rye, and brown rice.

4. Eat cooked vegetables twice daily. Eat few raw vegetables.

5. Use warming spices like ginger, garlic, and cayenne in foods.

6. Eat plenty of sea vegetables such as dulse, wakame, kombu, and nori, which are rich in trace minerals.

7. Proteins may include fresh fish, organic poultry and liver, tofu, soured-milk products, nuts and seeds.

Supplements

1. Liquid chlorophyll—three tablespoons twice daily in half a glass of water for magnesium.

2. Trace minerals, preferably powdered sea vegetables—three teaspoons daily—or a multivitamin mineral three times daily.

3. Potassium/magnesium capsules or calcium/magnesium capsules—four daily.

4. Vitamin B-12 (preferably in liquid form)—three times daily.

5. Manganese capsules—four to six daily for the nervous system.

6. B complex (non-yeast base)—1,000 mg three times daily.

7. Bioflavonoid capsule or tablet—1,000 mg three times daily.

ULCERS

Peptic ulcers may occur in the inner wall or lining of the stomach (gastric ulcers) or the duodenum (duodenal ulcers). This ulceration of the mucous membrane is caused by the action of the acid gastric juice. Symptoms include pain or a gnawing sensation in the abdominal area one to three hours after eating, often accompanied by gas and nausea.

If ulcers are untreated, bleeding can occur, leading to weakness and impaired health. The ulcer may also become perforated, allowing food to escape from the stomach and intestines into the peritoneal cavity, causing peritonitis.

Ulcers are found in three times as many men as women. Those who get ulcers have a great deal of stress and anxiety in their lives. They constantly worry and allow issues to "eat away at them." They need to learn to relax, let go of their problems, and change their life style.

Treatments

1. Stress-reduction therapies like biofeedback, autogenics, and meditation help to control the level of anxiety.

2. Exercise like yoga and tai chi relaxes the body and also slows down the breathing, leading to deeper states of awareness.

3. Cleansing the intestinal area through colonics and enemas with slippery elm powder (2 T. slippery elm to 1 qt. water) is most important.

Herbs

Internally, drinking tea from some of the mucilaginous herbs is soothing to the mucous membranes. These herbs include slippery elm root or powder, comfrey root or leaf, marshmallow root, borage, and mullein. For roots, simmer one teaspoon root to one cup water.

Externally, a compress of ginger root applied to the stomach and intestinal area is very soothing. Grate fresh ginger root and place in a cheesecloth or two small tea balls. Cook in two quarts of water for 20 minutes. Then apply to abdominal area with a towel or flannel as hot as one can handle.

For acute conditions, take comfrey-pepsin tablets several times a day. These provide an antacid effect.

Diet

1. Eat small amounts of food at frequent intervals; chew food well.

2. Avoid alcohol, cigarettes, sugars of all kinds, caffeine foods, and any preservatives and chemicals.

3. Avoid salt and foods high in sodium (soy sauce, miso soup).

4. Avoid foods that are irritating like tomatoes, citrus fruit, soured apples and pears, strawberries, cranberries, vinegar, nutritional yeast, raw spinach, and raw green pepper. Keep fruit to a minimum—one small portion on alternate days. Eliminate fruit juices except for small amounts of papaya.

5. Avoid heavy proteins that are difficult to digest like meats, shellfish, butter, cheese, and milk. Eliminate nuts and seeds except ground-up nuts occasionally.

6. Avoid beans and pasta, which are also difficult to break down.

7. Avoid highly spiced foods as they increase the digestive juices which irritate the stomach lining.

8. Include mucilaginous foods in the diet such as okra, ground-up chia seeds (in cereals or on salads), ground-up flaxseeds, and powdered slippery elm in cereals.

9. Eat whole grains, made into gruels in the morning by grinding and cooking in one cup boiling water (3 T. ground grain to 1 cup water). Especially include oats, barley, and buckwheat.

10. Eat plenty of steamed vegetables; avoid raw vegetables.

11. For fruit, eat baked apples and pears, bananas, cooked peaches, and stewed fruit.

12. Use soured-milk products like yogurt and kefir. Goat's milk may also be used as well as nut milks like almond milk and cashew milk. (Blend a small handful of nuts with one cup water and a small amount of barley malt syrup or rice syrup to sweeten.)

Supplements

1. Aloe vera juice—three to four tablespoons daily on an empty stomach is very soothing to the mucous membranes and helps to keep the colon clear.

2. Liquid chlorophyll—two to three tablespoons twice daily in half a glass of water provides magnesium and other minerals to the system.

3. Powdered trace minerals from sea vegetables—three tea-

spoons daily—or multivitamin/mineral capsules—three daily.

4. Potassium capsules or potassium/magnesium capsules to alkalinize the system—three daily.

5. Manganese capsules or tablets—three daily.

6. Vitamin B complex (non-yeast base)—1,000 mg three daily.

7. Bioflavonoid capsules—1,000 mg three daily.

8. Amino acid capsules—three daily help to keep up the blood sugar, which is often connected with ulcers.

VARICOSE VEINS

Varicose veins are swollen veins visible especially in the legs which result from a sluggish flow of blood in combination with defective valves and weakened walls of the veins.

Jobs that require constant standing, the conditions of being overweight and pregnancy, and a lack of exercise often cause varicosity. If not treated, more serious conditions like leg ulcers, swelling, and clots may result.

Emotional causes of varicose veins include feelings of restraint and the holding back of emotions in addition to the inability to circulate ideas.

Treatments

1. Elevate the legs at every opportunity. This allows blood to drain and fresh blood to take its place. Keep the feet active, and try to do some deep knee bends during the day.

2. Exercise of all kinds is a must, especially bicycling for about one hour a day. Swimming, running, walking, and other aerobic-type exercises will also keep the circulation going.

3. Yoga postures like the head stand and the shoulder stand are very important for getting the blood flowing. They should be done several times a day.

4. Since constipation is often a contributory cause of varicosity, making sure the colon is empty through regular colonic irrigations and high enemas is important.

5. Deep-massage techniques loosen the muscular structure and help circulate oxygen throughout the body.

6. Hydrotherapy—preferably in the ocean, but if not, in a pond or lake, walking forward and backward into the water, raising the

knees as high as possible—helps bring circulation to the legs.

Herbs

Internal—Blood-purifying teas like chaparral, red clover, yarrow, marigold flowers, and St. John's wort flowers are good as well as herbs that increase circulation and bring warmth to areas of the body like ginger root and Chinese cinnamon.

External—Rub St. John's wort oil on affected areas. Make white oak bark tea, and put compresses of this on the area for several hours if possible. Towels can be soaked in the tea and wrapped around the legs.

Diet

1. Avoid all heavy starchy foods like beans, tortillas, and pasta. Also sugars, caffeine foods, chemicals and preservatives.

2. Use figs, prunes, cherries, and fig, prune, and cherry juice to keep the bowels open.

3. Include mucilaginous herbs and foods like ground flaxseed, ground chia seed, slippery elm tea, and okra.

4. Include soured-milk products like yogurt, kefir, and other acidophilus products.

5. Add garlic and onion to foods since they are good blood purifiers.

6. Use cooked whole grains, especially buckwheat, which is high in rutin.

7. Include plenty of cooked steamed vegetables; keep salads to a minimum.

8. Include proteins like fresh fish (not shellfish), tofu or bean curd, organic poultry, and fertile eggs twice a week.

Supplements

1. Aloe vera juice—four tablespoons every other day to keep the colon cleansed.

2. Bioflavonoid complex—1,000 mg three times daily.

3. Liquid lecithin—two tablespoons on alternate days.

4. Vitamin E—600-1,000 i.u.'s in dry form, three times a day on alternate days.

5. Octacosanol—three capsules alternate days (alternate with vitamin E). This is very important in aiding circulation.

6. Trace minerals, preferably powdered from sea vegeta-

bles—three teaspoons daily—or a multivitamin mineral three times daily.

7. Pantothenic acid—1,000 mg on alternate days.

8. Potassium/magnesium or calcium/magnesium capsules—three daily.

NOTES

1. Victor H. Kallman, *Use of Blue-Green Algae in the Treatment of Alzheimer's Disease* (Wynelta Spence Publishing Services, 1982).
2. Richard Passwater, Ph.D. *Cancer and Its Nutritional Therapies.* (New Canaan, CT: Keats Publishing, 1983), p. 20.
3. Ibid.
4. Ibid.

◊ APPENDIX I ◊

CONSULTATION SERVICES AND HERBS

Health consultations utilizing nutrition, herbology, flower remedies, and medical astrology:

> Marcia Starck
> Earth Medicine Ways
> 6714 Manila Ave.
> El Cerrito, CA 94530
> (415) 236-0635

Information on Chinese herbs and health consultations utilizing medical astrology:

> Russell Klobas, L.Ac.
> 220 Water St., #2
> Hallowell, ME 04347
> (207) 621-0985

Herbs and herbal products used by Earth Medicine Ways:

> Earth Essences/Botanical Pharmaceuticals
> P.O. Box 1438
> Sedona, AZ 86336
> (602) 282-7136

Oak Valley Herb Farm
14648 Pear Tree Lane
Nevada City, CA 95959
(916) 265-9552

Simpler's Botanical Co.
P.O. Box 39-C
Forestville, CA 95436
(707) 887-2012

Other herbal distributors recommended by the American Herb Association:

Alexandra Avery
Purely Natural Body Care
Northrup Creek
Birkenfield, OR 97016

American Indian Herb Co.
P.O. Box 16684
San Diego, CA 92102

Attar Herbs & Spice Inc.
Playground Road
Box 245
New Ipswich, NH 03071

Avena Botanical
P.O. Box 365
W. Rockport, ME 04865

Bisbee Botanicals
P.O. Box 26
Bisbee, AZ 85603

Blue Heron Herbs
Mara Levin
Rt. 1, Box 26
Deadwood, OR 97430

The Herb Field
Box 125
Wendell, MA 01379

The Herb Shop
P.O. Box 352
Provo, UT 84603

Herbalist & Alchemist Inc.
P.O. Box 63
Franklin Park, NJ 08823

Herb-Pharm
P.O. Box 116-C
Williams, OR 97544
(503) 846-7178

Mountain Butterfly Herbs
Suzanne McDougal
106 Roosevelt Ln.
Hamilton, MT 59840

Weleda Inc.
841 S. Main St.
P.O. Box 769
Spring Valley, NY 10977

Willow Rain Herb Farm
P.O. Box 15
Grubville, MO 63041

For Chinese herbal formulas:

Health Concerns
2236 Mariner Square Drive
Alameda, CA 94501
(415) 521-7401

For first-aid kit containing Chinese herbal formulas and home-opathy:

> Charis
> 2512 9th St., #18
> Berkeley, CA 94710

For combinations of herbs, vitamins, and minerals:

> Rainbow Light Nutritional Systems
> 207 McPherson
> Santa Cruz, CA 95060

Other important addresses:

> American Herb Association
> P.O. Box 353
> Rescue, CA 95672
>
> California School of Herbal Studies
> 9309 Highway #116
> Forestville, CA 95436

◊ APPENDIX II ◊

HOMEOPATHIC REMEDIES

Homeopathic remedies and first-aid kits can be obtained from the following companies:

Dolisos America
3014 Rigel Ave.
Las Vegas, NV 89102
(800) 365-4767

Hahnemann Medical Clinic Pharmacy
1918 Bonita Ave.
Berkeley, CA 94704

Homeopathic Educational Services
2124 Kittredge St.
Berkeley, CA 94704
(800) 359-9051
(also has books and tapes on homeopathy)

Other homeopathic pharmacies (some carry first-aid kits; list taken from the directory of the National Center of Homeopathy):

Annandale Apothecary
3299 Woodburn Road
Annandale, VA 22003

Boericke & Taffel
1011 Arch St.
Philadelphia, PA 19074
(800) 272-2820

Boericke & Taffel
2381 Circadian Way
Santa Rosa, CA 95407
(800) 876-9505

Boiron/Borneman
1208 Amosland Road
Norwood, PA 19074
(800) blu-tube
(215) 532-2035

Boiron/Borneman
98C West Cochran St.
Simi Valley, CA 93065
(800) blu-tube
(805) 582-9091

City Pharmacy
1435 State St.
Santa Barbara, CA 93101
(800) 635-1227
(805) 962-8188

Drug Stop 22 Pharmacy
8468 Santa Monica Boulevard
Los Angeles, CA 90069
(213) 650-8284

Hanson Homeopathic
12332 Naomi Drive
Jacksonville, FL 32218
(904) 757-7920

Kelvin Levitt's Health Dept.
8719a Liberty Plaza Mall
Randallstown, MD 21133
(301) 655-6618

Longevity Pure Medicine
9595 Wilshire Boulevard, Suite 706
Beverly Hills, CA 90212
(800) 327-5519
(213) 273-7423

Luyties Pharmaceutical Company
4200 Laciede Ave.
St. Louis, MO 63108
(800) 325-8080

The Medicine Shoppe
6307 York Road
Baltimore, MD 21212
(301) 323-1515

Merz Apothecary
4716 North Lincoln Ave.
Chicago, IL 60625
(312) 989-0900

Mid America Homeopathic Medicine Shop
P.O. Box 1275
Berkley, MI 48072
(800) 552-4956

Santa Monica Drug Company
1513 Fourth St.
Santa Monica, CA 90401
(213) 395-1131

Standard Homeopathic Co.
P.O. Box 61067
Los Angeles, CA 90061
(800) 624-9659
(213) 321-4284

Washington Homeopathic Pharmacy Inc.
4914 Del Ray Ave.
Bethesda, MD 20814
(301) 656-1695

Weleda Pharmacy Inc.
841 S. Main Street
P.O. Box 769
Spring Valley, NY 10977
(914) 352-6145

Other important addresses:

International Foundation for the
Promotion of Homeopathy
4 Sherman Ave.
Fairfax, CA 94930

National Center for Homeopathy
1500 Massachusetts Ave. N.W., #41
Washington, D.C. 20005

◊ APPENDIX III ◊

FLOWER ESSENCES

Earth Medicine Ways uses the following essences:

Bach Flower Essences
Bach/Ellon Company
Box 320
Woodmere, NY 11598
or
Dr. Edward Bach Centre
Mt. Vernon, Sotwell
Wallingford, Oxon
England OX10 OPZ

Flower Essence Society
P.O. Box 1769
Nevada City, CA 95959
(800) 548-0075

Perelandra, Ltd.
Box 3603
Warrenton, VA 22186

The other addresses listed here are courtesy of *Shooting Star* magazine, 727 President St., Brooklyn, NY 11215.

Alaskan Flower Essences
1153 Donna Drive
Fairbanks, AK 99701
(907) 457-2440

Australian Bush Essences
Box 531
Spit Junction, NSW
Australia 2088

The Bailey Essences
Arthur Bailey, Ph.D.
7/8 Nelson Road
Ilkley, W. Yorkshire
England LS29 8HN

The Bailey Essences
In Sight Unlimited
707 S. Regester St.
Baltimore, MD 21231
(301) 675-8313

Desert Alchemy
Box 44189
Tucson, AZ 85733
(602) 325-1545

Deva
Natural Labs Co.
Box 229
Encinitas, CA 92024
(619) 944-2878

Earthfriends
116 Los Angeles Ave., NE
Atlanta, GA 30306
(404) 373-0111

Earthsong Herbs
Box 263
Little Falls, NJ 07424
(201) 256-4261

Harebell Remedies
Moneybuie, Corsock
Castle Douglas
Kirkcudbrightshire
S.W. Scotland DG7 3DY

Jade Mountain Essences
Box 125
Mt. Lakes, NY 07046

Laboratoires Deva
BP3
38880 Autrans
France

Living Essences
Box 355
Scarborough, W. Australia
Australia 6019

Master's Flower Essences
14618 Tyler Foote Road
Nevada City, CA 95959
(916) 292-3397

Ozark Flower Essences
HCR 73, Box 160
Drury, MO 65638
(417) 679-3391

Pacific Essences
Box 1624, Stn. E
Victoria, B.C.
Canada V8W 2X7
(604) 380-0840

Pegasus Products
Box 228
Boulder, CO 80306
(800) 527-6104

Petite Fleur Essences, Inc.
8524 Whispering Creek Trail
Fort Worth, TX 76134
(817) 293-5410

Santa Fe Flower Connection
Box 25
Torreon, NM 87061
(505) 384-5022

Vita Florum
Box 876
Banff, Alberta
Canada
(403) 762-2673

Vita Florum, Ltd.
Coombe Castle Elworthy
Taunton, Somerset
England TA4 3PX

◊ APPENDIX IV ◊

AYURVEDA, CRYSTALS AND AROMATHERAPY

Ayurveda

A correspondence course in Ayurveda and more information may be obtained from:

> The Ayurvedic Institute
> P.O. Box 6265
> Santa Fe, NM 87502

Crystals

To study crystals or obtain crystals through the mail, write to:

> The Crystal Academy
> P.O. Box 3208
> Taos, NM 87571

Aromatherapy

A correspondence course on aromatherapy as well as individual oils may be ordered from:

> Pacific Institute of Aromatherapy
> P.O. Box 606
> San Rafael, CA 94915

Individual oils may also be ordered from:

Ledet Oils
P.O. Box 2354
Fair Oaks, CA 95628

Oak Valley Herb Farm
14648 Pear Tree Lane
Nevada City, CA 95959

◊ APPENDIX V ◊

FOOD IRRADIATION

Food irradiation continues to be a highly controversial issue between individuals pursuing a healthy, ecologically sound life style and Big Business organizations promoting it for commercial value. Irradiating food not only destroys many essential nutrients but it also causes changes in the smell, taste, and texture of foods. Some of the worst side effects include the mutation of micro-organisms under radiation, which may create new species even more dangerous, and radiation-resistant bacteria (for example, those which cause botulism), which would make it harder for consumers to spot foods affected by botulism since other signs of spoilage might have been prevented by irradiation. Foods are not always labeled as being irradiated due to the FDA's desire not to scare people with the word *radiation*.

To become educated about food irradiation, and to protest it, the following addresses are helpful:

Center for Food Safety and Applied Nutrition
Food and Drug Administration
200 C St. S.W.
Washington, D.C. 20204
(202) 472-5740

Coalition to Stop Food Irradiation
44 Montgomery St.
San Francisco, CA 94104
(415) 776-8299

Committee for Nuclear Responsibility
P.O. Box 11207
San Francisco, CA 94101
(415) 776-8299

Consumers United for Food Safety
c/o Linda Copper
P.O. Box 22928
Seattle, WA 98122

Environmental Policy Institute
218 D St. S.E.
Washington, D.C. 20003
(202) 544-2600

Health and Energy Institute
236 Mass. Ave. N.E., #506
Washington, D.C. 20006
(202) 543-1070

Health Research Group
2000 P St. N.W.
Washington, D.C. 20036
(202) 872-0320

National Health Federation
5001 Seminary Rd., #1330
Alexandria, VA 22311
(703) 379-0589

Vermont Alliance to Protect Our Food
P.O. Box 237
Vergennes, VT 05491
(802) 877-3289

BIBLIOGRAPHY

General

Airola, Paavo, N.D. *How to Get Well.* Phoenix, AZ: Health Plus, Pubs., 1974.

Asimov, Isaac. *The Human Body—Its Structure and Operation.* New York: New American Library, 1963.

Ballantine, Rudolph, M.D. *Diet and Nutrition—A Holistic Approach.* Honesdale, PA: Himalayan International Institute, 1978.

A Barefoot Doctor's Manual. Seattle, WA: Madrona Publishers, Inc., 1977.

Bliss, Shepherd, ed. *The New Holistic Health Handbook: Living Well in a New Age.* Berkeley, CA: Berkeley Holistic Center, Stephen Greene Press, Inc., 1985.

Bricklin, Mark, ed. *The Practical Encyclopedia of Natural Healing.* Emmaus, PA: Rodale Press, Inc., 1983.

Carroll, David. *The Complete Book of Natural Medicines.* New York: Summit Books, 1980.

Clark, Linda. *Get Well Naturally.* New York: ARC Int'l, Ltd., 1965.

Cousins, Norman. *Anatomy of an Illness as Perceived by the Patient.* New York: W. W. Norton & Co., Inc., 1979.

Dextreit, Raymond. *Our Earth, Our Cure.* Ed. and tr. from French by Michel Abehsera. Secaucus, NJ: Citadel Press, 1986.

Haas, Elson. *Staying Healthy with the Seasons.* Berkeley, CA: Celestial Arts Pub. Co., 1981.

Hall, Manly Palmer. *Paracelsus: His Mystical and Medical Philosophy.* Los Angeles, CA: Philosophical Research Society, 1964.

Hay, Louise. *Heal Your Body—Metaphysical Causations for Physical Illness.* Los Angeles, CA: Louise Hay, 1976.

_____. *You Can Heal Your Life*. Santa Monica, CA: Hay House, Inc., 1988.

Heritage, Ford. *Composition and Facts about Foods*. Mokelumne Hill, CA: Health Research, 1971.

Hill, Ann, ed. *A Visual Encyclopedia of Unconventional Medicine*. New York: Crown Publishers, Inc., 1978.

Hunter, Beatrice Trum. *Consumer Beware!* Touchstone Books. New York: Simon and Schuster, Inc., 1971.

Jackson, Mildred, N.D. and Terri Teague. *The Handbook of Alternatives to Chemical Medicine*. Oakland, CA: Terri Teague and Mildred Jackson, 1974.

Jensen, Bernard. *World Keys to Health and Long Life*. Provo, UT: Bi World Industries, Inc., 1975.

Kirschmann, John D. *Nutrition Almanac*. New York: McGraw-Hill Pub. Co., 1979.

Kulvinskas, Viktoras. *Survival into the 21st Century*. Woodstock Valley, CT: O'Mawgo D Press, 1975.

Reilly, Harold J., M.D. *The Edgar Cayce Handbook for Health through Drugless Therapy*. New York: Macmillan Publishing Co., Inc., 1975.

Rohe, Fred. *The Complete Book of Natural Foods*. Boulder, CO: Shambhala Pubns., 1983.

Samuels, Mike, M.D. and Hal Bennett. *The Well Body Book*. New York: Random House, Inc., 1978.

Schneider, Meir. *Self-Healing: My Life and Vision*. New York & London: Routledge & Kegan Paul, Ltd., 1987.

Selye, Hans. *The Stress of Life*. New York: McGraw-Hill Pub. Co., 1956.

Siegel, Bernie, M.D. *Love, Medicine, and Miracles*. New York: Harper & Row Pubs., Inc., 1990.

_____. *Peace, Love, and Healing*. New York: Harper & Row Pubs., Inc., 1990.

Steadman, Alice. *Who's The Matter with Me?* Marina del Rey, CA: De Vorss & Co., 1966.

Vogel, Virgil. *American Indian Medicine*. Norman, OK: Univ. of Oklahoma Press, 1970.

Williams, Roger J. *Biochemical Individuality: The Basis for the Genetotrophic Concept*. Austin, TX: Univ. of Texas Press, 1956.

Chapter 3

Walker, Norman W. *Colon Health: The Key to a Vibrant Life*. Prescott, AZ: Norwalk Press, 1979.

Chapter 4

Aihara, Herman. *Acid and Alkaline*. Oroville, CA: George Ohsawa Macrobiotic Foundation, 1980.

Cousens, Gabriel, M.D. *Spiritual Nutrition and the Rainbow Diet*. Boulder, CO: Cassandra Press, 1986.

Kelley, W.D., D.D.S. *Metabolic Typing*. Winthrop, WA: International Health Institute, 1982, pamphlet.

Chapter 5

Kushi, Michio. *The Book of Macrobiotics: The Universal Way of Health and Happiness*. Tokyo: Japan Publications, Inc., 1977.

Lappe, Frances Moore. *Diet for a Small Planet*. New York: Ballantine Books, Inc., 1975.

Wigmore, Ann. *Why Suffer*. Boston, MA: Hippocrates Institute, 1964.

Chapter 9

Bliznakow, Emile G., M.D. and Gerald L. Hunt. *The Miracle Nutrient: Coenzyme Q-10*. New York: Bantam Books, Inc., 1987.

Passwater, Richard and Earl Mindell, eds. *Good Health Guides*. New Canaan, CT: Keats Publishing, Inc., 1982.

Russell-Manning, Betsy. *Wheatgrass Juice: Gift of Nature*. Calistoga, CA: Betsy Russell, 1979.

Chapter 12

Gladstar, Rosemary. *The Sage Healing Ways Series*. R. Gladstar, Box 420, E. Barre, VT 06649.

Green, James. *Herbs & Health Care for Males*. Forestville, CA: Simplers Botanicals, 1987.

Grieve, M. *A Modern Herbal*. Vols. I & II. Mineola, NY: Dover Publications, Inc., 1971.

Hoffman, David. *The Holistic Herbal*. Longmead, Shaftesbury, Dorset, England: Element Books, 1989.

Hutchens, Alma R. *Indian Herbology of North America*. Windsor, Ontario, Canada: Merco, 1969.

Kloss, Jethro. *Back to Eden*. Greenwich, CT: Benedict Lust Publications, 1971.

Lucas, Richard M. *Secrets of the Chinese Herbalists*. New York: Cornerstone Library, Inc., 1979.

Lust, John. *The Herb Book*. Greenwich, CT: Benedict Lust Publications, 1974.

Moore, Michael. *Medicinal Plants of the Mountain West*. Santa Fe, NM: Museum of New Mexico Press, 1980.

Parvati, Jeannine. *Hygeia—A Woman's Herbal*. Monroe, UT: Freestone Pub. Co., 1978.

Rose, Jeanne. *Herbs and Things*. New York: Grosset and Dunlap, 1972.

Santillo, Humbart. *Natural Healing with Herbs*. Prescott Valley, AZ: Hohm Press, 1984.

Tierra, Michael. *Planetary Herbology*. Santa Fe, NM: Lotus Press, 1988.

_____. *The Way of Herbs*. Berkeley, CA: Unity Press, 1980.

Weiner, Michael A. *Earth Medicine, Earth Food*. New York: Collier-Macmillan, 1980.

Wood, Matthew. *Seven Herbs: Plants as Teachers*. Berkeley, CA: North Atlantic Books, 1987.

Chapter 13

Chapman, J. B., M.D. *Dr. Schuessler's Biochemistry*. London: New Era Laboratories, 1961.

Cummings, Stephen and Dana Ullman. *Everybody's Guide to Homeopathic Medicines*. Los Angeles, CA: Jeremy P. Tarcher, Inc., 1984.

Kent, J. T. *Lectures on Homeopathic Materia Medica with New Remedies*. New Delhi: B. Jain Publishers, 1981.

_____. *Repertory of the Homeopathic Materia Medica*. New Delhi: B. Jain Publishers, 1986.

Panos, Maesimund B., M.D. and Jane Heimlich. *Homeopathic Medicine at Home*. Los Angeles, CA: Jeremy P. Tarcher, Inc., 1980.

Smith, Trevor. *The Homeopathic Treatment of Emotional Illness*. New York: Thorsons Publishers, Inc., 1984.

Ullmann, Dana. *Homeopathy: Medicine for the 21st Century*. Berkeley, CA: North Atlantic Books, 1988.

Vithoulkas, George. *Homeopathy: Medicine for the New Man*. New York: Prentice-Hall, Inc., 1987.

_____. *The Science of Homeopathy*. Athens: George Vithoulkas, Athenian School of Homeopathic Medicine, 1978.

Chapter 14

Bensky, Dan et al. *Chinese Herbal Medicine: Materia Medica*. Seattle, WA: Eastland Press, 1986.

Connelly, Diane M. *Traditional Acupuncture: The Law of the Five Elements*. Columbia, MD: Centre for Traditional Acupuncture.

Garvy, John W., Jr. *The Five Phases of Food: How to Begin*. Newtonville, MA: Well Being Books, 1985, pamphlet.

Hsu, Dr. Hong-Yen. *How to Treat Yourself with Chinese Herbs*. Long Beach, CA: Oriental Healing Arts Institute, 1980.

Kaptchuk, Ted J. *The Web That Has No Weaver: Understanding Chinese Medicine*. New York: Congdon & Weed, 1983.

Mann, Felix. *Acupuncture—The Ancient Chinese Art of Healing and How It Works Scientifically*. New York: Random House, Inc., 1962.

Porkert, Manfred. *The Essentials of Chinese Diagnostics*. Zurich: Chinese Medicine Publications, Ltd., 1983.

_____. *The Theoretical Foundations of Chinese Medicine*. Cambridge, MA: MIT Press, 1978.

Veith, Ilza, tr. *The Yellow Emperor's Classic of Internal Medicine*. Berkeley, CA: University of California Press, 1970.

Chapter 15

Frawley, David and Vasant Lad. *The Yoga of Herbs*. Santa Fe, NM: Lotus Press, 1986.

Heyn, Birgit. *Ayurvedic Medicine*. Wellingborough, Northants, England: Thorsons Publishing Group, 1983.

Lad, Vasant. *Ayurveda: The Science of Self-Healing*. Santa Fe, NM: Lotus Press, 1984.

Svoboda, Robert. *Prakruti: Your Ayurvedic Constitution*. Albuquerque, NM: Geocom, Ltd., 1988.

Chapter 16

Feltman, John, ed. *Hands-on Healing: Massage Remedies for Hundreds of Health Problems*. Emmaus, PA: Rodale Press, Inc., 1989.

Kaye, Anna. *Reflexology for Good Health*. No. Hollywood, CA: Hal Leighton Printing Co., 1978.

Masunaga, Shizuto and Waturu Ohashi. *Zen/Shiatsu: How to Harmonize Yin and Yang for Better Health*. Tokyo: Japan Publications, Inc., 1977.

Teegarden, Iona. *The Acupressure Way of Health—Jin Shin Do*. Tokyo: Japan Publications, Inc., 1978.

Chapter 17

Feldenkrais, Moshe. *Awareness through Movement: Health Exercises for Personal Growth*. New York: Harper & Row Pubs., Inc., 1972.

Man-ch'ing, Cheng and Robert Smith. *T'ai-Chi*. Tokyo: John Weatherhill Inc., 1966.

Pritikin, Nathan. *The Pritikin Program for Diet & Exercise*. New York: Bantam Books, Inc., 1979.

Russell, W. Scott. *Karate: The Energy Connection*. New York: Delacorte Press, 1976.

Sivananda, Swami Radha. *Hatha Yoga: The Hidden Language*. Boulder, CO: Shambhala Pubns., 1989.

Taylor, Louise and Betty Bryant. *Acupressure, Yoga, and You*. Tokyo: Japan Publications, Inc., 1984.

Vishnudevananda, Swami. *The Complete Illustrated Book of Yoga*. New York: Bell Publishing Co., 1960.

Chapter 18

Achterberg, Jeanne. *Imagery in Healing: Shamanism and Modern Medicine*. Boulder, CO: Shambhala Pubns., 1985.

Brown, Barbara. *Stress and the Art of Biofeedback*. New York: Bantam Books, Inc., 1978.

Finkelstein, Adrian, M.D. *Your Past Lives and the Healing Process*. Palatine, IL: Adrian Finkelstein, 1985.

Mason, L. John. *Guide to Stress Reduction*. Culver City, CA: Peace Press, 1980.

Moody, Raymond, M.D. *Life After Life*. New York: Bantam Books, Inc., 1975.

Pelletier, Kenneth R. *Mind as Healer, Mind as Slayer*. New York: Dell Publishing Co., 1977.

Simonton, O. Carl, Stephanie Simonton & James Creighton. *Getting Well Again*. New York: Bantam Books, Inc., 1981.

Chapter 19

Brennan, Barbara. *Hands of Light*. New York: Bantam Books, Inc., 1987.

Chancellor, Philip M. *Handbook of the Bach Flower Remedies*. London: C. W. Daniel Co., Ltd., 1971.

Chopra, Deepak, M.D. *Quantum Healing: Exploring the Frontiers of Mind-Body Medicine*. New York: Bantam Books, Inc., 1989.

Clark, Linda. *The Ancient Art of Color Therapy*. New York: Simon & Schuster, Inc., 1975.

Color Healing: An Exhaustive Survey Compiled by Health Research from the 21 Works of the Leading Practitioners of Chromotherapy. Mokelumne Hill, CA: Health Research, 1956.

David, William. *The Harmonics of Sound, Color, & Vibration*. Marina del Rey, CA: De Vorss & Co., 1980.

Dinshah, Darius. *The Spectro-Chrome System*. Malaga, NJ: Dinshah Health Society, 1979.

Flower Essence Repertory. Nevada City, CA: Flower Essence Society, 1986.

Gerber, Richard, M.D. *Vibrational Medicine: New Choices for Healing Ourselves*. Santa Fe, NM: Bear & Co., 1988.

Gimbel, Theo. *Healing Through Colour.* Saffron Walden, Essex, Great Britain: C. W. Daniel Co., Ltd., 1980.

Gurudas. *Flower Essences and Vibrational Healing.* Albuquerque, NM: Brotherhood of Life, Inc., 1983.

Heline, Corinne. *Healing and Regeneration through Color.* Santa Barbara, CA: J. F. Rowny Press, 1972.

_____. *Healing and Regeneration through Music.* Santa Barbara, CA: J.F. Rowny Press, 1968.

Isaacs, Thelma. *Gemstones, Crystals, & Healing.* Black Mountain, NC: Lorien House, 1982.

Keyes, Laurel. *Toning: The Creative Power of the Voice.* Marina del Rey, CA: De Vorss & Co., 1964.

Lingerman, Hal. *The Healing Energies of Music.* Wheaton, IL: Theosophical Publishing House, 1983.

Lorusso, Julia and Joel Glick. *Healing Stoned: The Therapeutic Use of Gems & Minerals.* Albuquerque, NM: Adobe Press, 1976.

Price, Shirley. *Practical Aromatherapy.* Wellingborough, Northamptonshire, England: Thorsons Publishers, Inc., 1983.

Raphaell, Katrina. *Crystal Enlightenment.* Vol. I. New York: Aurora Press, 1985.

_____. *Crystal Healing.* Vol. II. New York: Aurora Press, 1987.

_____. *The Crystalline Transmission.* Vol. III. Santa Fe, NM: Aurora Press, 1990.

Tame, David. *The Secret Power of Music: The Transformation of Self & Society through Musical Energy.* New York: Destiny Books, 1984.

Tisserand, Robert. *The Art of Aromatherapy.* New York: Destiny Books, 1977.

Uyldert, Mellie. *The Magic of Precious Stones.* Wellingborough, Northamptonshire, England: Turnstone Press, 1981.

Valnet, Jean, M.D. *The Practice of Aromatherapy: Holistic Health & Essential Oils of Flowers & Herbs.* New York: Destiny Books, 1980.

Wright, Machaelle Small. *Flower Essences.* Jeffersonton, VA: Perelandra, Ltd., 1988.

Chapter 20
Blackburn, Gabriele. *The Science and Art of the Pendulum: A Complete Course in Radiesthesia.* Ojai, CA: Idylwild Books, 1983.

Fairchild, Dennis. *The Handbook of Humanistic Palmistry.* Ferndale, MI: Thumbs Up, 1980.

Jensen, Bernard. *Iridology Simplified.* Bernard Jensen, Iridologists Int'l., Route 1, Escondido, CA, 1980.

Kushi, Michio. *How to See Your Health: The Book of Oriental Diagnosis.* Tokyo: Japan Publications, Inc., 1980.

Neilsen, Greg and Joseph Polansky. *Pendulum Power.* New York: Warner Destiny Books, 1977.

Starck, Marcia. *Astrology: Key to Holistic Health.* Birmingham, MI: Seek-it Pubns., 1982.

_____. *Earth Mother Astrology.* St. Paul, MN: Llewellyn Publications, 1989.

Tansley, David, D.C. *Radionics & the Subtle Anatomy of Man.* Devon, England: Health Science Press, 1972.

Westlake, Aubrey, M.D. *The Pattern of Health.* Boulder, CO: Shambhala Pubns., 1973.

Chapter 21

Abrahamson, E. M., M.D. and A. W. Pezet. *Body, Mind and Sugar.* New York: Holt, Rinehart, & Winston, Inc., 1951.

Adams, Ruth and Frank Murray. *All You Should Know about Arthritis.* New York: Larchmont Books, 1979.

Airola, Paavo, N.D. *Cancer: The Total Approach.* Phoenix, AZ: Health Plus Pubs., 1975.

_____. *Hypoglycemia: A Better Approach.* Phoenix, AZ: Health Plus Pubs., 1980.

Badgley, Laurence, M.D. *Healing AIDS Naturally.* San Bruno, CA: Human Energy Press, 1987.

Coca, Arthur F., M.D. *The Pulse Test—Easy Allergy Detection.* New York: Arco Publishers, 1959.

Gerson, Max, M.D. *A Cancer Therapy—Results of 50 Cases.* Del Mar, CA: Totality Books, 1977.

Greenwood, Sadja, M.D. *Menopause, Naturally.* Volcano, CA: Volcano Press, 1984.

Kelley, Wm. Donald, D.D.S. *One Answer to Cancer.* Kelley Foundation, 1974.

Kübler-Ross, Elisabeth, M.D. *AIDS: The Ultimate Challenge.* New York: Macmillan Publishing Co., Inc., 1987.

Kushi, Michio. *Cancer and Diet.* Boston, MA: East West Foundation, 1980.

Passwater, Richard, M.D. *Cancer and Its Nutritional Therapies.* New Canaan, CT: Keats Publishing, Inc., 1978.

Serinus, Jason. *Psychoimmunity and the Healing Process: A Holistic Approach to Immunity and AIDS.* Berkeley, CA: Celestial Arts Pub. Co., 1986.

Stoff, Jesse and Charles Pellegrino. *Chronic Fatigue Syndrome: The Hidden Epidemic.* New York: Random House, Inc., 1988.

Williams, Roger J. *Alcoholism: The Nutritional Approach.* Austin, TX: Univ. of Texas Press, 1978.

INDEX

A

AIDS, 257, 258, 259, 260

ARC, 257, 258, 260

acid, 6, 17, 21, 22, 23, 26, 29, 31,
33, 34, 39, 46, 49, 52, 61, 82,
88, 98, 107, 108, 117, 118, 119,
121, 129, 137, 148, 165, 184,
215, 259, 264, 265, 266, 267,
274, 277, 278, 281, 283, 289,
290, 291, 297, 299, 304, 306,
308, 309, 312, 325, 327, 328,
332, 333, 340, 342, 350, 353

acidophilus, 33, 67, 68, 259, 261,
265, 290, 293, 299, 301, 307,
309, 326, 328, 332, 356

acne, 68, 89, 98, 100, 101, 112, 121,
123, 149, 165, 185, 289

acupressure, 10, 191, 197, 198,
269, 271, 295, 303, 319, 338,
342, 352

acupuncture, 10, 157, 172, 173,
174, 197, 198, 217, 234, 249,
250, 257, 260, 265, 269, 277,
287, 290, 292, 294, 303, 306,
328, 342, 351

alcohol, 4, 26, 33, 67, 72, 74, 85, 97,
98, 121, 143, 145, 158, 163,
226, 231, 233, 262, 263, 267,
271, 278, 290, 299, 302, 304,
322, 342, 348, 351, 354

alcoholism, 5, 74, 85, 98, 123, 124,
255, 262, 263, 342

alkaline, 6, 16, 17, 21, 22, 23, 31,
53, 59, 77, 88, 107, 108, 117,
118, 119, 120, 121, 122, 129,
165, 281, 303, 304, 347, 355

allergies, 3, 10, 17, 33, 34, 40, 47,
48, 68, 69, 71, 73, 82, 98, 104,
107, 108, 113, 121, 126, 158,
162, 163, 164, 165, 185, 248,
250, 266, 267, 268, 269, 270,
278, 289, 290, 301, 311, 312,
313, 318, 327, 329, 330, 335,
338, 339, 340, 344, 349, 350

Alzheimer's disease, 78, 270, 271

amino acids, 34, 45, 46, 47, 48, 49,
68, 71, 82, 83, 84, 85, 86, 87,

I

J

N

O

P

STAY IN TOUCH

On the following pages you will find listed, with their current prices, some of the books and tapes now available on related subjects. Your book dealer stocks most of these, and will stock new titles in the Llewellyn series as they become available. We urge your patronage.

However, to obtain our full catalog, to keep informed of new titles as they are released and to benefit from informative articles and helpful news, you are invited to write for our bi-monthly news magazine/catalog. A sample copy is free, and it will continue coming to you at no cost as long as you are an active mail customer. Or you may keep it coming for a full year with a donation of just $2.00 in U.S.A. ($7.00 for Canada & Mexico, $20.00 overseas, first class mail). Many bookstores also have *The Llewellyn New Times* available to their customers. Ask for it.

Stay in touch! In *The Llewellyn New Times'* pages you will find news and reviews of new books, tapes and services, announcements of meetings and seminars, articles helpful to our readers, news of authors, advertising of products and services, special moneymaking opportunities, and much more.

The Llewellyn New Times
P.O. Box 64383-Dept. 742, St. Paul, MN 55164-0383, U.S.A.

• • •

TO ORDER BOOKS AND TAPES

If your book dealer does not have the books and tapes described on the following pages readily available, you may order them directly from the publisher by sending full price in U.S. funds, plus $1.50 for postage and handling for orders *under* $10.00; $3.00 for orders *over* $10.00. There are no postage and handling charges for orders over $50. UPS Delivery: We ship UPS whenever possible. Delivery guaranteed. Provide your street address as UPS does not deliver to P.O. Boxes. UPS to Canada requires a $50 minimum order. Allow 4-6 weeks for delivery. Orders outside the U.S.A. and Canada: Airmail—add retail price of book; add $5 for each non-book item (tapes, etc.); add $1 per item for surface mail.

FOR GROUP STUDY AND PURCHASE

Because there is a great deal of interest in group discussion and study of the subject matter of this book, we feel that we should encourage the adoption and use of this particular book by such groups by offering a special "quantity" price to group leaders or "agents."

Our Special Quantity Price for a minimum order of five copies of *The Complete Handbook of Natural Healing* is $38.85 cash-with-order. This price includes postage and handling within the United States. Minnesota residents must add 6% sales tax. For additional quantities, please order in multiples of five. For Canadian and foreign orders, add postage and handling charges as above. Credit card (VISA, Master Card, American Express) orders are accepted. Charge card orders only may be phoned free ($15.00 minimum order) within the U.S.A. or Canada by dialing 1-800-THE-MOON. Customer service calls dial 1-612-291-1970. Mail orders to:

LLEWELLYN PUBLICATIONS
P.O. Box 64383-Dept. 742 / St. Paul, MN 55164-0383, U.S.A.

EARTH MOTHER ASTROLOGY
by Marcia Starck

Now, for the first time, a book that combines the science of astrology with current New Age interest in crystals, herbs, aromas, and holistic health. With this book and a copy of your astrological birth chart (readily available from sources listed in the book) you can use your horoscope to benefit your total being—body, mind and spirit. Learn, for example, what special nutrients you need during specific planetary cycles, or what sounds or colors will help you transform emotional states during certain times of the year.

This is a compendium of information for the New Age astrologer and healer. For the beginner, it explains all the astrological signs, planets and houses in a simple and yet new way, physiologically as well as symbolically.

This is a book of modern alchemy, showing the reader how to work with Earth energies to achieve healing and transformation, thereby creating a sense of the cosmic unity of all Earth's elements.

0-87542-741-3, 294 pgs., 5 1/4 x 8 $12.95

DOWSING FOR HEALTH
by Arthur Bailey

This is the first comprehensive and authoritative guide into the "how to's" of dowsing or "divining" in health, healing and complementary medicine. The techniques in *Dowsing for Health* are proven, based on the author's personal experiences.

Dowsing for Health presents simple exercises for the beginner to build confidence, appreciation and understanding, before outlining the applications to holistic health. The tools of dowsing are fully described. There are also details of scientific work into the mechanics of dowsing and how it relates to brain activity.

Dowsers are split into two camps: one group believes that dowsing has a direct physical effect on the dowser; the second group believes that dowsing is under the control of the dowser. The author explores the whole matter thoroughly, employing a unified approach with practical applications in the field of holistic health and healing.

0-87542-059-1, 176 pgs., 6 x 9, illus. $9.95

THE WOMEN'S BOOK OF HEALING
by Diane Stein

Women's healing, which is healing for the benefit of women and men, children, animals and the planet alike, includes such skills as aura and chakra work, color and vibrational therapy, creative visualization, meditation states, laying on of hands, psychic healing and crystals and gemstones. This ancient and universal knowledge is elemental, and though long submerged, it has never been lost. Receiving increasing attention in the New Age and Women's Spirituality movements, healing is being re-learned and re-claimed. This book takes healing out of the exclusive domain of professionals and gives it back to the people.

The Women's Book of Healing demystifies, explains and teaches healing skills in ways that anyone can learn and use. Healing and well-being are within choice and reach, for the good of all.

0-87542-759-6, 317 pgs., 6 x 9, illus. $12.95

THE INNER WORLD OF FITNESS
by Melita Denning

Because the artificialities and the daily hassles of routine living tend to turn our attention from the real values, *The Inner World of Fitness* leads us back by means of those natural factors in life which remain to us: air, water, sunlight, the food we eat, the world of nature, meditations, sexual love and the power of our wishes—so that through these things we can re-link ourselves in awareness to the great non-material forces of life and being which underline them.

The unity and interaction of inner and outer, keeping body and psyche open to the great currents of life and of the natural forces, is seen as the essential secret of youthfulness and hence of radiant fitness. Regardless of our physical age, so long as we are within the flow of these great currents, we have the vital quality of youthfulness: but if we begin to close off or turn away from those contacts, in the same measure we begin to lose youthfulness. Also included is a metaphysical examination of AIDS.

This book will help you to experience the total energy of abundant health.

0-87542-165-2, 240 pgs., 5 1/4 x 8, illus. $7.95

THE ART OF SPIRITUAL HEALING
by Keith Sherwood

Each of us has the potential to be a healer; to heal ourselves and to become a channel for healing others. Healing energy is always flowing through you. Learn how to recognize and tap this incredible energy source. You do not need to be a victim of disease or poor health. Rid yourself of negativity and become a channel for positive healing.

Become acquainted with your three auras and learn how to recognize problems and heal them on a higher level before they become manifested in the physical body as disease.

Special techniques make this book a "breakthrough" to healing power, but you are also given a concise, easy-to-follow regimen of good health to follow in order to maintain a superior state of being. This is a practical guide to healing.

0-87542-720-0, 224 pgs., 5 1/4 x 8, illus.   **$7.95**

CHAKRA THERAPY
by Keith Sherwood

Keith Sherwood presents another excellent how-to book on healing. His previous book, *The Art of Spiritual Healing*, has helped many people learn how to heal themselves and others.

Chakra Therapy follows in the same direction: understand yourself, know how your body and mind function and learn how to overcome negative programming so that you can become a free, healthy, self-fulfilled human being.

This book fills in the missing pieces of the human anatomy system left out by orthodox psychological models. It serves as a superb workbook. Within its pages are exercises and techniques designed to increase your level of energy, to transmute unhealthy frequencies of energy into healthy ones, to bring you back into balance and harmony with your self, your loved ones and the multidimensional world in which you live. Finally, it will help bring you back into union with the universal field of energy and consciousness.

Chakra Therapy will teach you how to heal yourself by healing your energy system because it is actually energy in its myriad forms which determines a person's level of consciousness and physical, emotional, and mental health.

0-87542-721-9, 270 pgs., 5 1/4 x 8, illus.   **$7.95**

CRYSTAL HEALING: The Next Step
by Phyllis Galde

Discover the secrets of quartz crystal! Now modern research and use have shown that crystals have even more healing and therapeutic properties than has been realized. Learn why polished, smoothed crystal is better to use to heighten your intuition, improve creativity and for healing.

Learn to use crystals for reprogramming your subconscious to eliminate problems and negative attitudes that prevent success. Here are techniques that people have successfully used—not just theories.

This book reveals newly discovered abilities of crystal now accessible to all, and is a sensible approach to crystal use. *Crystal Healing* will be your guide to improve the quality of your life and expand your consciousness.

0-87542-246-2, 224 pgs., mass market, illus.   **$3.95**

WHEELS OF LIFE: A User's Guide to the Chakra System
by Anodea Judith

An instruction manual for owning and operating the inner gears that run the machinery of our lives. Written in a practical, down-to-earth style, this fully-illustrated book will take the reader on a journey through aspects of consciousness, from the bodily instincts of survival to the processing of deep thoughts.

Discover this ancient metaphysical system under the new light of popular Western metaphors—quantum physics, elemental magick, Kabalah, physical exercises, poetic meditations, and visionary art. Learn how to open these centers in yourself, and see how the chakras shed light on the present world crises we face today. And learn what you can do about it!

This book is a vital resource for: Magicians, Witches, Pagans, Mystics, Yoga practitioners, Martial Arts people, psychologists, medical people, and all those who are concerned with holistic growth techniques.

The modern picture of the chakras was introduced to the West largely in the context of Hatha and Kundalini Yoga and through the theosophical writings of Leadbeater and Besant. But the chakra system is *equally* innate to Western Magick: all psychic development, spiritual growth, and practical attainment is fully dependent upon the opening of the chakras!

0-87542-320-5, 544 pgs., 6 x 9, illus.   **$12.95**